プロメテウス
解剖学アトラス
コンパクト版 第2版

PROMETHEUS
LernKarten der Anatomie 5. Auflage

プロメテウス
解剖学アトラス
コンパクト版 第2版

PROMETHEUS
LernKarten der Anatomie 5. Auflage

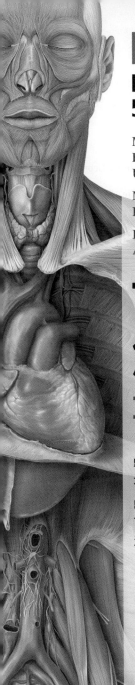

PROMETHEUS
LernKarten der Anatomie
5.Auflage

Michael Schünke
Erik Schulte
Udo Schumacher

Markus Voll
Karl Wesker

Bearbeitet von
Anne M.Gilroy

プロメテウス
解剖学アトラス
コンパクト版　第2版

監訳
坂井 建雄　　　順天堂大学医学部教授

訳
市村 浩一郎　　順天堂大学医学部准教授
澤井 直　　　　順天堂大学医学部助教

医学書院

Copyright © of the original German language edition 2016 by Georg Thieme Verlag KG, Stuttgart, Germany.
Original title : Prometheus LernKarten der Anatomie., 5/e, by Michael Schünke, Erik Schulte, Udo Schumacher, with illustrations by Markus Voll and Karl H. Wesker, edited by Anne M. Gilroy.
© Second Japanese edition 2019 by Igaku-Shoin Ltd., Tokyo
Printed and bound in Japan

プロメテウス解剖学アトラス コンパクト版

発　行	2011年3月1日	第1版第1刷
	2017年12月1日	第1版第5刷
	2019年3月15日	第2版第1刷
	2023年3月15日	第2版第3刷

監訳者　　坂井建雄
さかい　たつお

発行者　　株式会社　医学書院

　　　　　代表取締役　金原　俊

　　　　　〒113-8719　東京都文京区本郷 1-28-23

　　　　　電話　03-3817-5600（社内案内）

印刷・製本　横山印刷

本書の複製権・翻訳権・上映権・譲渡権・貸与権・公衆送信権（送信可能化権を含む）は株式会社医学書院が保有します．

ISBN978-4-260-03698-6

本書を無断で複製する行為（複写，スキャン，デジタルデータ化など）は，「私的使用のための複製」など著作権法上の限られた例外を除き禁じられています．大学，病院，診療所，企業などにおいて，業務上使用する目的（診療，研究活動を含む）で上記の行為を行うことは，その使用範囲が内部的であっても，私的使用には該当せず，違法です．また私的使用に該当する場合であっても，代行業者等の第三者に依頼して上記の行為を行うことは違法となります．

JCOPY　〈出版者著作権管理機構　委託出版物〉

本書の無断複製は著作権法上での例外を除き禁じられています．複製される場合は，そのつど事前に，出版者著作権管理機構（電話 03-5244-5088，FAX 03-5244-5089，info@jcopy.or.jp）の許諾を得てください．

第2版 監訳者序

　『プロメテウス解剖学アトラス』は，21世紀を代表する解剖学アトラスである．オリジナルの3冊本は2005～2006年に出版され，その精細で迫真の解剖図は世界中の人々に強烈な印象を与え，数多くの国々で翻訳・出版されている．その日本語版も2007～2009年に出版され，わが国の医療関係者と学生に広く迎え入れられて改訂を重ねている．1冊本の『プロメテウス解剖学 コア アトラス』も，オリジナルが2008年に出版され，日本語版が2010年に出版されて多くの読者に支持され，現在は第3版が刊行されている．

　本書『プロメテウス解剖学アトラス コンパクト版 第2版』は，このように広がり続ける「プロメテウス」シリーズから生み出された，きらりと輝く小品である．「プロメテウス」のすばらしい解剖図が，解剖学の学習に手軽に利用できるように編まれている．今回の日本語版第2版は，ドイツ語版第5版の翻訳である．原書は箱入りのカードという形式で出版されたが，日本語版の製作にあたっては読者の便を考えてポケット版の冊子体を採用した．原書のカードは初版で367枚だったものが，今回は460枚と大幅に増えている．新規カードの多くには，筋の起始・停止・神経支配・作用の表がつくなど，学習に役立つように工夫されている．

　本書には，解剖学の学習に役立つさまざまな工夫が凝らされている．見開きの左に解剖図，右に用語解説という構成にしているが，これにより必要な情報をひと目で見つけ出し，的確に理解することができる．さらに，原書にはない巻末の索引を利用することにより，必要なときに必要な図をすばやく探し出すことができる．また，臨床的なコメントや，理解を深めるためのQ&Aを随所で頁の下部に挿入し，アイコンをつけて表示している．より深い学習への足がかりにしていただけるとありがたい．

翻訳にあたっては，若手の優秀な解剖学者である市村と澤井が日本語訳の作業を行い，坂井が全体に目を通して監訳を担当した．特に「プロメテウス」シリーズの既刊本および解剖学用語との内容および用語の整合性に配慮した．日本語訳にあたっては瑕疵がないように細心の注意をしたつもりではあるが，至らぬところは監訳者の責である．

　本書『プロメテウス解剖学アトラス コンパクト版 第2版』が，解剖学の学習の場で多くの学生たちに役立てていただけることを願うものである．

2019年1月31日
八王子の寓居にて

坂井建雄

目次

背部

脊柱 1-3 ……………………………………… 2
椎骨の構成要素 ……………………………… 8
頸椎 1-4 ……………………………………… 10
胸椎 …………………………………………… 18
腰椎 …………………………………………… 20
仙骨と尾骨 1, 2 ……………………………… 22
脊柱の関節 …………………………………… 26
頸部脊柱の靱帯 1, 2 ………………………… 28
胸腰部脊柱の靱帯 1-3 ……………………… 32
背部の筋の概観 1-4 ………………………… 38
背部の筋の区分 1-10 ……………………… 46
背部の動脈 …………………………………… 66
背部の静脈 …………………………………… 68
背部の神経 …………………………………… 70
項部の神経・血管 (局所解剖) …………… 72
背部の神経・血管 (局所解剖) …………… 74
背部の体表解剖 ……………………………… 76

胸部

胸部の骨格 …………………………………… 80
胸部の構造 …………………………………… 82
胸骨 …………………………………………… 84
胸部の筋肉の概観 …………………………… 86
胸部の筋 1-3 ………………………………… 88
原位置の横隔膜 1, 2 ………………………… 94
横隔膜の各部 ………………………………… 98
横隔膜の開口部 ……………………………… 100
胸壁の動脈 …………………………………… 102
胸壁の静脈 …………………………………… 104
胸壁の神経 …………………………………… 106
肋間神経の経路 ……………………………… 108
横隔膜の神経・血管 ………………………… 110
女性の乳房への栄養血管 …………………… 112
女性の乳房のリンパ管 ……………………… 114
女性の乳房の構造 …………………………… 116
縦隔の区分 …………………………………… 118
胸部の CT …………………………………… 120
胸大動脈 ……………………………………… 122
奇静脈系 ……………………………………… 124
胸腔のリンパ管 ……………………………… 126
胸腔の神経 …………………………………… 128
縦隔 1-4 ……………………………………… 130
心膜の折れ返り 1, 2 ………………………… 138
原位置の心臓 ………………………………… 142
心臓の胸肋面 ………………………………… 144
心臓の底面 …………………………………… 146
心臓の部屋 1-3 ……………………………… 148
心臓弁 ………………………………………… 154
心臓の動脈と静脈 1, 2 ……………………… 156
心臓刺激伝導系 ……………………………… 160
心臓の自律神経 ……………………………… 162
心臓の X 線像 1, 2 …………………………… 164
水平断面での心臓 …………………………… 168
出生前の循環 ………………………………… 170
出生後の循環 ………………………………… 172
壁側胸膜 ……………………………………… 174
原位置の肺 …………………………………… 176
右肺 …………………………………………… 178
左肺 …………………………………………… 180
気管 …………………………………………… 182
気管支樹の区分 ……………………………… 184
気管支樹の呼吸部 …………………………… 186
肺動脈と肺静脈 ……………………………… 188
胸膜腔のリンパ節 …………………………… 190
胸部の体表解剖 ……………………………… 192

腹部・骨盤部

寛骨 …………………………………………… 196
下肢帯 ………………………………………… 198

骨盤部の靱帯 1, 2	200
腹壁の筋の概観 1-3	204
腹壁の筋 1-5	210
鼡径部 1, 2	220
骨盤底の筋の概観 1-3	224
骨盤底の筋 1-3	230
腹腔・骨盤腔	236
腹膜腔	238
網嚢	240
腸間膜と臓器	242
腹膜腔の後壁	244
男性骨盤部の内容	246
女性骨盤部の内容	248
腹部の水平断面	250
原位置の胃	252
十二指腸	254
大腸	256
原位置の直腸	258
直腸と肛門管	260
肝臓の表面 1, 2	262
肝外胆管	266
原位置の胆路	268
膵臓	270
原位置の腎臓と尿管	272
女性の膀胱と尿道	274
膀胱三角	276
子宮と卵管 1, 2	278
女性の外生殖器	282
女性の勃起組織	284
女性会陰の神経・血管	286
陰茎の横断面	288
陰茎	290
精巣と精巣上体	292
精巣の被膜	294
男性の付属生殖腺	296
原位置の前立腺	298
男性会陰の神経・血管	300
腹大動脈	302
腎動脈	304
腹腔動脈 1, 2	306
上腸間膜動脈	310
下腸間膜動脈	312
下大静脈の支脈	314
腎動脈・静脈	316
門脈の分布	318
原位置の門脈	320
女性骨盤部の血管	322
直腸の血管	324
男性生殖器の血管	326
壁側リンパ節	328
自律神経叢	330
女性骨盤部の神経支配	332
男性骨盤部の神経支配	334
腹部・骨盤部の体表解剖	336

上肢

上肢の骨格	340
鎖骨	342
肩甲骨 1, 2	344
上腕骨 1, 2	348
上肢帯の関節	352
胸鎖関節	354
肩関節 (肩甲上腕関節) 1, 2	356
肩の冠状断面	360
肩と上腕の筋 (前面) 1-4	362
肩と上腕の筋 (後面) 1-3	370
上肢帯の筋の区分 1-5	376
肩関節の筋の区分 1-4	386
上腕の筋の区分 1, 2	394
橈骨と尺骨	398
肘関節 1, 2	400
前腕の筋 (前面) 1-3	404
前腕の筋 (後面) 1, 2	410
前腕の筋の区分 1-7	414
手首と手の骨格 1, 2	428
手首と手の関節	432
手の筋 1-4	434
手背	442
手の筋の区分 1-5	444
上肢の動脈	454
上肢の皮静脈	456
腕神経叢の構造	458
腕神経叢の走行	460
腕神経叢からの神経 1-5	462
肩の後部における神経・血管 1, 2	472

腋窩の神経・血管 1-3	476
上腕の神経・血管	482
前腕の神経・血管	484
手根管	486
浅掌動脈弓	488
深掌動脈弓	490
解剖学的嗅ぎタバコ入れ	492
手における感覚神経の分布 1, 2	494
上腕の横断面	498
前腕の横断面	500
手の体表解剖	502

下肢

下肢の骨格	506
寛骨の構成	508
大腿骨	510
股関節 1, 2	512
股関節の靱帯 1, 2	516
骨盤と大腿の筋 1-8	520
骨盤と殿部の筋の区分 1-7	536
大腿の筋の区分 1-4	550
脛骨と腓骨	558
膝関節 1, 2	560
膝関節の靱帯 1-3	564
下腿の筋 1-5	570
下腿の筋の区分 1-4	580
足の骨格 1, 2	588
足首と足の関節 1-3	592
足首と足の靱帯 1-3	598
足底の筋 1-4	604
足首と足	612
足の筋の区分 1-7	614
下肢の動脈 1, 2	628
腰仙骨神経叢 1, 2	632
腰神経叢からの神経 1, 2	636
仙骨神経叢からの神経 1, 2	640
皮静脈と皮神経	644
鼠径部	646
坐骨孔	648
大腿前面の神経・血管	650
大腿後面の神経・血管	652
下腿後面の神経・血管	654
足根管	656
下腿外側の神経・血管	658
下腿前面の神経・血管	660
足背の神経・血管	662
足底の神経・血管	664
大腿の横断面	666
下腿の横断面	668
下肢の体表解剖	670

頭頸部

頭蓋の骨 1-3	674
頭蓋底 1-3	680
表情筋	686
頭部の筋の区分 1-3	688
脳神経 1-10	694
感覚神経支配	714
頭蓋と顔面の動脈 1, 2	716
頭頸部の静脈 1, 2	720
顔面浅層の神経・血管 1, 2	724
耳下腺咬筋部 1, 2	728
側頭下窩 1-3	732
翼口蓋窩	738
眼窩の骨	740
眼窩の筋	742
眼窩の神経 1, 2	744
眼窩の局所解剖 1, 2	748
眼瞼と結膜	752
涙器	754
眼球の構造	756
鼻腔の骨 1-3	758
鼻腔の神経・血管 1, 2	764
外耳	768
耳介の構造	770
鼓室	772
耳小骨連鎖	774
内耳	776
下顎骨	778
口腔の三叉神経	780
舌背	782
舌の筋	784

舌の感覚性神経支配と味覚神経支配	786
舌の神経と血管	788
口腔の区分 1, 2	790
唾液腺 1, 2	794
咽頭筋 1, 2	798
咽頭の神経・血管	802
頸部の筋の概観	804
頸部の筋 1-6	806
頸部の動脈	818
頸部の神経	820
甲状腺	822
甲状腺の位置	824
喉頭の構造	826
喉頭腔	828
喉頭の神経・血管 1, 2	830
頸部の部位	834
胸郭上口 1, 2	836
外側頸三角部の局所解剖 1, 2	840
頭頸部の体表解剖	844

神経解剖

成人の脳 1-3	848
髄膜 1, 2	854
硬膜中隔	858
脳脊髄液の循環	860
脳室系	862
脳の動脈	864
静脈洞交会	866
頭蓋底にある硬膜静脈洞	868
終脳 1-6	870
間脳 1, 2	882
脳の内部構造 1-3	886
脳幹 1-4	892
小脳 1, 2	900
脊髄 1-10	904
脊髄の動脈	924
脊髄の静脈流出路	926
感覚系と運動系	928
視覚系	930
自律神経系	932
索引	935

アイコン一覧

本書のアイコンは，それぞれ下記を意味しています．

Q クエスチョン   解説

A アンサー   臨床

背部 Back

脊柱 1-3 ･････････････････････････････････ 2
椎骨の構成要素 ･････････････････････････ 8
頸椎 1-4 ･････････････････････････････････ 10
胸椎 ････････････････････････････････････ 18
腰椎 ････････････････････････････････････ 20
仙骨と尾骨 1, 2 ････････････････････････ 22
脊柱の関節 ･････････････････････････････ 26
頸部脊柱の靱帯 1, 2 ･･･････････････････ 28
胸腰部脊柱の靱帯 1-3 ･････････････････ 32

背部の筋の概観 1-4 ････････････････････ 38
背部の筋の区分 1-10 ･･･････････････････ 46
背部の動脈 ･････････････････････････････ 66
背部の静脈 ･････････････････････････････ 68
背部の神経 ･････････････････････････････ 70
項部の神経・血管（局所解剖） ･････････ 72
背部の神経・血管（局所解剖） ･････････ 74
背部の体表解剖 ････････････････････････ 76

Vertebral Column I

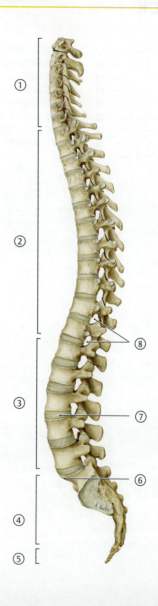

脊柱 1

左外側面

① ☐ 第 1-7 頸椎 ☐ C1-C7 vertebrae
② ☐ 第 1-12 胸椎 ☐ T1-T12 vertebrae
③ ☐ 第 1-5 腰椎 ☐ L1-L5 vertebrae
④ ☐ 仙骨（第 1-5 仙椎） ☐ Sacrum (S1-S5 vertebrae)
⑤ ☐ 尾骨 ☐ Coccyx
⑥ ☐ 岬角 ☐ Promontory
⑦ ☐ 椎間円板 ☐ Intervertebral disc
⑧ ☐ 椎間孔 ☐ Intervertebral foramen

解説

成人では脊柱に特徴的な弯曲（4ヵ所）が見られる．この弯曲は生後の発達過程で形成される．新生児では胸部脊柱の後弯のみが見られる．腰部脊柱の前弯は生後に発達し，思春期に安定化する．

Vertebral Column II

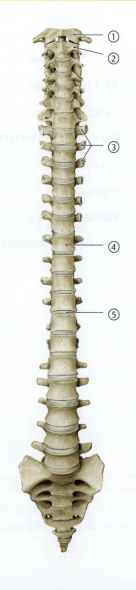
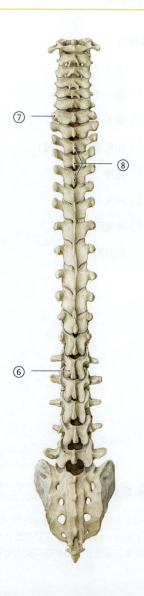

脊柱 2

左：前面，右：後面

① □ 環椎（第1頸椎） □ Atlas (C1)
② □ 軸椎（第2頸椎） □ Axis (C2)
③ □ 横突起 □ Transverse processes
④ □ 椎体 □ Vertebral body
⑤ □ 椎間円板 □ Intervertebral disc
⑥ □ 第1腰椎 □ L1 vertebra
⑦ □ 隆椎（第7頸椎） □ Vertebra prominens (C7)
⑧ □ 棘突起 □ Spinous processes

臨床

脊柱は骨格の退行性疾患（例えば，変形性関節症や骨粗鬆症）によって最も侵されやすい部位である．骨粗鬆症では，骨吸収が骨形成を上回り，骨量が減少する．この疾患では椎体の圧迫骨折により背部痛を生じる場合がある．

Vertebral Column III

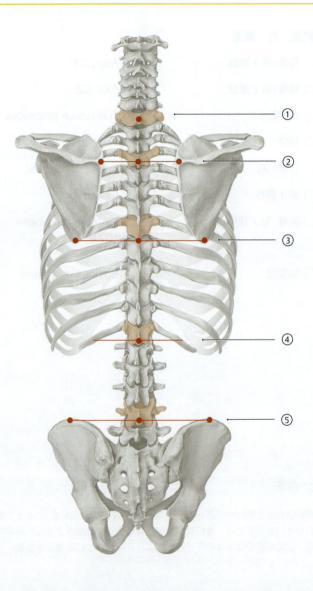

脊柱 3

指標としての棘突起 Spinous processes, 後面

① □ 頸椎と胸椎の移行部 　　□ Cervicothoracic junction
　　　〔第7頸椎(隆椎)〕　　　　　　(C7 prominent vertebra)

② □ 肩甲棘(第3胸椎)　　　　□ Scapular spine(T3)

③ □ 肩甲骨の下角(第7胸椎)　□ Inferior scapular angle(T7)

④ □ 第12肋骨(第12胸椎)　　□ 12th rib(T12)

⑤ □ 腸骨稜(第4腰椎)　　　　□ Iliac crest(L4)

臨床

棘突起は体表から容易に触知することができ，理学的診察の際に特定の位置を表す指標として役立つ．

Structural Elements of a Vertebra

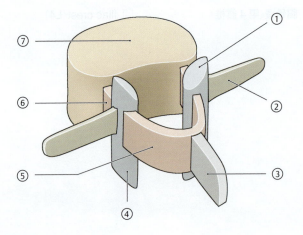

椎骨の構成要素

左後上面

① □ 上関節突起 　　□ Superior articular process
② □ 横突起 　　　　□ Transverse process
③ □ 棘突起 　　　　□ Spinous process
④ □ 下関節突起 　　□ Inferior articular process
⑤ □ 椎弓板 　　　　□ Lamina of vertebral arch
⑥ □ 椎弓根 　　　　□ Pedicle of vertebral arch
⑦ □ 椎体 　　　　　□ Vertebral body

解説

　環椎(C1)と軸椎(C2)以外の椎骨は，共通した構成要素(椎弓，椎体，棘突起，横突起，関節突起)からなる．椎弓は椎弓根と椎弓板からなり，椎体とともに椎孔を形成する．すべての椎骨の椎孔が縦に連なり，脊柱管が形成される．

Cervical Vertebrae I

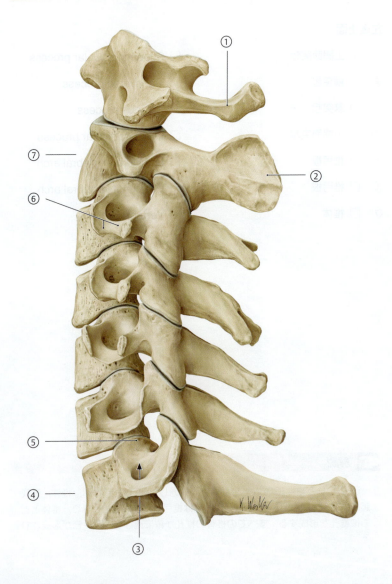

頸椎 1

左外側面

① □ 環椎後弓 □ Posterior arch of atlas
② □ 棘突起 □ Spinous process
③ □ 横突孔 □ Foramen transverse
④ □ 第7頸椎（隆椎） □ C7 (vertebra prominens)
⑤ □ 鈎状突起 □ Uncinate process
⑥ □ 脊髄神経溝 □ Groove for spinal nerve
⑦ □ 第2頸椎（軸椎） □ C2 (axis)

臨床

頸部脊柱は過伸展による損傷（いわゆる"むち打ち症"）を受けやすい部位であり、頭部が通常の可動域を大きく越えて後方に伸展した場合に生じる。頸部脊柱で見られる最も多い外傷は、歯突起骨折、外傷性脊椎すべり症（椎体の前方への偏位）、環椎骨折である。これらの患者の予後は、損傷を受けた脊髄の高さにほぼ依存する。

Cervical Vertebrae II

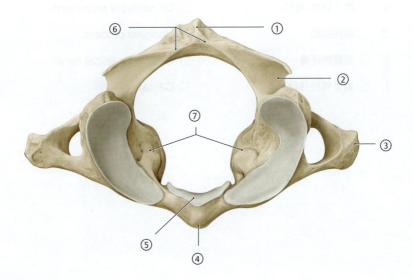

環椎（C1）の基本構造は，典型的な頸椎（C3-C7）とどのように異なるか？

頸椎 2

環椎（第1頸椎）〔Atlas（C1）〕，上面

① □ 後結節　　　　　　　□ Posterior tubercle
② □ 椎骨動脈溝　　　　　□ Groove for vertebral artery
③ □ 横突起　　　　　　　□ Transverse process
④ □ 前結節　　　　　　　□ Anterior tubercle
⑤ □ 歯突起窩　　　　　　□ Facet for dens
⑥ □ 後弓　　　　　　　　□ Posterior arch
⑦ □ 外側塊　　　　　　　□ Lateral masses

A 環椎は典型的な頸椎（C3-C7）で見られるような椎体と棘突起を欠く．環椎は上方では頭蓋（後頭骨）の後頭顆と関節をなす．

Cervical Vertebrae III

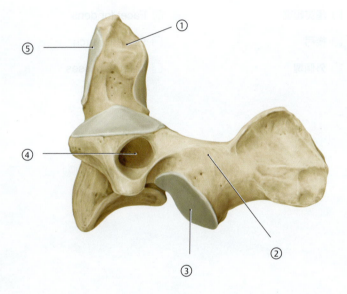

頸椎 3

軸椎(第2頸椎)〔Axis(C2)〕，左外側面

① □ 歯突起　　　　　□ Dens
② □ 椎弓　　　　　　□ Vertebral arch
③ □ 下関節面　　　　□ Inferior articular facet
④ □ 横突孔　　　　　□ Foramen transverse
⑤ □ 前関節面　　　　□ Anterior articular facet

解説

軸椎は上方に突出する特有の突起(歯突起)を有する．歯突起は環椎の前弓と関節をなす．

Cervical Vertebrae IV

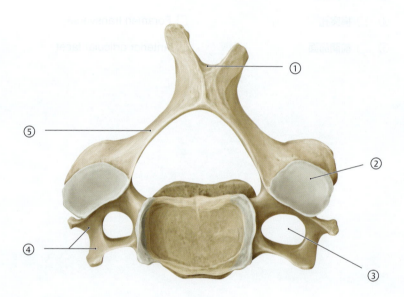

Q 頸椎の横突孔を通る構造は何か？

頸椎 4

第 4 頸椎〔Cervical vertebra(C4)〕，上面

① □ 棘突起　　　　　　　　□ Spinous process
② □ 上関節面　　　　　　　□ Superior articular facet
③ □ 横突孔　　　　　　　　□ Foramen transverse
④ □ 横突起，脊髄神経溝　　□ Transverse process with sulcus for spinal nerve
⑤ □ 椎弓板　　　　　　　　□ Lamina of vertebral arch

椎骨動脈が C1-C6 の横突孔を通る．

Thoracic Vertebrae

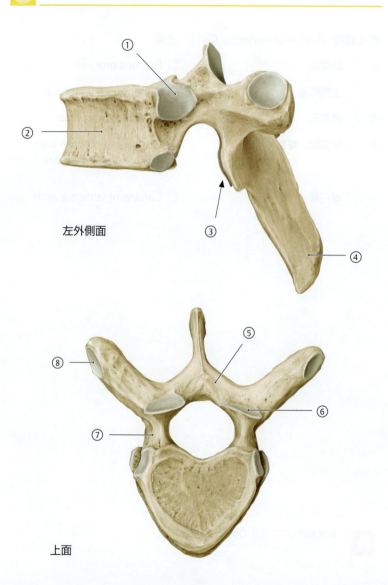

左外側面

上面

胸椎

**典型的な胸椎（第6胸椎）〔Thoracic vertebra (T6)〕，
上：左外側面，下：上面**

① □ 上肋骨窩　　　　　□ Superior costal facet
② □ 椎体　　　　　　　□ Vertebral body
③ □ 下関節面　　　　　□ Inferior articular facet
④ □ 棘突起　　　　　　□ Spinous process
⑤ □ 椎弓板　　　　　　□ Lamina of vertebral arch
⑥ □ 上関節面　　　　　□ Superior articular facet
⑦ □ 椎弓根　　　　　　□ Pedicle of vertebral arch
⑧ □ 横突肋骨窩　　　　□ Transverse costal facet

Lumbar Vertebrae

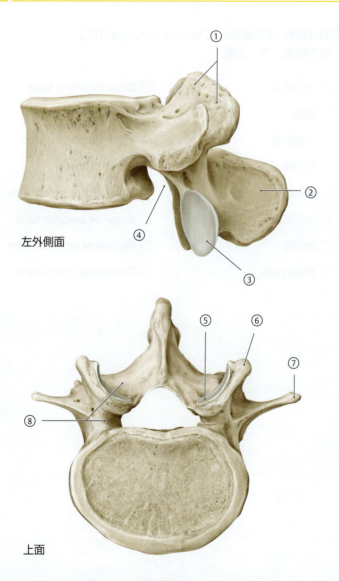

左外側面

上面

腰椎

**第4腰椎〔Lumbar vertebra(L4)〕,
上:左外側面,下:上面**

① □ 上関節突起　　　　　□ Superior articular process
② □ 棘突起　　　　　　　□ Spinous process
③ □ 下関節面　　　　　　□ Inferior articular facet
④ □ 下椎切痕　　　　　　□ Inferior vertebral notch
⑤ □ 上関節面　　　　　　□ Superior articular facet
⑥ □ 乳頭突起　　　　　　□ Mammillary process
⑦ □ 横突起　　　　　　　□ Transverse process
⑧ □ 椎弓　　　　　　　　□ Vertebral arch

Sacrum & Coccyx I

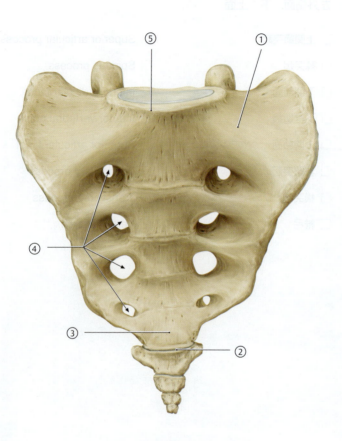

Q 前仙骨孔を通る構造は何か？

仙骨と尾骨 1

前面

① □ 仙骨翼　　　　　□ Ala of sacrum
② □ 仙尾関節　　　　□ Sacrococcygeal joint
③ □ 仙骨尖　　　　　□ Apex of sacrum
④ □ 前仙骨孔　　　　□ Anterior sacral foramina
⑤ □ 岬角　　　　　　□ Promontory

仙骨神経の前枝が前仙骨孔を通過し，仙骨神経叢を形成する．

Sacrum & Coccyx II

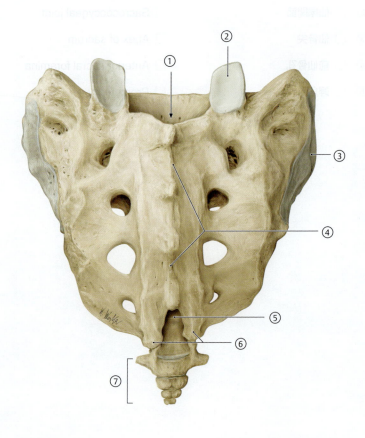

仙骨と尾骨 2

後面

① □ 仙骨管　　　　□ Sacral canal
② □ 上関節面　　　□ Superior articular facet
③ □ 耳状面　　　　□ Auricular surface
④ □ 正中仙骨稜　　□ Median sacral crest
⑤ □ 仙骨裂孔　　　□ Sacral hiatus
⑥ □ 仙骨角　　　　□ Sacral horn
⑦ □ 尾骨　　　　　□ Coccyx

解説

仙骨は生後に癒合した5つの仙椎からなる．仙骨底はL5と，仙骨尖は尾骨と，それぞれ関節をなす．仙骨裂孔は仙骨角の間にできる裂隙であり，仙骨管内に麻酔薬を投与する経路として利用される．

Joints of the Vertebral Column

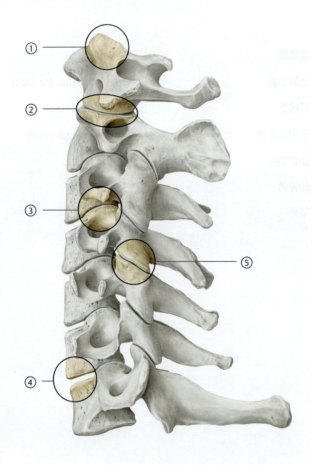

頸部脊柱に特有の関節はどれか？

脊柱の関節

左外側面

① □ 環椎後頭関節　　□ Atlanto-occipital joint
② □ 環軸関節　　　　□ Atlantoaxial joint
③ □ 鈎椎関節　　　　□ Uncovertebral joint
④ □ 椎体間関節　　　□ Intervertebral joint
⑤ □ 椎間関節　　　　□ Zygapophyseal joint

　環椎後頭関節（頭蓋-C1 間），環軸関節（C1-C2 間），鈎椎関節（C3-C7 間）が頸部脊柱に特有の関節である．椎間関節はすべての椎骨間で見られる．椎体間関節（椎間円板を伴う）は C1-C2 間を除くすべての椎骨間で見られる．

Cervical Spine Ligaments I

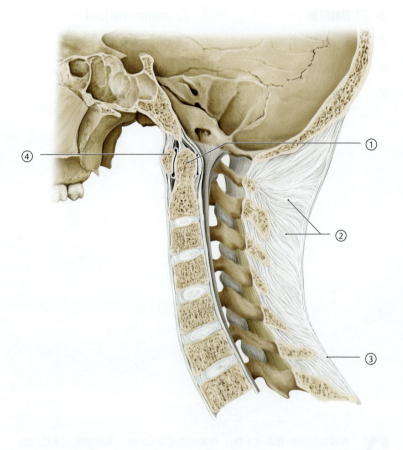

頸部脊柱の靱帯 1

正中矢状断面，左外側面

① □ 軸椎（第2頸椎）の歯突起　　□ Dens of axis（C2）
② □ 項靱帯　　□ Nuchal ligament
③ □ 棘上靱帯　　□ Supraspinous ligament
④ □ 環椎（第1頸椎）の前弓　　□ Anterior arch of atlas（C1）

臨床

項靱帯は棘上靱帯が矢状方向に広がったものであり，隆椎（C7）の棘突起と後頭骨の外後頭隆起の間に存在する．

Cervical Spine Ligaments II

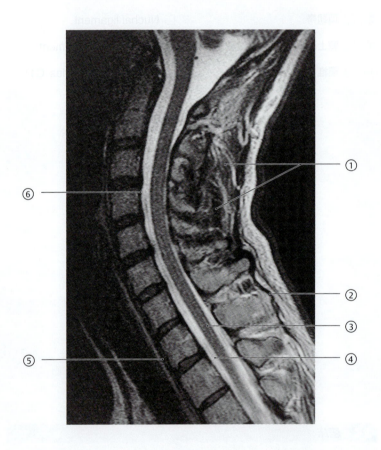

頸部脊柱の靱帯 2

T2 強調 MR 像（正中矢状断面），左外側面

① □ 項靱帯 　　　　　　　　□ Nuchal ligament
② □ 棘上靱帯 　　　　　　　□ Supraspinous ligament
③ □ 脊髄 　　　　　　　　　□ Spinal cord
④ □ クモ膜下腔 　　　　　　□ Subarachnoid space
⑤ □ 前縦靱帯 　　　　　　　□ Anterior longitudinal ligament
⑥ □ 後縦靱帯 　　　　　　　□ Posterior longitudinal ligament

Thoracolumbar Spine Ligaments I

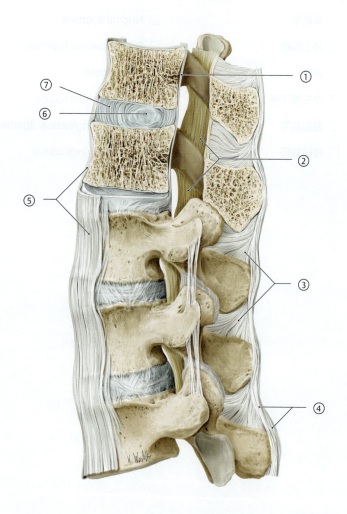

胸腰部脊柱の靱帯 1

胸腰部の連結．
T11-L3 の左外側面，T11-T12 は正中矢状断面が見えている

①	□ 後縦靱帯	□	Posterior longitudinal ligament
②	□ 黄色靱帯	□	Ligamenta flava
③	□ 棘間靱帯	□	Interspinous ligaments
④	□ 棘上靱帯	□	Supraspinous ligament
⑤	□ 前縦靱帯	□	Anterior longitudinal ligament
⑥	□ 椎間円板の髄核	□	Nucleus pulposus of intervertebral disc
⑦	□ 椎間円板の線維輪	□	Anulus fibrosus of intervertebral disc

解説

脊椎の靱帯は椎骨どうしをしっかりと連結し，大きな荷重やせん断ストレスから脊柱を保護している．

Thoracolumbar Spine Ligaments II

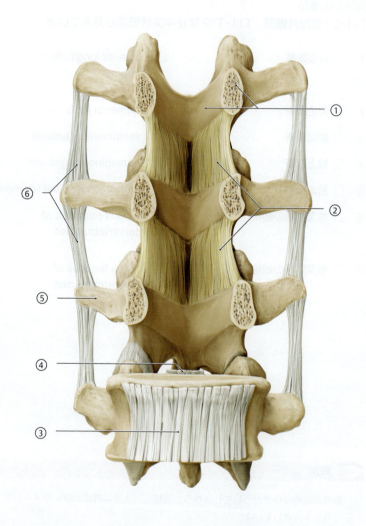

胸腰部脊柱の靱帯 2

脊柱管を開放したところ，前面

① □ 椎弓板　　　　　　　□ Lamina of vertebral arch
② □ 黄色靱帯　　　　　　□ Ligamenta flava
③ □ 前縦靱帯　　　　　　□ Anterior longitudinal ligament
④ □ 後縦靱帯　　　　　　□ Posterior longitudinal ligament
⑤ □ 肋骨突起　　　　　　□ Costal process
⑥ □ 横突間靱帯　　　　　□ Intertransverse ligaments

解説

黄色靱帯は主に弾性線維からなる．この靱帯は弾性線維を豊富に含むため特有の色（黄色）をしている．

Thoracolumbar Spine Ligaments III

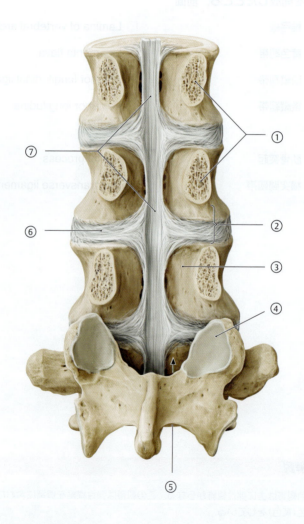

胸腰部脊柱の靱帯 3

脊柱管を開放したところ，後面

① □ 椎弓根　　　　　□ Pedicles of vertebral arches
② □ 椎間孔　　　　　□ Intervertebral foramen
③ □ 椎体　　　　　　□ Vertebral body
④ □ 上関節面　　　　□ Superior articular facet
⑤ □ 脊柱管　　　　　□ Vertebral canal
⑥ □ 椎間円板　　　　□ Intervertebral disc
⑦ □ 後縦靱帯　　　　□ Posterior longitudinal ligament

Muscles of the Back : Overview

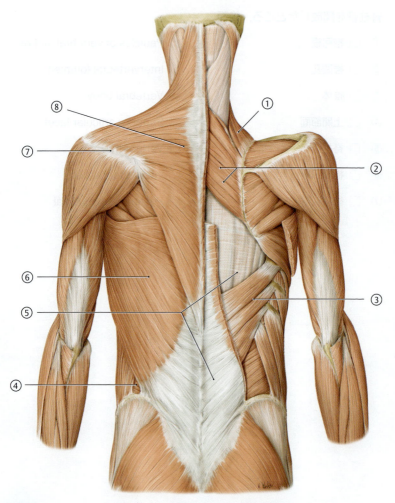

 描かれている筋肉のうち，どの筋肉が呼吸補助筋として働くか？

背部の筋の概観 1

後面

① ☐ 肩甲挙筋　　　　　　　　　☐ Levator scapulae

② ☐ 大菱形筋　　　　　　　　　☐ Rhomboid major

③ ☐ 下後鋸筋　　　　　　　　　☐ Serratus posterior inferior

④ ☐ 腰三角，内腹斜筋　　　　　☐ Lumbar triangle, internal oblique

⑤ ☐ 胸腰筋膜の浅葉　　　　　　☐ Superficial layer of thoracolumbar fascia

⑥ ☐ 広背筋　　　　　　　　　　☐ Latissimus dorsi

⑦ ☐ 肩甲棘　　　　　　　　　　☐ Scapular spine

⑧ ☐ 僧帽筋の横行部（水平部）　☐ Transverse part of trapezius

A 胸鎖乳突筋，外肋間筋，外腹斜筋，内腹斜筋，下後鋸筋．

Muscles of the Back : Overview II

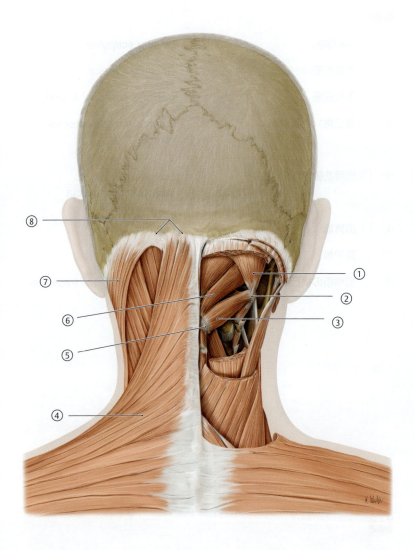

背部の筋の概観 2

項部の固有筋

① ☐ 上頭斜筋 ☐ Obliquus capitis superior
② ☐ 環椎（第1頸椎），横突起 ☐ Atlas(C1), transverse process
③ ☐ 下頭斜筋 ☐ Obliquus capitis inferior
④ ☐ 僧帽筋 ☐ Trapezius
⑤ ☐ 軸椎（第2頸椎），棘突起 ☐ Axis(C2), spinous process
⑥ ☐ 大後頭直筋 ☐ Rectus capitis posterior major
⑦ ☐ 胸鎖乳突筋 ☐ Sternocleidomastoid
⑧ ☐ 上項線 ☐ Superior nuchal line

Muscles of the Back : Overview III

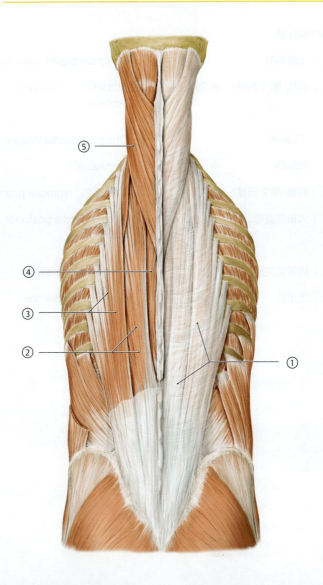

背部の筋の概観 3

固有筋，外側部，後面

① □ 胸腰筋膜の浅葉　　　　□ Superficial layer of thoracolumbar fascia

② □ 最長筋　　　　　　　　□ Longissimus

③ □ 腸肋筋　　　　　　　　□ Iliocostalis

④ □ 棘筋　　　　　　　　　□ Spinalis

⑤ □ 頸板状筋　　　　　　　□ Splenius cervicis

解説

脊柱起立筋の外側部には，腸肋筋および最長筋（いわゆる仙棘筋系）ならびに頸板状筋および頭板状筋（いわゆる棘横突筋系）が属する．肋骨挙筋および横突間筋も，外側部に含まれ（いわゆる横突間筋系），腸肋筋および最長筋によって覆われている（pp.46-49を参照）．

Muscles of the Back : Overview IV

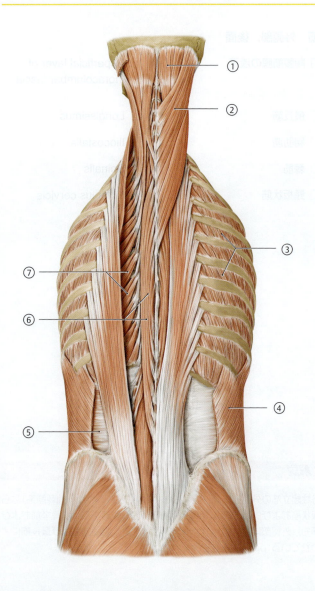

背部の筋の概観 4

固有筋，内側部，後面

① □ 頭半棘筋　　　　　　□ Semispinalis capitis

② □ 頭板状筋　　　　　　□ Splenius capitis

③ □ 外肋間筋　　　　　　□ External intercostal muscles

④ □ 内腹斜筋　　　　　　□ Internal oblique

⑤ □ 腹横筋　　　　　　　□ Transversus abdominis

⑥ □ 棘筋　　　　　　　　□ Spinalis

⑦ □ 肋骨挙筋　　　　　　□ Levatores costarum

解説

脊柱起立筋の内側部には棘間筋および棘筋（いわゆる棘筋系）ならびに短回旋筋，長回旋筋，多裂筋および半棘筋（いわゆる横突棘筋系）が属する．

System of the Muscles of the Back I

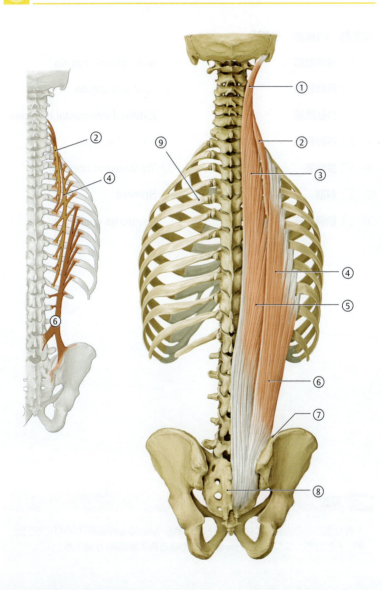

背部の筋の区分 1

固有筋，外側部：腸肋筋

① ☐ 頭最長筋　　　　　　☐ Longissimus capitis
② ☐ 頸腸肋筋　　　　　　☐ **Iliocostalis cervicis**
③ ☐ 頸最長筋　　　　　　☐ Longissimus cervicis
④ ☐ 胸腸肋筋　　　　　　☐ **Iliocostalis thoracis**
⑤ ☐ 胸最長筋　　　　　　☐ Longissimus thoracis
⑥ ☐ 腰腸肋筋　　　　　　☐ **Iliocostalis lumborum**
⑦ ☐ 腸骨稜　　　　　　　☐ Iliac crest
⑧ ☐ 仙骨　　　　　　　　☐ Sacrum
⑨ ☐ 第5肋骨　　　　　　☐ 5th rib

筋	起始	停止	作用	神経支配
腰腸肋筋	・仙骨 ・腸骨稜 ・胸腰筋膜（浅葉）	・第6-12肋骨 ・胸腰筋膜（深葉） ・上位腰椎（横突起）	・両側：脊柱を伸展させる ・片側：脊柱を同側に側屈させる	C8-L1（後枝の外側枝）
胸腸肋筋	第7-12肋骨	第1-6肋骨		
頸腸肋筋	第3-7肋骨	C4-C6（横突起）		

解説

腸肋筋は固有背筋の外側部のいわゆる仙棘筋系に属する．

System of the Muscles of the Back II

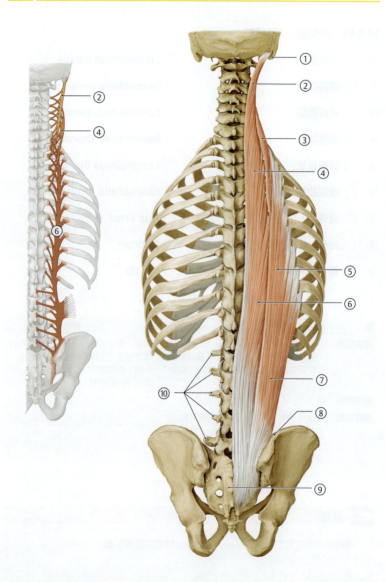

背部の筋の区分 2

固有筋,外側部:最長筋

① □ 乳様突起　　　　　　　□ Mastoid process
② □ **頭最長筋**　　　　　　□ **Longissimus capitis**
③ □ 頸腸肋筋　　　　　　　□ Iliocostalis cervicis
④ □ **頸最長筋**　　　　　　□ **Longissimus cervicis**
⑤ □ 胸腸肋筋　　　　　　　□ Iliocostalis thoracis
⑥ □ **胸最長筋**　　　　　　□ **Longissimus thoracis**
⑦ □ 腰腸肋筋　　　　　　　□ Iliocostalis lumborum
⑧ □ 腸骨稜　　　　　　　　□ Iliac crest
⑨ □ 仙骨　　　　　　　　　□ Sacrum
⑩ □ 肋骨突起(第1-5腰椎)　□ Costal process(L1-L5)

筋	起始	停止	作用	神経支配
胸最長筋	・仙骨 ・腸骨稜(腸肋筋と共通の起始腱) ・腰椎(肋骨突起) ・下位胸椎(横突起)	・第2-12肋骨 ・腰椎(肋骨突起) ・胸椎(横突起)	・両側:脊柱を伸展させる ・片側:脊柱を同側に側屈させる	C1-L5(後枝の外側枝)
頸最長筋	T1-T6(横突起)	C2-C5(横突起)		
頭最長筋	・T1-T3(横突起) ・C4-C7(横突起,関節突起)	側頭骨(乳様突起)	・両側:頭部を後屈させる ・片側:頭部を同側に側屈・回旋させる	

解説

最長筋は腸肋筋と同様に,固有背筋の外側部のいわゆる仙棘筋系に属する.

System of the Muscles of the Back III

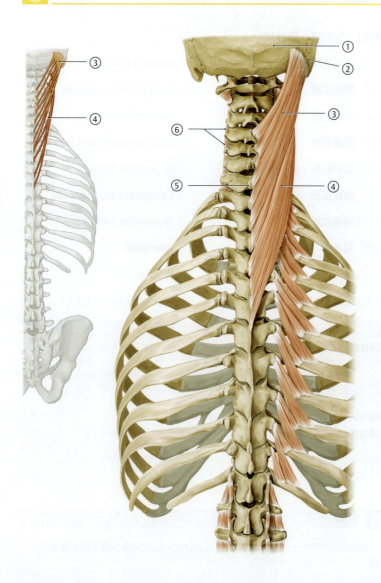

背部の筋の区分 3

固有筋，外側部：板状筋

① □ 上項線 　　　　　　　□ Superior nuchal line
② □ 乳様突起 　　　　　　□ Mastoid process
③ □ 頭板状筋 　　　　　　□ **Splenius capitis**
④ □ 頸板状筋 　　　　　　□ **Splenius cervicis**
⑤ □ 第7頸椎（隆椎）の棘突起 　□ Spinous process of C7 (vertebra prominens)
⑥ □ 頸後横突間筋 　　　　□ Posterior cervical intertransversarii

筋	起始	停止	作用	神経支配
頸板状筋	T3-T6（棘突起）	C1-C2（横突起）	・両側：頭部と頸部脊柱を後屈させる ・片側：頭部を同側に側屈・回旋させる	C1-C6（後枝の外側枝）
頭板状筋	C3-T3（棘突起）	・上項線の外側 ・乳様突起		

解説

板状筋は固有背筋の外側部のいわゆる棘横突筋系に属する．

System of the Muscles of the Back IV

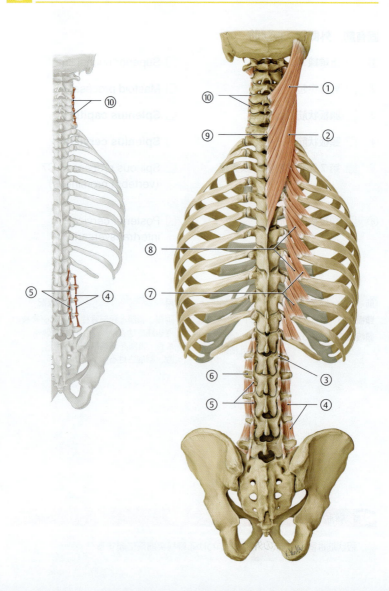

背部の筋の区分 4

固有筋, 外側部：横突間筋

① ☐ 頭板状筋　　　　　　　　☐ Splenius capitis
② ☐ 頸板状筋　　　　　　　　☐ Splenius cervicis
③ ☐ 乳頭突起　　　　　　　　☐ Mammillary process
④ ☐ 腰外側横突間筋　　　　　☐ **Intertransversarii lateralis lumborum**
⑤ ☐ 腰内側横突間筋　　　　　☐ **Intertransversarii mediales lumborum**
⑥ ☐ 肋骨突起　　　　　　　　☐ Costal process
⑦ ☐ 長肋骨挙筋　　　　　　　☐ Levatores costarum longi
⑧ ☐ 短肋骨挙筋　　　　　　　☐ Levatores costarum breves
⑨ ☐ 第7頸椎（隆椎）の棘突起　☐ Spinous process of C7 (vertebra prominens)
⑩ ☐ 頸後横突間筋　　　　　　☐ **Posterior cervical intertransversarii**

筋	起始・停止	作用	神経支配
腰内側横突間筋	隣接する腰椎の乳頭突起を結ぶ	・両側：頸部と腰部の脊柱を伸展，安定化させる ・片側：頸部と腰部の脊柱を同側に側屈させる	脊髄神経の後枝
腰外側横突間筋	隣接する腰椎の肋骨突起を結ぶ		脊髄神経の前枝
頸後横突間筋	C2-C7（隣接する頸椎の後結節を結ぶ）		脊髄神経の後枝
頸前横突間筋	C2-C7（隣接する頸椎の前結節を結ぶ）		脊髄神経の前枝

解説

横突間筋は固有背筋の外側部のいわゆる横突間筋系に属する．

System of the Muscles of the Back V

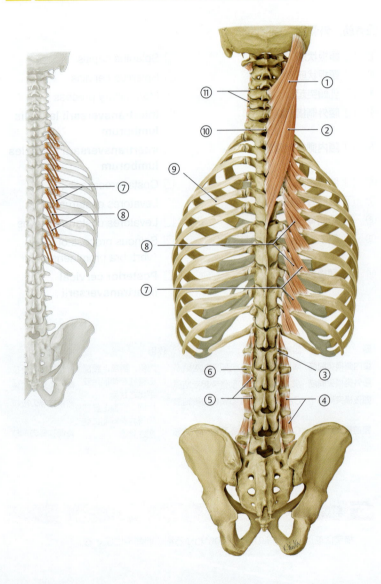

背部 55

背部の筋の区分 5

固有筋，外側部：肋骨挙筋

① ☐ 頭板状筋　　　　　　　　　☐ Splenius capitis
② ☐ 頸板状筋　　　　　　　　　☐ Splenius cervicis
③ ☐ 乳頭突起　　　　　　　　　☐ Mammillary process
④ ☐ 腰外側横突間筋　　　　　　☐ Intertransversarii lateralis lumborum
⑤ ☐ 腰内側横突間筋　　　　　　☐ Intertransversarii mediales lumborum
⑥ ☐ 肋骨突起　　　　　　　　　☐ Costal process
⑦ ☐ **長肋骨挙筋**　　　　　　　☐ **Levatores costarum longi**
⑧ ☐ **短肋骨挙筋**　　　　　　　☐ **Levatores costarum breves**
⑨ ☐ 第5肋骨　　　　　　　　　☐ 5th rib
⑩ ☐ 第7頸椎（隆椎）の棘突起　☐ Spinous process of C7 (vertebra prominens)
⑪ ☐ 頸後横突間筋　　　　　　　☐ Posterior cervical intertransversarii

筋	起始	停止	作用	神経支配
短肋骨挙筋	C7-T11（横突起）	1つ下位の肋骨の肋骨角	・両側：胸部脊柱を伸展させる ・片側：胸部脊柱を同側に側屈させ，反対側に回旋させる	脊髄神経の前枝・後枝
長肋骨挙筋	C7-T10（横突起）	2つ下位の肋骨の肋骨角		

解説

　肋骨挙筋は横突間筋と同様に，固有背筋の外側部のいわゆる横突間筋系に属する．

System of the Muscles of the Back VI

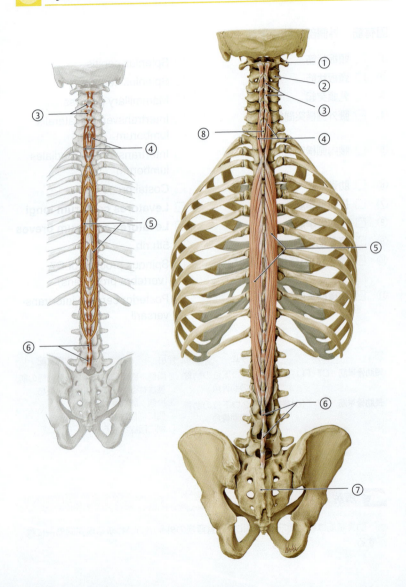

背部の筋の区分 6

固有筋，内側部：棘間筋と棘筋

① ☐ 第 1 頸椎（環椎）　☐ C1（atlas）
② ☐ 第 2 頸椎（軸椎）　☐ C2（axis）
③ ☐ 頸棘間筋　☐ **Interspinales cervicis**
④ ☐ 頸棘筋　☐ **Spinalis cervicis**
⑤ ☐ 胸棘筋　☐ **Spinalis thoracis**
⑥ ☐ 腰棘間筋　☐ **Interspinales lumborum**
⑦ ☐ 仙骨　☐ Sacrum
⑧ ☐ 第 7 頸椎（隆椎）の棘突起　☐ Spinous process of C7 （vertebra prominens）

筋	起始	停止	作用	神経支配
頸棘間筋	隣接する頸椎の棘突起を結ぶ		頸部と腰部の脊柱を伸展させる	脊髄神経の後枝
腰棘間筋	隣接する腰椎の棘突起を結ぶ		・両側：頸胸部の脊柱を伸展させる ・片側：頸胸部の脊柱を同側に側屈させる	
胸棘筋	T10-L3（棘突起の外側面）	T2-T8（棘突起）		
頸棘筋	C5-T2（棘突起）	C2-C4（棘突起）		

 解説

棘間筋と棘筋は固有背筋の内側部のいわゆる棘筋系に属する．

System of the Muscles of the Back VII

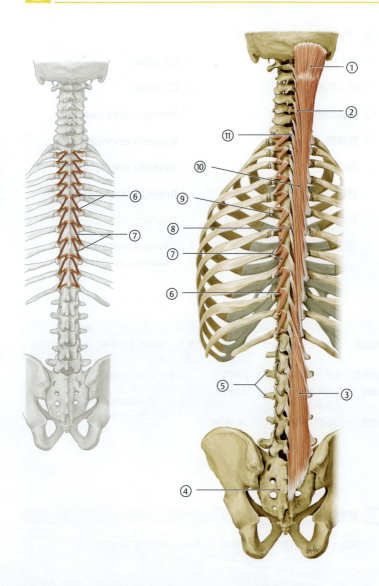

背部の筋の区分 7

固有筋，内側部：短回旋筋と長回旋筋

① ☐ 頭半棘筋 — ☐ Semispinalis capitis
② ☐ 頸半棘筋 — ☐ Semispinalis cervicis
③ ☐ 多裂筋 — ☐ Multifidus
④ ☐ 仙骨 — ☐ Sacrum
⑤ ☐ 肋骨突起 — ☐ Costal processes
⑥ ☐ **短回旋筋** — ☐ **Rotatores breves**
⑦ ☐ **長回旋筋** — ☐ **Rotatores longi**
⑧ ☐ 棘突起 — ☐ Spinous process
⑨ ☐ 横突起 — ☐ Transverse process
⑩ ☐ 胸半棘筋 — ☐ Semispinalis thoracis
⑪ ☐ 第7頸椎（隆椎）の棘突起 — ☐ Spinous process of C7 (vertebra prominens)

筋	起始	停止	作用	神経支配
短回旋筋	胸椎の横突起	1つ上位の胸椎の棘突起	・両側：胸部の脊柱を伸展させる ・片側：胸部の脊柱を反対側に回旋させる	脊髄神経の後枝
長回旋筋	胸椎の横突起	2つ上位の胸椎の棘突起		

 解説

短回旋筋と長回旋筋は固有背筋の内側部のいわゆる横突棘筋系に属する．

System of the Muscles of the Back VIII

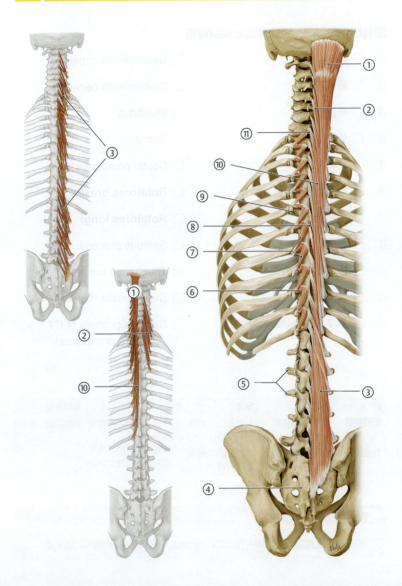

背部の筋の区分 8

固有筋，内側部：多裂筋と半棘筋

① ☐ 頭半棘筋　　　　　　　☐ **Semispinalis capitis**
② ☐ 頸半棘筋　　　　　　　☐ **Semispinalis cervicis**
③ ☐ 多裂筋　　　　　　　　☐ **Multifidus**
④ ☐ 仙骨　　　　　　　　　☐ Sacrum
⑤ ☐ 肋骨突起　　　　　　　☐ Costal processes
⑥ ☐ 短回旋筋　　　　　　　☐ Rotatores breves
⑦ ☐ 長回旋筋　　　　　　　☐ Rotatores longi
⑧ ☐ 棘突起　　　　　　　　☐ Spinous process
⑨ ☐ 横突起　　　　　　　　☐ Transverse process
⑩ ☐ 胸半棘筋　　　　　　　☐ **Semispinalis thoracis**
⑪ ☐ 第7頸椎（隆椎）の棘突起　☐ Spinous process of C7 (vertebra prominens)

筋	起始	停止	作用	神経支配
多裂筋（脊柱内全体で2〜4個の椎骨をまたぐ）	C2-仙骨（横突起）	C2-仙骨（棘突起）	・両側：脊柱を伸展させる ・片側：脊柱を同側に側屈させる	脊髄神経の後枝
胸半棘筋	T6-T12（横突起）	C6-T4（棘突起）	・両側：頸胸部の脊柱を伸展させる，また頭部を後屈させる（頭椎関節を安定化させる） ・片側：頭部と頸胸部の脊柱を同側に側屈させ，反対側に回旋させる	
頸半棘筋	T1-T6（横突起）	C2-C7（棘突起）		
頭半棘筋	C3-T6（横突起）	後頭骨（上項線と下項線の間）		

解説

多裂筋と半棘筋は，短回旋筋と長回旋筋と同様に，固有背筋の内側部のいわゆる横突棘筋系に属する．

System of the Muscles of the Back IX

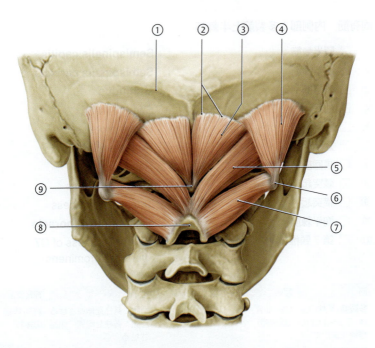

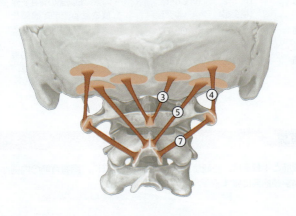

背部の筋の区分 9

固有筋，短い項筋：後頭直筋と頭斜筋

① □ 上項線　　　　　　　　　　□ Superior nuchal line
② □ 下項線　　　　　　　　　　□ Inferior nuchal line
③ □ 小後頭直筋　　　　　　　　□ **Rectus capitis posterior minor**
④ □ 上頭斜筋　　　　　　　　　□ **Obliquus capitis superior**
⑤ □ 大後頭直筋　　　　　　　　□ **Rectus capitis posterior major**
⑥ □ 第1頸椎（環椎）の横突起　　□ Transverse process of C1 (atlas)
⑦ □ 下頭斜筋　　　　　　　　　□ **Obliquus capitis inferior**
⑧ □ 第2頸椎（軸椎）の棘突起　　□ Spinous process of C2 (axis)
⑨ □ 第1頸椎（環椎）の後結節　　□ Posterior tubercle of C1 (atlas)

筋	起始	停止	作用	神経支配
大後頭直筋	C2の棘突起	下項線の中央1/3	・両側：頭部を後屈させる ・片側：頭部を同側に回旋させる	C1の後枝（後頭下神経）
小後頭直筋	C1の後結節	下項線の内側1/3		
上頭斜筋	C1の横突起	大後頭直筋の停止の上方	・両側：頭部を後屈させる ・片側：頭部を同側に傾けるとともに反対側に回旋させる	
下頭斜筋	C2の棘突起	環椎の横突起	・両側：頭部を後屈させる ・片側：頭部を同側に回旋させる	

解説

　後頭骨下に位置している短い項筋と頭部関節筋（このため，これらは後頭下筋と呼ばれている）は，脊髄神経後枝によって支配されていることから，固有背筋に分類される．前頭直筋や外側頭直筋も同様に後頭骨下に位置しているが，脊髄神経前枝によって支配されているため，固有背筋には分類されない．

System of the Muscles of the Back X

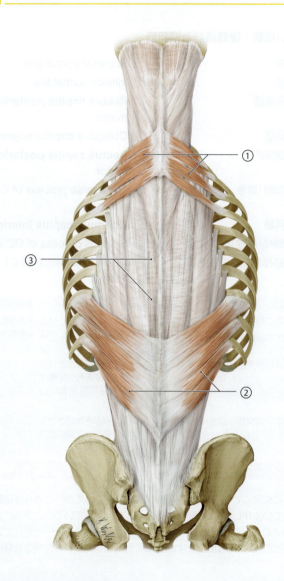

背部の筋の区分 10

二次的に入り込んだ背筋：後鋸筋

① □ 上後鋸筋　　　　　□ **Serratus posterior superior**

② □ 下後鋸筋　　　　　□ **Serratus posterior inferior**

③ □ 胸腰筋膜　　　　　□ Thoracolumbar fascia

筋	起始	停止	作用	神経支配
上後鋸筋	C6-T2（棘突起）	第2-5肋骨（肋骨角付近）	肋骨を引き上げ吸息の補助を行う	肋間神経（T1-T4）
下後鋸筋	・T11-L2（棘突起） ・胸腰筋膜	第9-12肋骨（下縁）	胸部下口（横隔膜の起始部）の狭窄を防ぎ，吸息の補助も行う	肋間神経（T9-T11），肋下神経（T12）

解説

後鋸筋は，二次的に背部に入り込んだ筋であり，固有背筋には含まれない．

Arteries of the Back

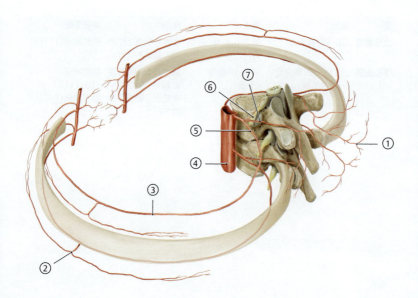

背部 67

背部の動脈

左後上面

① ☐ 内側皮枝 ☐ Medial cutaneous branch

② ☐ 外側皮枝 ☐ Lateral cutaneous branch

③ ☐ 肋間動脈 ☐ Posterior intercostal artery

④ ☐ 胸大動脈 ☐ Thoracic aorta

⑤ ☐ 前枝 ☐ Anterior ramus

⑥ ☐ 脊髄枝 ☐ Spinal branch

⑦ ☐ 後枝 ☐ Posterior ramus

解説

背部の構造には肋間動脈の後枝が分布する．肋間動脈は胸大動脈もしくは鎖骨下動脈から起こる．肋間動脈の後枝は，皮枝，筋枝，脊髄枝に分かれる．

Veins of the Back

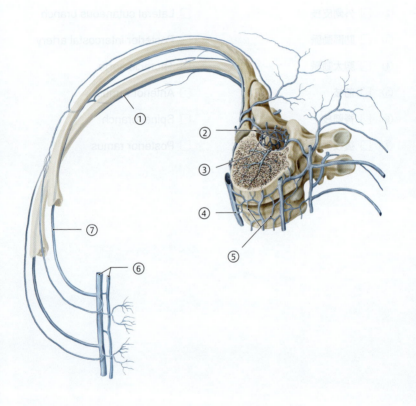

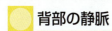
背部の静脈

肋間静脈と椎骨静脈叢(Intercostal veins and vertebral venous plexus), 右前上面

① □ 肋間静脈　　　　　　　□ Posterior intercostal vein

② □ 後内椎骨静脈叢　　　　□ Posterior internal vertebral venous plexus

③ □ 前内椎骨静脈叢　　　　□ Anterior internal vertebral venous plexus

④ □ 奇静脈　　　　　　　　□ Azygos vein

⑤ □ 前外椎骨静脈叢　　　　□ Anterior external vertebral venous plexus

⑥ □ 内胸静脈　　　　　　　□ Internal thoracic veins

⑦ □ 前肋間静脈　　　　　　□ Anterior intercostal vein

解説

　背部の静脈は，半奇静脈，副半奇静脈，上行腰静脈を介して奇静脈に流入する．脊柱の内部からの静脈は，脊柱に沿って存在する椎骨静脈叢を介して流出する．

Nerves of the Back

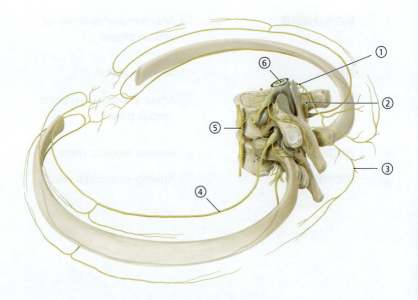

背部の神経

脊髄神経の枝（Spinal nerve branches），左後上面

① □ 後枝　　　　　　　　　　□ Posterior ramus
② □ 関節枝　　　　　　　　　□ Articular branch
③ □ 内側枝　　　　　　　　　□ Medial branch
④ □ 前枝　　　　　　　　　　□ Anterior ramus
⑤ □ 交感神経幹神経節　　　　□ Sympathetic ganglion
⑥ □ 脊髄　　　　　　　　　　□ Spinal cord

 解説

　背部の構造には脊髄神経の後枝が分布する．脊髄神経の後枝は皮枝，筋枝，関節枝（椎間関節に分布する）に分かれる．後枝からの筋枝は固有背筋に分布する．外来背筋には脊髄神経の前枝が分布する．

Neurovascular Topography of the Nuchal Region

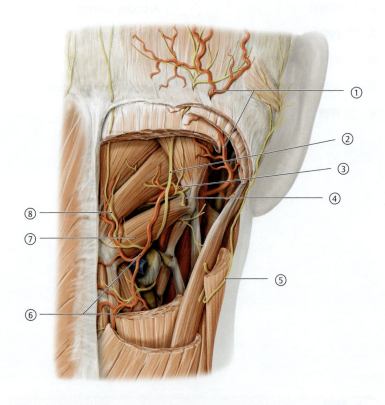

項部の神経・血管（局所解剖）

項部の神経と動脈（Neurovasculature of the nuchal region），後面

① ☐ 後頭動脈　　　　　☐ Occipital artery
② ☐ 大後頭神経　　　　☐ Greater occipital nerve（C2）
③ ☐ 椎骨動脈　　　　　☐ Vertebral artery
④ ☐ 後頭下神経　　　　☐ Suboccipital nerve（C1）
⑤ ☐ 大耳介神経　　　　☐ Great auricular nerve
⑥ ☐ 深頸動脈　　　　　☐ Deep cervical artery
⑦ ☐ 下頭斜筋　　　　　☐ Obliquus capitis inferior
⑧ ☐ 第3後頭神経　　　☐ 3rd occipital nerve（C3）

解説

項部の構造には脊髄神経の後枝が分布する．C1-C3の後枝には特に名称が付けられている：後頭下神経（C1），大後頭神経（C2），第3後頭神経（C3）．小後頭神経と大耳介神経は脊髄神経の前枝（C1-C4）から起こり，頭頸部の前外側の皮膚に分布する．

Neurovascular Topography of the Back

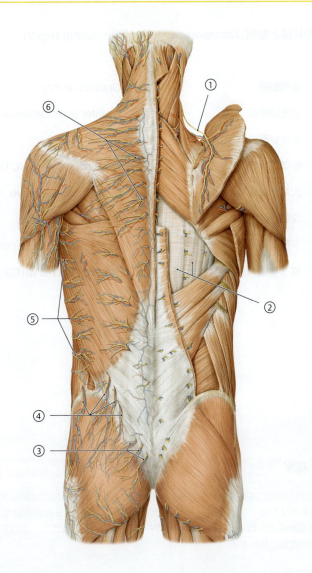

背部の神経・血管（局所解剖）

後面

① ☐ 副神経　　　　　　　　　　☐ Accessory nerve (CN XI)
② ☐ 胸腰筋膜　　　　　　　　　☐ Thoracolumbar fascia
③ ☐ 中殿皮神経　　　　　　　　☐ Middle cluneal nerves
④ ☐ 上殿皮神経　　　　　　　　☐ Superior cluneal nerves
⑤ ☐ 肋間神経と肋間動脈・静脈，それぞれの外側皮枝　　☐ Intercostal nerves and posterior intercostal arteries and veins, lateral cutaneous branches
⑥ ☐ 脊髄神経の後枝（内側皮枝）　☐ Posterior rami (medial cutaneous branches) of spinal nerves

Surface Anatomy

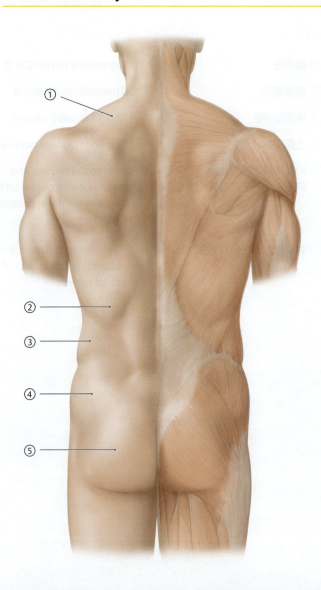

背部の体表解剖

背部の浅層の筋（Musculature of the back），後面

① □ 僧帽筋　　　　　　　　　□ Trapezius
② □ 広背筋　　　　　　　　　□ Latissimus dorsi
③ □ 外腹斜筋　　　　　　　　□ External oblique
④ □ 中殿筋　　　　　　　　　□ Gluteus medius
⑤ □ 大殿筋　　　　　　　　　□ Gluteus maximus

背部の体表解剖

胸部 Thorax

胸部の骨格 ……………………… 80	心膜の折れ返り 1, 2 …………… 138
胸部の構造 ……………………… 82	原位置の心臓 …………………… 142
胸骨 ……………………………… 84	心臓の胸肋面 …………………… 144
胸部の筋の概観 ………………… 86	心臓の底面 ……………………… 146
胸部の筋 1-3 …………………… 88	心臓の部屋 1-3 ………………… 148
原位置の横隔膜 1, 2 …………… 94	心臓弁 …………………………… 154
横隔膜の各部 …………………… 98	心臓の動脈と静脈 1, 2 ………… 156
横隔膜の開口部 ………………… 100	心臓刺激伝導系 ………………… 160
胸壁の動脈 ……………………… 102	心臓の自律神経 ………………… 162
胸壁の静脈 ……………………… 104	心臓のX線像 1, 2 ……………… 164
胸壁の神経 ……………………… 106	水平断面での心臓 ……………… 168
肋間神経の経路 ………………… 108	出生前の循環 …………………… 170
横隔膜の神経・血管 …………… 110	出生後の循環 …………………… 172
女性の乳房への栄養血管 ……… 112	壁側胸膜 ………………………… 174
女性の乳房のリンパ管 ………… 114	原位置の肺 ……………………… 176
女性の乳房の構造 ……………… 116	右肺 ……………………………… 178
縦隔の区分 ……………………… 118	左肺 ……………………………… 180
胸部のCT ……………………… 120	気管 ……………………………… 182
胸大動脈 ………………………… 122	気管支樹の区分 ………………… 184
奇静脈系 ………………………… 124	気管支樹の呼吸部 ……………… 186
胸腔のリンパ管 ………………… 126	肺動脈と肺静脈 ………………… 188
胸腔の神経 ……………………… 128	胸膜腔のリンパ節 ……………… 190
縦隔 1-4 ………………………… 130	胸部の体表解剖 ………………… 192

Thoracic Skeleton

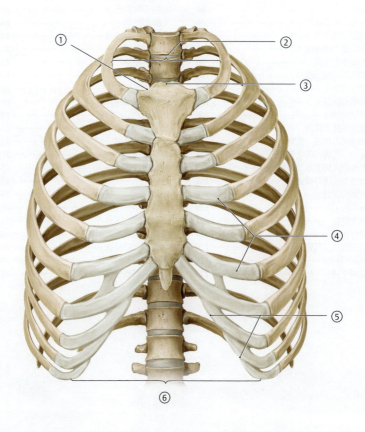

Q 肋軟骨を介して胸骨に連結する真肋は何番目から何番目の肋骨か？

胸部の骨格

前面

① ☐ 鎖骨切痕　　　　　　　☐ Clavicular notch

② ☐ 胸郭上口　　　　　　　☐ Superior thoracic aperture

③ ☐ 頸切痕　　　　　　　　☐ Jugular notch

④ ☐ 肋軟骨　　　　　　　　☐ Costal cartilage

⑤ ☐ 肋骨弓　　　　　　　　☐ Costal margin（arch）

⑥ ☐ 胸郭下口　　　　　　　☐ Inferior thoracic aperture

A 第1-7肋骨の肋軟骨は直接胸骨と連結する．第8-10肋骨は胸骨に間接的に連結し，仮肋と呼ばれる．第11・12肋骨は胸骨に連結せず，浮遊肋と呼ばれる．

Structure of a Thoracic Segment

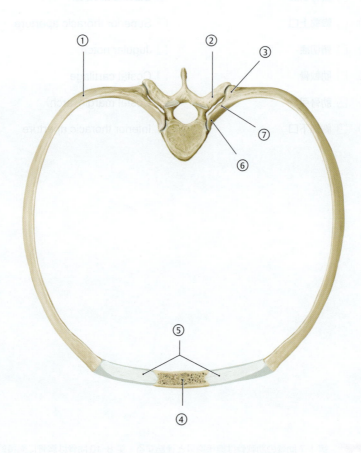

胸部の構造

第6肋骨（6th rib pair），上面

① □ 肋骨角　　　　　□ Costal angle

② □ 横突起　　　　　□ Transverse process

③ □ 肋骨結節　　　　□ Tubercle of rib

④ □ 胸骨　　　　　　□ Sternum

⑤ □ 肋軟骨　　　　　□ Costal cartilage

⑥ □ 肋骨頭　　　　　□ Head of rib

⑦ □ 肋骨頸　　　　　□ Neck of rib

Sternum

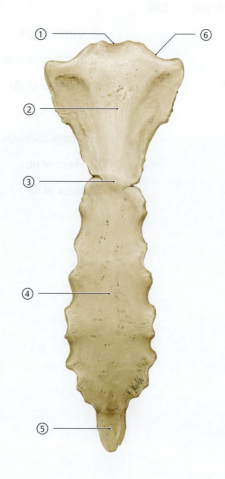

Q 胸骨角で胸骨に連結するのは通常どの肋骨か？

胸骨

前面

① ☐ 頸切痕　　　　　　　　☐ Jugular notch

② ☐ 胸骨柄　　　　　　　　☐ Manubrium of sternum

③ ☐ 胸骨角　　　　　　　　☐ Sternal angle of sternum

④ ☐ 胸骨体　　　　　　　　☐ Body of sternum

⑤ ☐ 剣状突起　　　　　　　☐ Xiphoid process

⑥ ☐ 鎖骨切痕　　　　　　　☐ Clavicular notch

A 胸骨角は第2肋骨の高さにある．

Thoracic Muscles

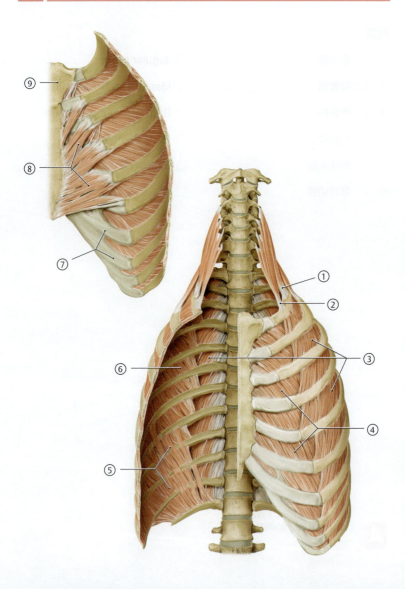

胸部の筋の概観

前面，胸郭を開き，前壁の後面を見せる

① ☐ 中斜角筋　　　　　　　　　☐ Middle scalene

② ☐ 前斜角筋　　　　　　　　　☐ Scalenus anterior
　　　　　　　　　　　　　　　　　（anterior scalene）

③ ☐ 外肋間筋　　　　　　　　　☐ External intercostal muscle

④ ☐ 内肋間筋　　　　　　　　　☐ Internal intercostal muscle

⑤ ☐ 肋下筋　　　　　　　　　　☐ Subcotales

⑥ ☐ 最内肋間筋　　　　　　　　☐ Innermost intercostal muscle

⑦ ☐ 肋軟骨　　　　　　　　　　☐ Costal cartilage

⑧ ☐ 胸横筋　　　　　　　　　　☐ Transversus thoracis

⑨ ☐ 胸骨柄　　　　　　　　　　☐ Manubrium of sternum

解説

　胸壁の筋肉は胸式呼吸の主要筋であり，努力呼吸時には他の筋肉も働き，肋骨の挙上・下制および胸郭を安定させる．内肋間筋のうち1個または2個の肋骨を越えて付くもの(特に第6-11肋骨の領域で)は肋下筋と呼ばれる．最内肋間筋は内肋間の一部であり，内肋間筋と同じ走行と作用をもつ．

System of the Thoracic Muscles I

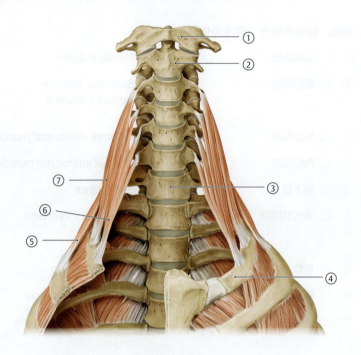

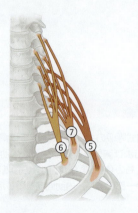

胸部の筋 1

斜角筋

① □ 第1頸椎（環椎）　　　　□ C1（atlas）

② □ 第2頸椎（軸椎）　　　　□ C2（axis）

③ □ 第7頸椎　　　　　　　　□ C7（7th cervical vertebra）

④ □ 第1肋骨　　　　　　　　□ 1st rib

⑤ □ 後斜角筋　　　　　　　　□ Scalenus posterior （posterior scalene）

⑥ □ 前斜角筋　　　　　　　　□ Scalenus anterior （anterior scalene）

⑦ □ 中斜角筋　　　　　　　　□ Scalenus medius （middle scalene）

筋	起始	停止	作用	神経支配
前斜角筋	C3-C6の横突起の前結節	第1肋骨の前斜角筋結節	・肋骨可動時は，上位の肋骨を挙上する（吸息時） ・肋骨の動きを固定すると，（片側の収縮は）同側に頸椎を屈曲し，（両側の収縮は）頸を屈曲する	頸・腕神経叢（C3-C6）の枝
中斜角筋	C3-C7の横突起の後結節	第1肋骨の鎖骨下動脈溝の後ろ側		
後斜角筋	C5-C7の横突起の後結節	第2肋骨の外側面		

System of the Thoracic Muscles II

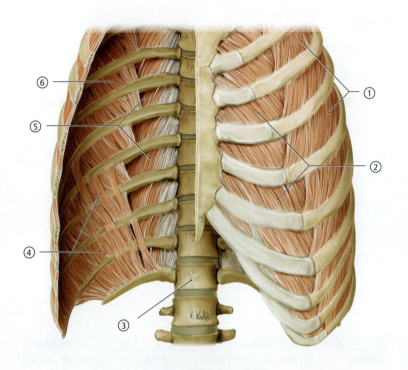

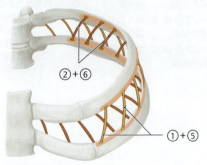

胸部の筋 2

肋間筋

① ☐ 外肋間筋　　　　　☐ **External intercostal muscles**

② ☐ 内肋間筋　　　　　☐ **Internal intercostal muscles**

③ ☐ 第12胸椎　　　　　☐ T12

④ ☐ 肋下筋　　　　　　☐ Subcostal muscles

⑤ ☐ 外肋間筋　　　　　☐ External intercostal muscles

⑥ ☐ 内肋間筋　　　　　☐ Internal intercostal muscles

筋	起始	停止	作用	神経支配
外肋間筋（肋骨結節から骨軟骨性接合部まで；後上から前下に向けて走行）	肋骨の下縁	隣接する下位の肋骨の上縁	・肋骨を挙上する（吸息時） ・肋間隙を支持する ・胸郭を安定する	肋間神経（T1-T11）
内肋間筋（肋骨角から胸骨まで，後下から前上に向けて走行）	肋骨の上縁	隣接する上位の肋骨の下縁	・肋骨を引き下げる（呼気時） ・肋間隙を支持する ・胸郭を安定する	

解説

　最内肋間筋は内肋間筋から分かれたものであり，このため，その走行と機能は内肋間筋に等しい。

System of the Thoracic Muscles III

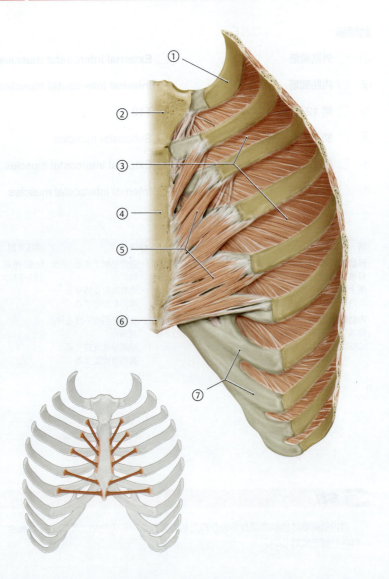

胸部の筋 3

胸横筋．後方から見たところ（胸横筋の右半分）

① □ 第 1 肋骨　　　　　　　□ 1st rib
② □ 胸骨柄　　　　　　　　□ Manubrium of sternum
③ □ 内肋間筋　　　　　　　□ Internal intercostal muscles
④ □ 胸骨体　　　　　　　　□ Body of sternum
⑤ □ **胸横筋**　　　　　　　□ **Transversus thoracis**
⑥ □ 剣状突起　　　　　　　□ Xiphoid process
⑦ □ 肋軟骨　　　　　　　　□ Costal cartilage

筋	起始	停止	作用	神経支配
胸横筋	胸骨体と剣状突起（内側面）	第2-6肋骨（肋軟骨の内側面）	肋骨を引き下げる（呼気時）	肋間神経（T2-T6）

Diaphragm in situ I

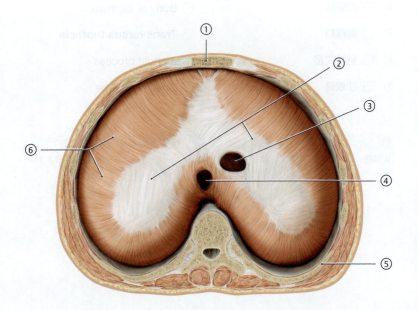

原位置の横隔膜 1

上面

① □ 胸骨　　　　　　　□ Sternum
② □ 腱中心　　　　　　□ Central tendon
③ □ 大静脈孔　　　　　□ Caval aperture
④ □ 食道裂孔　　　　　□ Esophageal aperture
⑤ □ 肋骨　　　　　　　□ Rib
⑥ □ 横隔膜の肋骨部　　□ Costal part of diaphragm

解説

横隔膜は，呼吸の主要筋であり，胸腔と腹腔を隔てている．肋間縁と腰椎から起始するが，腱中心は T8 の高さまで盛り上がったドームになっている．

Diaphragm in situ II

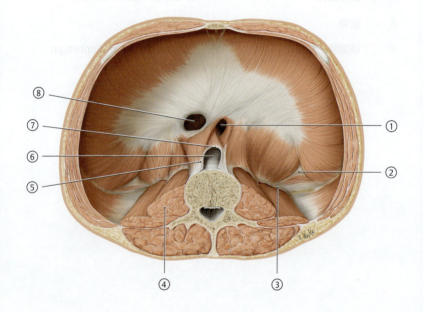

原位置の横隔膜 2

下面

① □ 食道裂孔 — □ Esophageal hiatus
② □ 腰肋三角（ボクダレク三角） — □ Lumbocostal triangle (Bochdalek's triangle)
③ □ 外側弓状靱帯 — □ Lateral arcuate ligament
④ □ 大腰筋 — □ Psoas major
⑤ □ 右脚 — □ Right crus
⑥ □ 大動脈裂孔 — □ Aortic aperture
⑦ □ 正中弓状靱帯 — □ Median arcuate ligament
⑧ □ 大静脈孔 — □ Caval aperture

臨床

胸腔出口は横隔膜によって閉ざされているが，通常横隔膜の開口部が胸部と腹部の間にある構造の通路となっている（pp.100-101 参照）．この開口部は臨床的に重要であり，穴が拡張して腹部の構造が胸腔に脱出することもある．脱出は食道裂孔においてよく起こる（裂孔ヘルニア）．

System of the Muscles of the Diaphragm

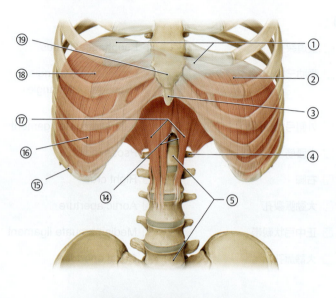
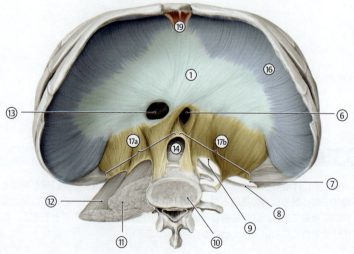

横隔膜の各部

横隔膜

① □ 腱中心 □ Central tendon
② □ 横隔膜の左天蓋 □ Left dome of diaphragm
③ □ 剣状突起 □ Xiphoid process
④ □ 第1腰椎の肋骨突起 □ Costal process of L1
⑤ □ 第1-5腰椎体 □ Vertebral bodies, L1-5
⑥ □ 食道裂孔 □ Esophageal hiatus
⑦ □ 方形筋弓 □ Quadratus arcade
⑧ □ 第12肋骨 □ 12th rib
⑨ □ 腰筋弓 □ Psoas arcade
⑩ □ 第3腰椎 □ L3
⑪ □ 大腰筋 □ Psoas major
⑫ □ 腰方形筋 □ Quadratus lumborum
⑬ □ 大静脈孔 □ Caval opening
⑭ □ 大動脈裂孔 □ Aortic hiatus
⑮ □ 第10肋骨 □ 10th rib
⑯ □ 横隔膜の肋骨部 □ **Costal part of diaphragm**
⑰ □ 横隔膜の腰椎部 □ **Lumbar part of diaphragm**
　　（a：右脚, b：左脚）　　　　（a：Right crus, b：Left crus）
⑱ □ 横隔膜の右天蓋 □ Right dome of diaphragm
⑲ □ 横隔膜の胸骨部 □ **Sternal part of diaphragm**

筋	起始	停止	作用	神経支配
横隔膜の肋骨部	第7-12肋骨（肋骨弓の下縁の内面）	腱中心	・呼吸（横隔膜・胸郭呼吸運動）の最も重要な筋である ・腹腔内臓への加圧を助ける（腹圧負荷）	頸神経叢の横隔神経（C3-5）
横隔膜の腰椎部（右脚・左脚），**内側部**	・L1-3椎体 ・L2-3間の椎間円板，前縦靱帯			
横隔膜の腰椎部（右脚・左脚），**外側部**	・腰筋弓の腱弓（内側弓状靱帯），L2からこれに所属する肋骨突起まで ・方形筋弓腱弓（外側弓状靱帯），L2の肋骨突起から第12肋骨先端まで			
横隔膜の胸骨部	剣状突起の後面			

Diaphragmatic Apertures

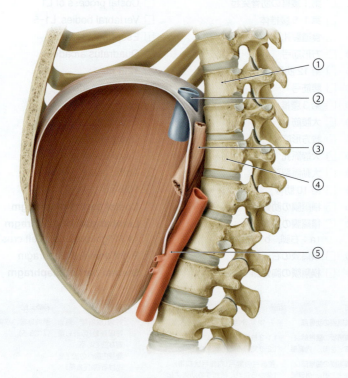

横隔膜の開口部

左外側面

① □ 第8胸椎 □ T8 vertebra
② □ 下大静脈 □ Inferior vena cava
③ □ 食道 □ Esophagus
④ □ 第10胸椎 □ T10 vertebra
⑤ □ 大動脈 □ Aorta

Arteries of Thoracic Wall

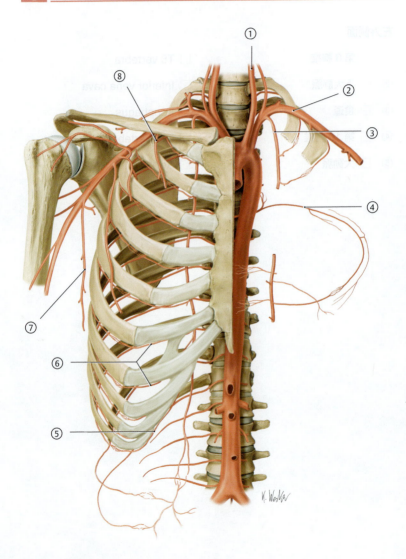

胸壁の動脈

前面

① □ 総頸動脈 □ Common carotid artery

② □ 鎖骨下動脈 □ Subclavian artery

③ □ 内胸動脈 □ Internal thoracic artery

④ □ 肋間動脈 □ Posterior intercostal artery

⑤ □ 筋横隔動脈 □ Musculophrenic artery

⑥ □ 内胸動脈の前肋間枝 □ Anterior intercostal branches of internal thoracic artery

⑦ □ 胸背動脈 □ Thoracodorsal artery

⑧ □ 最上胸動脈 □ Superior thoracic artery

 解説

　肋間動脈は内胸動脈の前肋間枝と吻合し，胸壁の構造を栄養する．肋間動脈は胸大動脈から分岐するが，第1および第2肋間動脈は肋頸動脈の枝の最上肋間動脈から起こる．

Veins of the Thoracic Wall

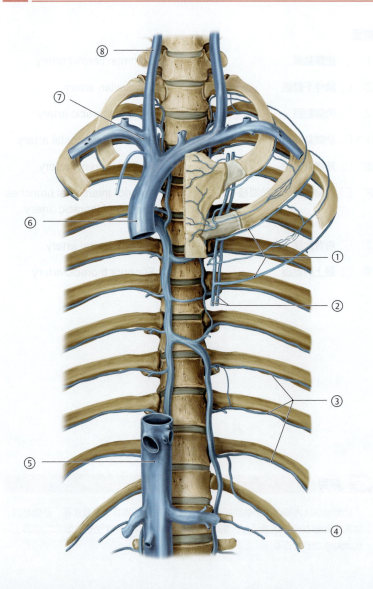

胸壁の静脈

前面

① □ 前肋間静脈　　　　　　　□ Anterior intercostal veins
② □ 内胸静脈　　　　　　　　□ Internal thoracic veins
③ □ 肋間静脈　　　　　　　　□ Posterior intercostal veins
④ □ 第1腰静脈　　　　　　　□ 1st lumbar vein
⑤ □ 下大静脈　　　　　　　　□ Inferior vena cava
⑥ □ 上大静脈　　　　　　　　□ Superior vena cava
⑦ □ 右腕頭静脈　　　　　　　□ Right brachiocephalic vein
⑧ □ 内頸静脈　　　　　　　　□ Internal jugular vein

 解説

・肋間静脈は主に奇静脈系へと連絡するが，内胸静脈にも注ぐ．血液は最終的には上大静脈を介して心臓に戻る．肋間静脈は肋間動脈と同様の位置に分布するが，脊柱の静脈は脊椎を全長にわたって横切る前・後外椎骨静脈叢を作る．

Nerves of the Thoracic Wall

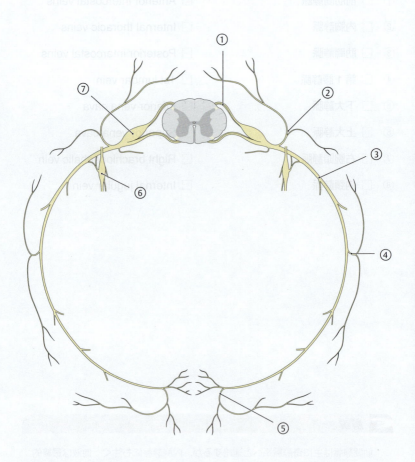

胸壁の神経

脊髄神経の枝（Spinal nerve branches），上面

① □ 後根　　　　　　　　　□ Dorsal root

② □ 後枝　　　　　　　　　□ Posterior (dorsal) ramus

③ □ 前枝（肋間神経）　　　　□ Anterior (ventral) ramus (intercostal nerve)

④ □ 外側皮枝　　　　　　　□ Lateral cutaneous branch

⑤ □ 前皮枝　　　　　　　　□ Anterior cutaneous branch

⑥ □ 交感神経幹神経節　　　□ Sympathetic ganglion

⑦ □ 脊髄神経節　　　　　　□ Spinal ganglion

解説

　後根（感覚性）と前根（運動性）からなる1cm足らずの脊髄神経が椎間孔を通過し，脊柱管の外に出る．脊髄神経の後枝は背部の皮膚と固有背筋を支配し，前枝は肋間神経をなす．

Course of the Intercostal Nerves

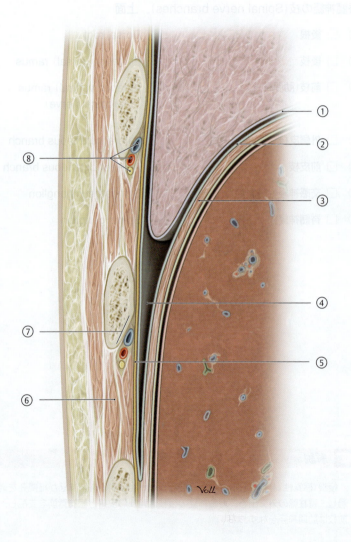

肋間神経の経路

冠状断面，前面

① □ 臓側胸膜（肺胸膜）　　　　□ Visceral pleura
② □ 壁側胸膜の横隔部　　　　　□ Diaphragmatic part of
　　　（横隔胸膜）　　　　　　　　 parietal pleura
③ □ 横隔膜　　　　　　　　　　□ Diaphragm
④ □ 肋骨横隔洞　　　　　　　　□ Costodiaphragmatic recess
⑤ □ 胸内筋膜　　　　　　　　　□ Endothoracic fascia
⑥ □ 外肋間筋　　　　　　　　　□ External intercostal muscles
⑦ □ 肋骨溝　　　　　　　　　　□ Costal groove
⑧ □ 肋間静脈・動脈・神経　　　□ Intercostal vein, artery,
　　　　　　　　　　　　　　　　　and nerve

臨床

気管支癌に起因する胸水のような，胸膜腔に貯留する過剰な滲出液には胸腔チューブが必要である．一般に，座位で最も有効な穿刺部位は後腋窩線沿いの第7-8肋間だとされる．チューブは肋骨上縁で挿入される．これは肋間動脈・静脈・神経を傷つけないためである．

Neurovasculature of the Diaphragm

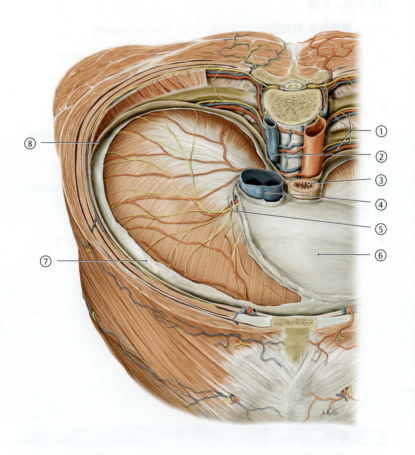

　横隔膜の支配神経はどの高さの脊髄から起こるか？

横隔膜の神経・血管

横断面, 前上面

① ☐ 肋間動脈・静脈 　　　　　☐ Posterior intercostal arteries and veins

② ☐ 奇静脈 　　　　　☐ Azygos vein

③ ☐ 食道 　　　　　☐ Esophagus

④ ☐ 下大静脈 　　　　　☐ Inferior vena cava

⑤ ☐ 横隔神経, 心膜横隔動脈・静脈 　　　　　☐ Phrenic nerve, pericardiacophrenic artery and vein

⑥ ☐ 心膜 　　　　　☐ Pericardium

⑦ ☐ 壁側胸膜の肋骨部（肋骨胸膜） 　　　　　☐ Costal part of parietal pleura

⑧ ☐ 胸内筋膜 　　　　　☐ Endothoracic fascia

横隔神経は C3-C5 の前枝から起こる.

Blood Supply to the Female Breast

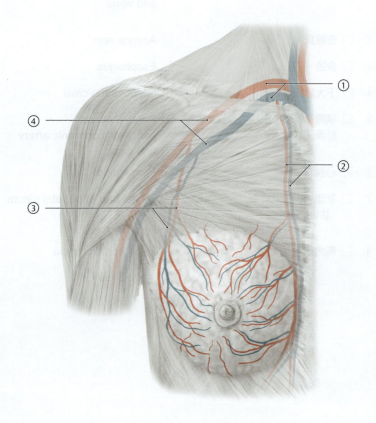

女性の乳房への栄養血管

前面

① □ 鎖骨下動脈・静脈　　　　　□ Subclavian artery and vein

② □ 内胸動脈・静脈　　　　　　□ Internal thoracic artery and vein

③ □ 外側胸動脈・静脈　　　　　□ Lateral thoracic artery and vein

④ □ 腋窩動脈・静脈　　　　　　□ Axillary artery and vein

Lymphatics of the Female Breast

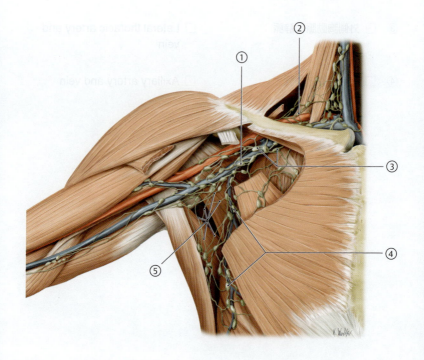

女性の乳房のリンパ管

前面

① □ 中心腋窩リンパ節　　　□ Central axillary node
② □ 鎖骨上リンパ節　　　　□ Supraclavicular node
③ □ 上腋窩リンパ節　　　　□ Apical axillary node
④ □ 胸筋腋窩リンパ節　　　□ Pectoral axillary node
⑤ □ 腋窩リンパ叢　　　　　□ Axillary lymphatic plexus

臨床

乳房腫瘍はリンパ管を通して広がる．胸骨傍リンパ節を経て正中線を越えて反対側に広がることもあるが，深リンパ管系（レベルⅢ）が特に重要である．乳癌の生存率は，腋窩リンパ節各レベルの転移したリンパ節の数と強く相関している．

Structures of the Female Breast

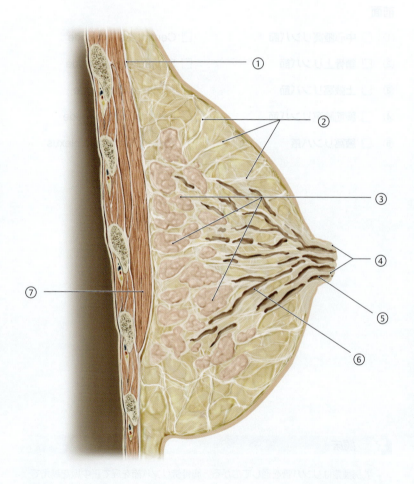

乳房のリンパ管は主にどのリンパ節群に注ぐか？

女性の乳房の構造

矢状断面

① □ 胸筋筋膜　　　　　　　　□ Pectoral fascia
② □ 乳房提靱帯（クーパー靱帯）　□ Suspensory (Cooper's) ligaments
③ □ 乳腺葉　　　　　　　　　□ Mammary lobes
④ □ 乳頭　　　　　　　　　　□ Nipple
⑤ □ 乳管洞　　　　　　　　　□ Lactiferous sinus
⑥ □ 乳管　　　　　　　　　　□ Lactiferous duct
⑦ □ 大胸筋　　　　　　　　　□ Pectoralis major

乳房のリンパ管は75%が腋窩リンパ節に注ぐ．

Divisions of the Mediastinum

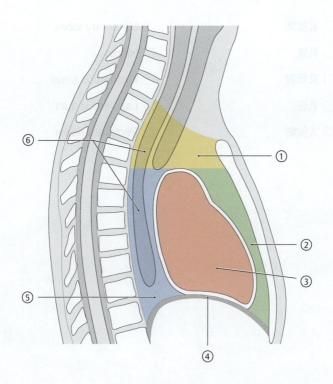

縦隔の区分

外側面

① □ 上縦隔　　□ Superior mediastinum
② □ 前縦隔　　□ Anterior mediastinum
③ □ 中縦隔　　□ Middle mediastinum
④ □ 横隔膜　　□ Diaphragm
⑤ □ 後縦隔　　□ Posterior mediastinum
⑥ □ 食道の胸部　□ Thoracic part of esophagus

解説

縦隔は両肺の胸膜嚢の間に挟まれた胸部の空間で，上縦隔と下縦隔に分けられる．下縦隔はさらに前縦隔，中縦隔，後縦隔に分けられる．

CT Scan of the Thorax

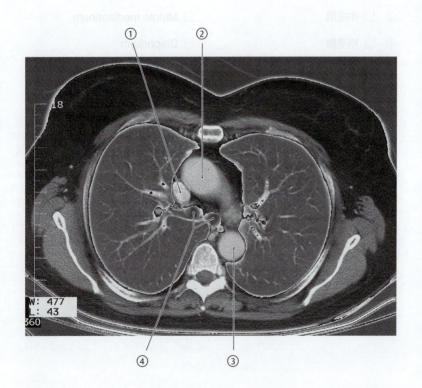

胸部の CT

水平断面, 下面

① □ 上大静脈　　　　　　　□ Superior vena cava

② □ 上行大動脈　　　　　　□ Ascending aorta

③ □ 下行大動脈　　　　　　□ Descending aorta

④ □ 右・左主気管支　　　　□ Right and left main bronchii

臨床

　大動脈の内膜裂傷によって血液が大動脈壁の層を分離させることで偽腔が生じ，潜在的に生死に関わる大動脈破裂につながる．急性大動脈解離は上行大動脈でよく起こり，一般的に外科手術が必要である．これより遠位の動脈解離は合併症がない場合は，保存的に治療される．冠状動脈分岐部での大動脈解離は心筋梗塞を引き起こす．

Thoracic Aorta

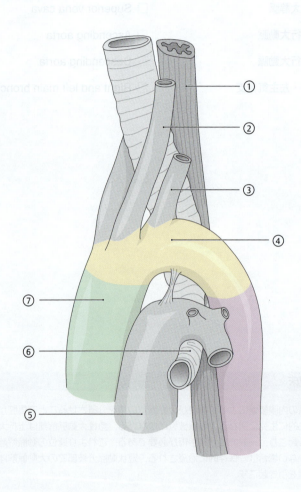

胸大動脈

左外側面

① □ 食道　　　　　□ Esophagus
② □ 左総頸動脈　　□ Left common carotid artery
③ □ 左鎖骨下動脈　□ Left subclavian artery
④ □ 大動脈弓　　　□ Aortic arch
⑤ □ 肺動脈幹　　　□ Pulmonary trunk
⑥ □ 左主気管支　　□ Left main bronchus
⑦ □ 上行大動脈　　□ Ascending aorta

 解説

　大動脈弓からは，腕頭動脈，左総頸動脈，左鎖骨下動脈の3つの大きな枝が分かれる．大動脈弓を経て大動脈は下行し，胸骨角の高さで胸大動脈となり，横隔膜の大動脈裂孔を通過後に腹大動脈となる．

Azygos System

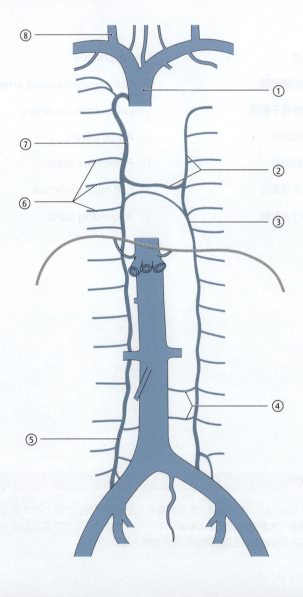

奇静脈系

前面

① □ 上大静脈 □ Superior vena cava
② □ 副半奇静脈 □ Accessory hemi-azygos vein
③ □ 半奇静脈 □ Hemi-azygos vein
④ □ 腰静脈 □ Lumbar veins
⑤ □ 右上行腰静脈 □ Right ascending lumbar vein
⑥ □ 肋間静脈 □ Posterior intercostal veins
⑦ □ 奇静脈 □ Azygos vein
⑧ □ 右内頸静脈 □ Right internal jugular vein

> **解説**
>
> 奇静脈系は頭部・頸部・上肢の静脈系と上大静脈によって連絡し，腹部・下肢の静脈系と下大静脈によって連絡する．

Lymphatics of the Thoracic Cavity

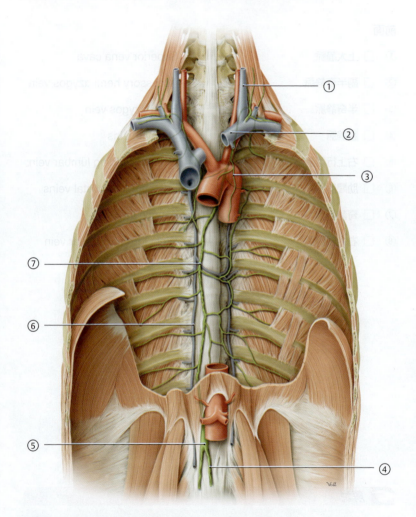

Q どの領域のリンパ管が胸管に注ぐか？

胸腔のリンパ管

前面

① □ 内頸静脈　　　　　□ Internal jugular vein
② □ 左腕頭静脈　　　　□ Left brachiocephalic vein
③ □ 気管支縦隔リンパ本幹　□ Bronchomediastinal trunk
④ □ 左腰リンパ本幹　　□ Left lumbar trunk
⑤ □ 乳ビ槽　　　　　　□ Cisterna chyli
⑥ □ 奇静脈　　　　　　□ Azygos vein
⑦ □ 胸管　　　　　　　□ Thoracic duct

 人体の最も主要なリンパ管は胸管である．胸管は，腹部の乳ビ槽から始まり，横隔膜より下の両側のリンパ，および左側の頭部・頸部・左肺下葉を除く胸部・上肢からのリンパが注ぐ．これ以外の領域では右リンパ本幹に注ぐ．

Nerves of the Thoracic Cavity

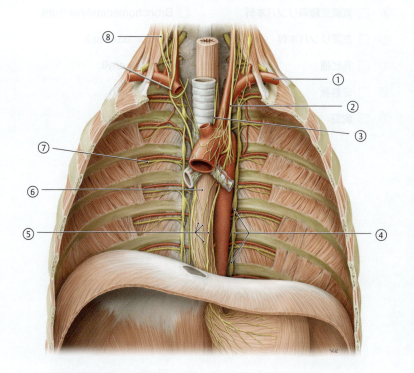

胸腔の神経

前面

① □ 左鎖骨下動脈 — □ Left subclavian artery
② □ 左迷走神経 — □ Left vagus nerve
③ □ 左反回神経 — □ Left recurrent laryngeal nerve
④ □ 交感神経幹 — □ Sympathetic trunk
⑤ □ 前迷走神経幹と食道神経叢 — □ Anterior vagal trunk (with esophageal plexus)
⑥ □ 食道の胸部 — □ Thoracic part of esophagus
⑦ □ 肋間神経 — □ Intercostal nerve
⑧ □ 交感神経幹，中頸神経節 — □ Sympathetic trunk, middle cervical ganglion

 解説

　胸部の神経支配はほとんどが自律神経で，交感神経幹と副交感性の迷走神経に由来する．例外は，心膜と横隔膜を支配する横隔神経と胸壁を支配する肋間神経の2つである．

Mediastinum I

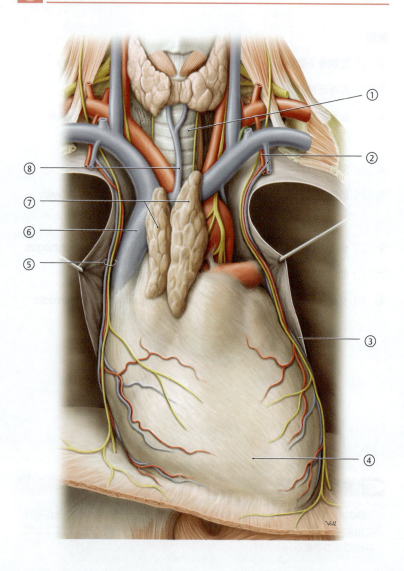

縦隔 1

前面

① ☐ 気管 — ☐ Trachea
② ☐ 内胸動脈・静脈 — ☐ Internal thoracic artery and vein
③ ☐ 壁側胸膜の縦隔部（縦隔胸膜） — ☐ Mediastinal part of parietal pleura
④ ☐ 線維性心膜 — ☐ Fibrous pericardium
⑤ ☐ 心膜横隔動脈・静脈, 横隔神経 — ☐ Pericardiacophrenic artery and vein, phrenic nerve
⑥ ☐ 上大静脈 — ☐ Superior vena cava
⑦ ☐ 胸腺 — ☐ Thymus
⑧ ☐ 下甲状腺静脈 — ☐ Inferior thyroid vein

Mediastinum II

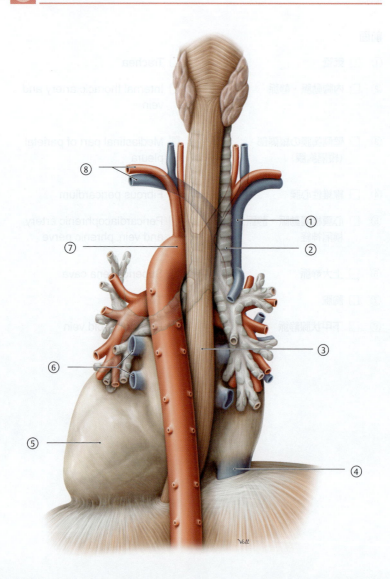

縦隔 2

縦隔の内容，後面

① □ 上大静脈　　　　　　　　　□ Superior vena cava
② □ 気管　　　　　　　　　　　□ Trachea
③ □ 食道の胸部　　　　　　　　□ Thoracic part of esophagus
④ □ 下大静脈（大静脈孔の中の）　□ Inferior vena cava (in caval aperture)
⑤ □ 線維性心膜，左心室　　　　□ Fibrous pericardium, left ventricle
⑥ □ 左肺静脈　　　　　　　　　□ Left pulmonary veins
⑦ □ 大動脈弓　　　　　　　　　□ Aortic arch
⑧ □ 左鎖骨下動脈・静脈　　　　□ Left subclavian artery and vein

Mediastinum III

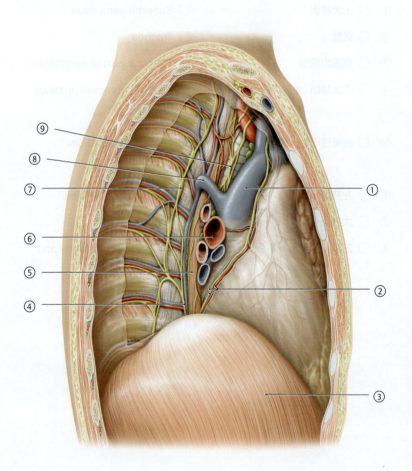

縦隔 3

傍矢状断面，右側面

① ☐ 上大静脈 — ☐ Superior vena cava
② ☐ 横隔神経，心膜横隔動脈・静脈 — ☐ Phrenic nerve, pericardiacophrenic artery and vein
③ ☐ 横隔膜 — ☐ Diaphragm
④ ☐ 大内臓神経 — ☐ Greater splanchnic nerve
⑤ ☐ 食道 — ☐ Esophagus
⑥ ☐ 右肺動脈 — ☐ Right pulmonary artery
⑦ ☐ 交感神経幹，胸神経節 — ☐ Sympathetic trunk, thoracic ganglion
⑧ ☐ 奇静脈 — ☐ Azygos vein
⑨ ☐ 右迷走神経 — ☐ Right vagus nerve

Mediastinum IV

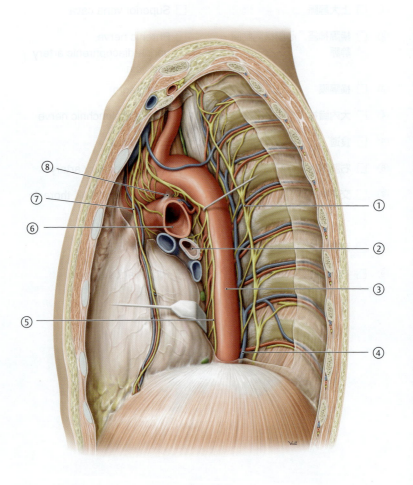

縦隔 4

傍矢状断面，左外側面

① ☐ 交感神経幹　　　　　　　　☐ Sympathetic trunk
② ☐ 左主気管支　　　　　　　　☐ Left main bronchus
③ ☐ 胸大動脈（下行大動脈）　　☐ Thoracic aorta (descending aorta)
④ ☐ 半奇静脈　　　　　　　　　☐ Hemi-azygos vein
⑤ ☐ 左迷走神経　　　　　　　　☐ Left vagus nerve
⑥ ☐ 左肺動脈　　　　　　　　　☐ Left pulmonary artery
⑦ ☐ 左横隔神経　　　　　　　　☐ Left phrenic nerve
⑧ ☐ 動脈管索　　　　　　　　　☐ Ligamentum arteriosum

Pericardial Reflections I

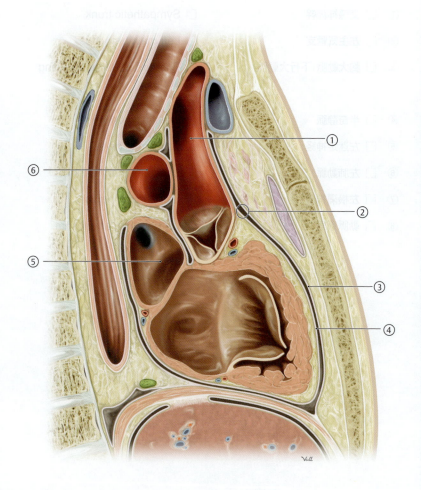

心膜の折れ返り 1

縦隔の矢状断面

① □ 上行大動脈　　　　　　　□ Ascending aorta
② □ 心膜腔　　　　　　　　　□ Pericardial cavity
③ □ 漿膜性心膜の壁側板　　　□ Parietal layer of serous pericardium
④ □ 漿膜性心膜の臓側板　　　□ Visceral layer of serous pericardium
⑤ □ 左心房　　　　　　　　　□ Left atrium
⑥ □ 右肺動脈　　　　　　　　□ Right pulmonary artery

解説

漿膜性心膜の臓側板と壁側板は心臓の大血管周囲で連続している．動脈の折れ返り部と静脈の折れ返り部の間にある空洞が心膜横洞である．

140　Thorax

Pericardial Reflections II

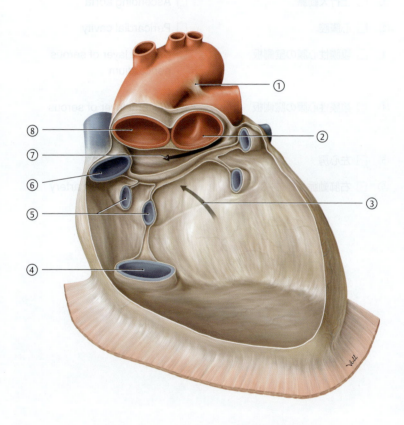

① Ascending aorta
② Pericardial cavity
⑧ Parietal layer of serous pericardium

Q 心膜横洞とは何か？

心膜の折れ返り 2

心臓を取り除いた心膜，前面

① □ 動脈管索　　　　□ Ligamentum arteriosum
② □ 肺動脈幹　　　　□ Pulmonary trunk
③ □ 心膜斜洞　　　　□ Oblique pericardial sinus
④ □ 下大静脈　　　　□ Inferior vena cava
⑤ □ 右肺静脈　　　　□ Right pulmonary veins
⑥ □ 上大静脈　　　　□ Superior vena cava
⑦ □ 心膜横洞　　　　□ Transverse pericardial sinus
⑧ □ 上行大動脈　　　□ Ascending aorta

A 心膜横洞は心臓の流入路（上・下大静脈と肺静脈）と流出路（大動脈と肺動脈幹）を隔てている．

Heart in situ

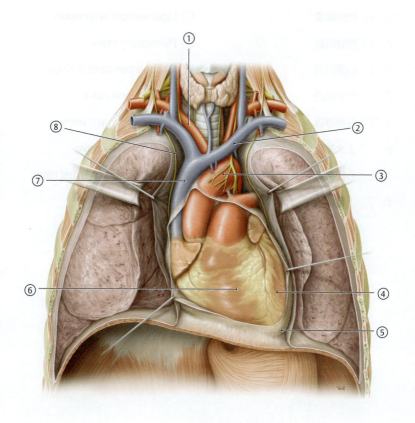

胸郭の骨に対する心臓の位置はどこか？

胸部 143

原位置の心臓

前面

① □ 腕頭動脈 　　　　　□ Brachiocephalic trunk
② □ 左腕頭静脈 　　　　□ Left brachiocephalic vein
③ □ 大動脈弓 　　　　　□ Aortic arch
④ □ 左心室 　　　　　　□ Left ventricle
⑤ □ 心尖 　　　　　　　□ Apex of heart
⑥ □ 右心室 　　　　　　□ Right ventricle
⑦ □ 上大静脈 　　　　　□ Superior vena cava
⑧ □ 右横隔神経 　　　　□ Right phrenic nerve

A 　心臓は胸骨体の後方で第2-6肋軟骨の間にある．心臓は下縦隔の中縦隔にあり，胸腔左側に投影される．

Sternocostal Surface of the Heart

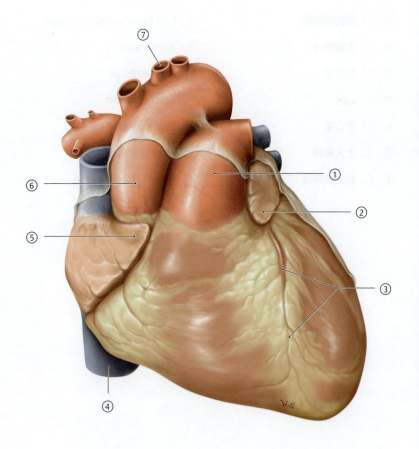

心臓の胸肋面

前面

① □ 肺動脈幹　　　　　　　　□ Pulmonary trunk

② □ 左心耳　　　　　　　　　□ Left auricle

③ □ 前室間溝　　　　　　　　□ Anterior interventricular sulcus

④ □ 下大静脈　　　　　　　　□ Inferior vena cava

⑤ □ 右心耳　　　　　　　　　□ Right auricle

⑥ □ 上行大動脈　　　　　　　□ Ascending aorta

⑦ □ 左総頸動脈　　　　　　　□ Left common carotid artery

Base of the Heart

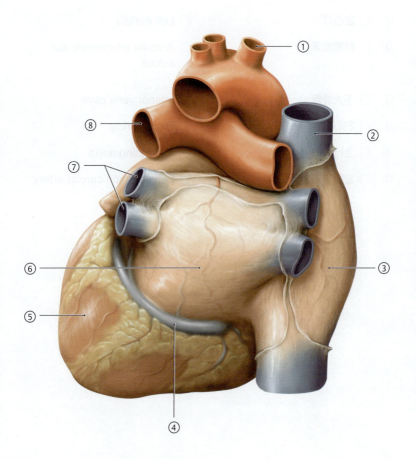

心臓の底面

後面

① ☐ 腕頭動脈　　　　　　　☐ Brachiocephalic trunk

② ☐ 上大静脈　　　　　　　☐ Superior vena cava

③ ☐ 右心房　　　　　　　　☐ Right atrium

④ ☐ 冠状静脈洞　　　　　　☐ Coronary sinus

⑤ ☐ 左心室　　　　　　　　☐ Left ventricle

⑥ ☐ 左心房　　　　　　　　☐ Left atrium

⑦ ☐ 左肺静脈　　　　　　　☐ Left pulmonary veins

⑧ ☐ 左肺動脈　　　　　　　☐ Left pulmonary artery

Chambers of the Heart I

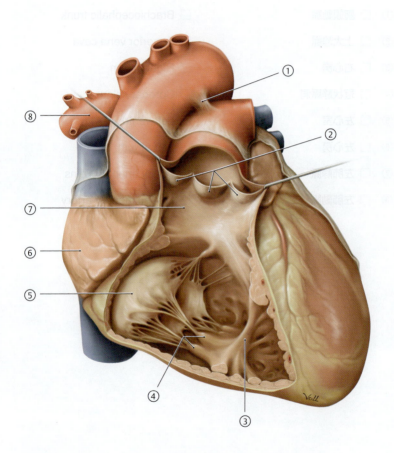

Q 肺動脈弁と大動脈弁が閉じるのは心周期のどのときか？

心臓の部屋 1

前面

① ☐ 動脈管索　　　　　　　　☐ Ligamentum arteriosum
② ☐ 肺動脈弁　　　　　　　　☐ Pulmonary valve
③ ☐ 中隔縁柱　　　　　　　　☐ Septomarginal trabecula
④ ☐ 前乳頭筋　　　　　　　　☐ Anterior papillary muscle
⑤ ☐ 右房室弁の前尖　　　　　☐ Anterior cusp of right atrioventricular valve
⑥ ☐ 右心房　　　　　　　　　☐ Right atrium
⑦ ☐ 動脈円錐　　　　　　　　☐ Conus arteriosus
⑧ ☐ 右肺動脈　　　　　　　　☐ Right pulmonary artery

動脈弁は拡張期（心室弛緩期）に閉じる．

Chambers of the Heart II

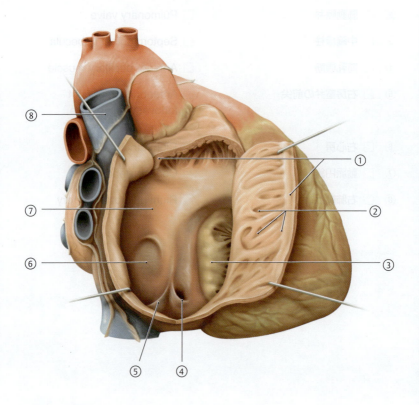

Q 右心房において胎児期に右心房と左心房を連絡していた構造の遺残物はどれか？

心臓の部屋 2

右外側面

① ☐ 分界稜 — ☐ Crista terminalis
② ☐ 櫛状筋 — ☐ Pectinate muscles
③ ☐ 右房室口と右房室弁 — ☐ Right atrioventricular orifice with atrioventricular valve
④ ☐ 冠状静脈口と冠状静脈弁 — ☐ Valved orifice of coronary sinus
⑤ ☐ 下大静脈口と下大静脈弁 — ☐ Valved orifice of inferior vena cava
⑥ ☐ 卵円窩 — ☐ Oval fossa
⑦ ☐ 心房中隔 — ☐ Interatrial septum
⑧ ☐ 上大静脈 — ☐ Superior vena cava

心房壁の浅い陥凹である卵円窩は，胎児期の心臓の卵円孔の遺残物である．

Chambers of the Heart III

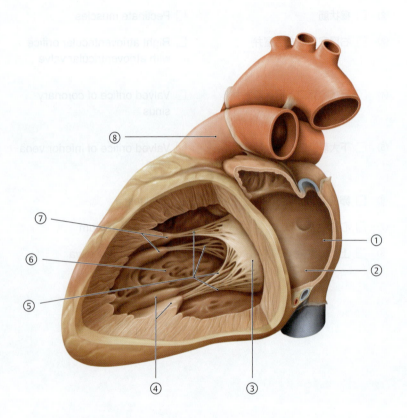

Q この絵はどの心周期のときの心臓か？

心臓の部屋 3

左外側面

① ☐ 左心房　　　　　　☐ Left atrium
② ☐ 心房中隔　　　　　☐ Interatrial septum
③ ☐ 左房室弁　　　　　☐ Left atrioventricular valve
④ ☐ 後乳頭筋　　　　　☐ Posterior papillary muscle
⑤ ☐ 腱索　　　　　　　☐ Tendinous cords
⑥ ☐ 心室中隔の肉柱　　☐ Trabeculae carneae of interventricular septum
⑦ ☐ 前乳頭筋　　　　　☐ Anterior papillary muscle
⑧ ☐ 肺動脈幹　　　　　☐ Pulmonary trunk

A 収縮期（心室収縮期）．

Heart Valves

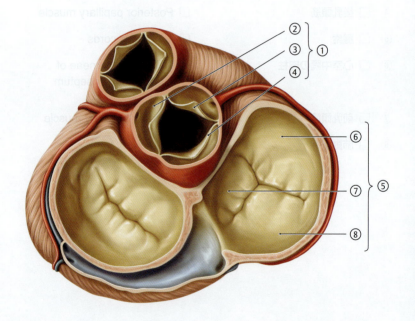

心臓弁

心室収縮期 Ventricular systole（contraction of the ventricles），上面

① □ 大動脈弁　　　　　□ Aortic valve
② □ 左半月弁　　　　　□ Left semilunar cusp
③ □ 右半月弁　　　　　□ Right semilunar cusp
④ □ 後半月弁　　　　　□ Posterior semilunar cusp
⑤ □ 右房室弁　　　　　□ Right atrioventricular valve
⑥ □ 前尖　　　　　　　□ Anterior cusp
⑦ □ 中隔尖　　　　　　□ Septal cusp
⑧ □ 後尖　　　　　　　□ Posterior cusp

解説

　心臓弁は半月弁と房室弁の2種類に分類される．半月弁には大動脈弁と肺動脈弁の2つがあり，心臓の2本の大血管基部で心室から大動脈と肺動脈幹への血流を調節する．2つの房室弁（左房室弁と右房室弁）は心房と心室の境界にある．

Arteries & Veins of the Heart I

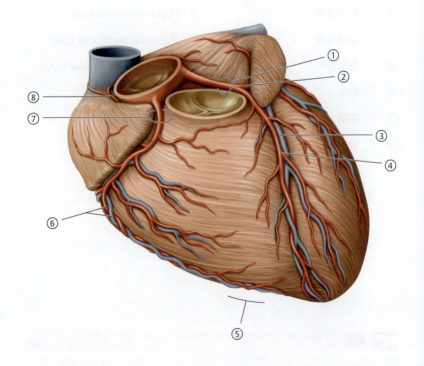

心臓の動脈と静脈 1

前面

① □ 左冠状動脈 　　　　　　　□ Left coronary artery
② □ 回旋枝 　　　　　　　　　□ Circumflex branch
③ □ 大心臓静脈 　　　　　　　□ Great cardiac vein
④ □ 前室間枝（前下行枝） 　　□ Anterior interventricular branch
⑤ □ 右心室 　　　　　　　　　□ Right ventricle
⑥ □ 右縁枝（鋭角縁枝）と右辺縁静脈 　□ Right marginal branch and vein
⑦ □ 右冠状動脈 　　　　　　　□ Right coronary artery
⑧ □ 洞房結節枝 　　　　　　　□ Sinu-atrial nodal branch

臨床

冠状動脈は吻合によって互いに連絡しているが，機能の面では終動脈である．血流不足の原因として最も多いのはアテローム性動脈硬化症であり，血管壁に斑点が沈着して血管腔が狭くなる．血管狭窄が亢進した場合には，冠血流が阻害される．心筋梗塞は血流不足によって心筋組織が壊死して起こる．梗塞の部位と広がりは障害された血管によって決まる．

Arteries & Veins of the Heart II

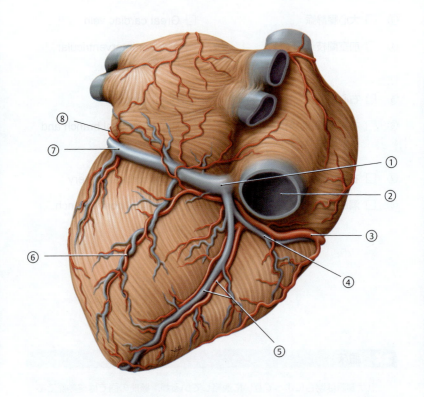

心臓の動脈と静脈 2

後下面

① □ 冠状静脈洞　　　　□ Coronary sinus

② □ 下大静脈　　　　　□ Inferior vena cava

③ □ 右冠状動脈　　　　□ Right coronary artery

④ □ 小心臓静脈　　　　□ Small cardiac vein

⑤ □ 後室間枝（後下行枝）と　□ Posterior interventricular
　　後室間静脈（中心臓静脈）　　(descending) branch and vein

⑥ □ 右後側壁枝　　　　□ Right posterolateral branch

⑦ □ 大心臓静脈　　　　□ Great cardiac vein

⑧ □ 回旋枝　　　　　　□ Circumflex branch

解説

右冠状動脈と左冠状動脈は，一般には左心房と左心室の後方で吻合する．

Cardiac Conduction System

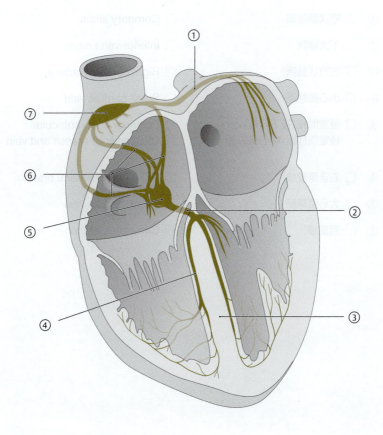

Q 洞房結節に血液を供給するのはどの血管か？

心臓刺激伝導系

前面

① □ 心房間束　　　　　□ Interatrial bundle
② □ 房室束（ヒス束）　□ Atrioventricular bundle（of His）
③ □ 心室中隔　　　　　□ Interventricular septum
④ □ 右脚　　　　　　　□ Right bundle branch
⑤ □ 房室結節　　　　　□ Atrioventricular（AV）node
⑥ □ 前・中・後結節間束　□ Anterior, middle, and posterior internodal bundles
⑦ □ 洞房結節　　　　　□ Sinu-atrial node

A 通常は右冠状動脈から洞房結節へ動脈が向かう．

Autonomic Nerves of the Heart

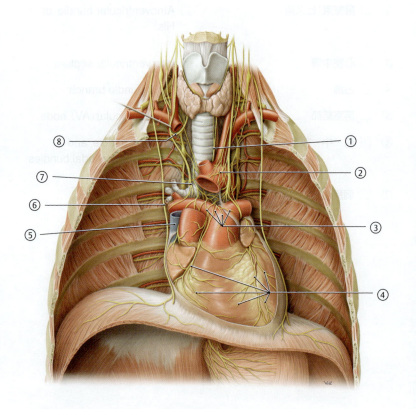

心臓の自律神経

前面，胸郭を開く

① ☐ 左反回神経　　☐ Left recurrent laryngeal nerve

② ☐ 胸大動脈神経叢　☐ Thoracic aortic plexus

③ ☐ 肺神経叢　　　☐ Pulmonary plexus

④ ☐ 心臓神経叢　　☐ Cardiac plexus

⑤ ☐ 上大静脈　　　☐ Superior vena cava

⑥ ☐ 右横隔神経　　☐ Right phrenic nerve

⑦ ☐ 右迷走神経　　☐ Right vagus nerve

⑧ ☐ 右反回神経　　☐ Right recurrent laryngeal nerve

解説

　心臓に分布する交感神経は，3本の頸心臓神経とT1-T6の胸神経節からの胸心臓枝である．副交感神経は迷走神経からの頸心臓枝と胸心臓枝である．交感神経と副交感神経はどちらも心臓神経叢，大動脈神経叢，肺神経叢に枝を出す．

Radiographic Appearance of the Heart I

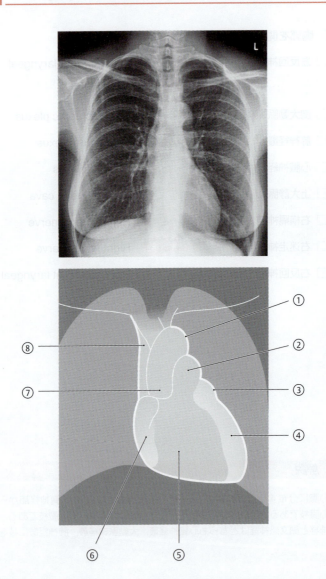

心臓のX線像 1

上:胸部X線前後像,下:前面

①	☐ 大動脈弓("大動脈隆起")	☐ Aortic arch ("aortic knob")
②	☐ 肺動脈幹	☐ Pulmonary trunk
③	☐ 左心房	☐ Left atrium
④	☐ 左心室	☐ Left ventricle
⑤	☐ 右心室	☐ Right ventricle
⑥	☐ 右心房	☐ Right atrium
⑦	☐ 上行大動脈	☐ Ascending aorta
⑧	☐ 上大静脈	☐ Superior vena cava

Radiographic Appearance of the Heart II

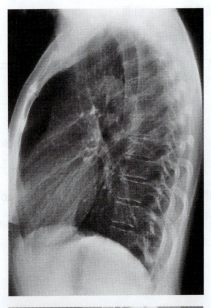

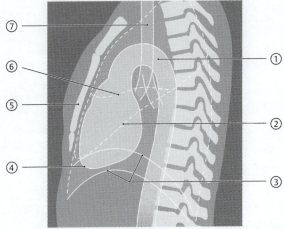

心臓のX線像 2

上:胸部X線左側面像,下:外側面

① ☐ 大動脈弓　　　　　　　　☐ Aortic arch
② ☐ 右肺の斜裂　　　　　　　☐ Oblique fissure of right lung
③ ☐ 左・右の横隔膜円蓋　　　☐ Left and right diaphragm leaflets
④ ☐ 心尖　　　　　　　　　　☐ Apex of heart
⑤ ☐ 胸骨体　　　　　　　　　☐ Body of sternum
⑥ ☐ 右肺の水平裂　　　　　　☐ Horizontal fissure of right lung
⑦ ☐ 気管　　　　　　　　　　☐ Trachea

Heart in Transverse Section

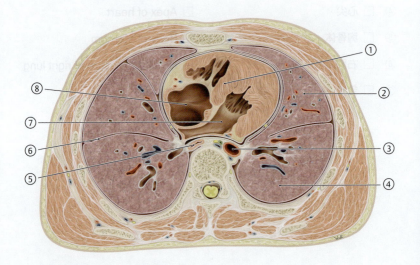

水平断面での心臓

第8胸椎（T8）の高さにおける水平断面，下面

① □ 心室中隔　　　　　　　　　□ Interventricular septum

② □ 左肺の上葉　　　　　　　　□ Superior lobe of left lung

③ □ 胸大動脈（下行大動脈）　　　□ Thoracic aorta (descending aorta)

④ □ 左肺の下葉　　　　　　　　□ Inferior lobe of left lung

⑤ □ 食道　　　　　　　　　　　□ Esophagus

⑥ □ 右肺の斜裂　　　　　　　　□ Oblique fissure of right lung

⑦ □ 左心房　　　　　　　　　　□ Left atrium

⑧ □ 右心房　　　　　　　　　　□ Right atrium

Prenatal Circulation

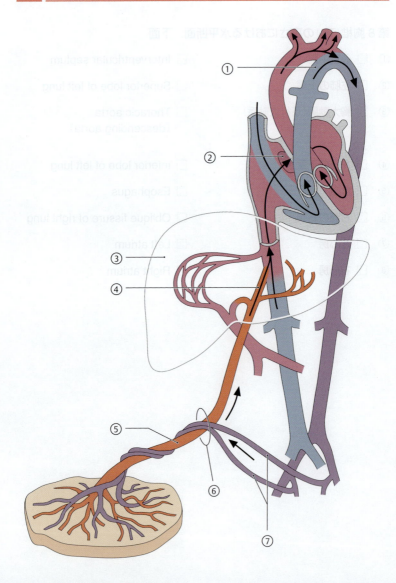

出生前の循環

① □ 動脈管（開いている）　□ Ductus arteriosus（patent）
② □ 卵円孔（開いている）　□ Foramen ovale（patent）
③ □ 肝臓　□ Liver
④ □ 静脈管　□ Ductus venosus
⑤ □ 臍静脈　□ Umbilical vein
⑥ □ 臍　□ Umbilicus
⑦ □ 臍動脈　□ Umbilical arteries

解説

注意：血管の色は運ばれている血液の酸素飽和度に従う．
赤＝酸素量が多い，青＝酸素量が少ない，紫＝混合．
pp.172, 173 と比較すること．

Postnatal Circulation

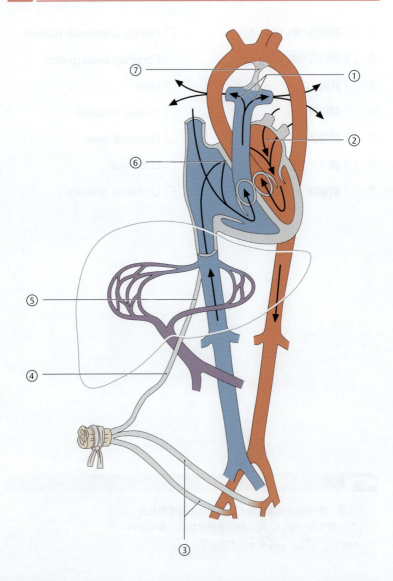

① ☐ Ductus arteriosus (patent)
  ☐ Foramen ovale (patent)
② ☐ Liver
⑥ ☐ Ductus venosus
  ☐ Umbilical vein
⑦ ☐ Urachus
  ☐ Umbilical arteries

出生後の循環

① ☐ 肺動脈(血流が豊富)　☐ Pulmonary arteries (perfused)
② ☐ 左心房　☐ Left atrium
③ ☐ 臍動脈の遺残(内側臍索)　☐ Obliterated umbilical arteries (medial umbilical ligaments)
④ ☐ 肝円索(臍静脈の遺残)　☐ Round ligament of liver (obliterated umbilical vein)
⑤ ☐ 静脈管索(静脈管の遺残)　☐ Ligamentum venosum (obliterated ductus venosus)
⑥ ☐ 卵円孔(閉じている)　☐ Foramen ovale (closed)
⑦ ☐ 動脈管索(動脈管の遺残)　☐ Ligamentum arteriosum (obliterated ductus arteriosus)

臨床

　先天的な心臓疾患のなかで最も一般的な中隔欠損症では,収縮期に左心の血液が右心へと流入してしまう.心室中隔欠損症(VSD)は最も一般的な型である.心房中隔欠損症(ASD)の最も一般的な型は,卵円孔開存症であり,胎児期のシャントの閉鎖が不完全であったことで生じる.

解説

注意:血管の色は運ばれている血液の酸素飽和度に従う.
　赤=酸素量が多い,青=酸素量が少ない.
　胎児循環(pp.170, 171)とは異なり生後循環には混合血は存在しない.ここでは紫は門脈の流域を表し,この血管は酸素量が低く栄養物質量の高い消化管からの血液を運ぶ.

Parietal Pleura

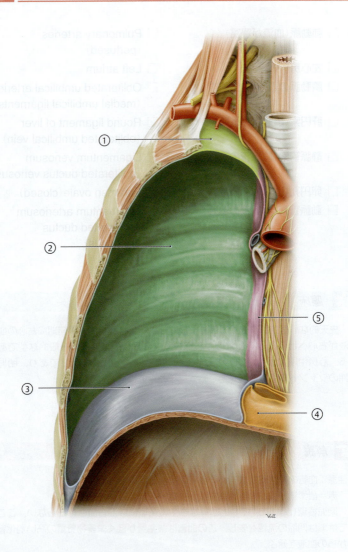

壁側胸膜

右胸膜腔を開く，前面

① □ 胸膜頂
② □ 肋骨部（肋骨胸膜）
③ □ 横隔部（横隔胸膜）
④ □ 線維性心膜
⑤ □ 縦隔部（縦隔胸膜）

□ Cervical pleura
□ Costal part
□ Diaphragmatic part
□ Fibrous pericardium
□ Mediastinal part

解説

　胸膜腔は2つの漿膜で囲まれる．臓側胸膜（肺胸膜）は肺を包み，壁側胸膜は胸腔の内面を覆う．壁側胸膜の4つの部分である肋骨胸膜，横隔胸膜，縦隔胸膜，胸膜頂は連続している．

Lungs in situ

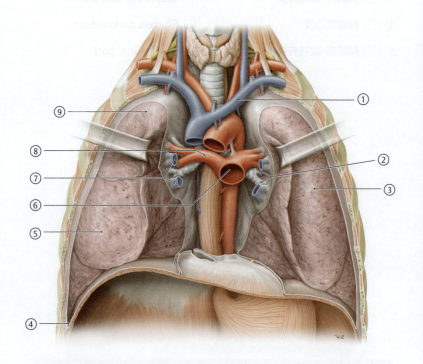

原位置の肺

前面

① □ 左腕頭静脈 □ Left brachiocephalic vein
② □ 上・下葉気管支 □ Superior and inferior lobar bronchi
③ □ 左肺の上葉 □ Superior lobe of left lung
④ □ 肋骨横隔洞 □ Costodiaphragmatic recess
⑤ □ 右肺の中葉 □ Middle lobe of right lung
⑥ □ 肺動脈幹 □ Pulmonary trunk
⑦ □ 右肺静脈 □ Right pulmonary veins
⑧ □ 右肺動脈 □ Right pulmonary artery
⑨ □ 肺尖 □ Apex of lung

 解説

　両肺は胸膜腔全体を占めている．心臓の位置のズレのために，左肺は右肺よりもわずかに小さい．
注意：血管の色は血管タイプに従う．
　赤＝動脈，青＝静脈．
　輸送される血液の酸素飽和度とは無関係．

Right Lung

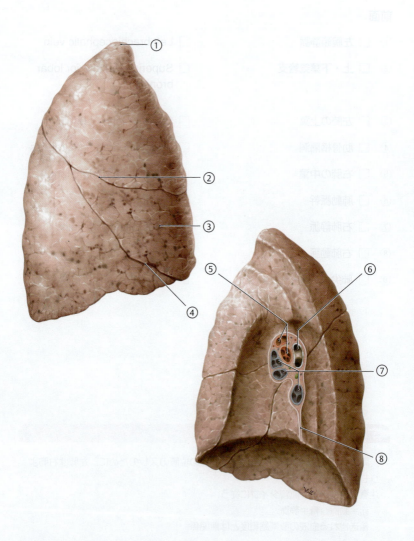

右肺

上:外側面,下:内側面

① □ 肺尖　　　　　　　□ Apex of lung

② □ 水平裂　　　　　　□ Horizontal fissure

③ □ 中葉　　　　　　　□ Middle lobe

④ □ 斜裂　　　　　　　□ Oblique fissure

⑤ □ 右肺動脈の枝　　　□ Branches of right pulmonary artery

⑥ □ 上葉気管支　　　　□ Superior lobar bronchus

⑦ □ 右肺静脈の枝　　　□ Branches of right pulmonary veins

⑧ □ 肺間膜　　　　　　□ Pulmonary ligament

 解説

　右肺は斜裂と水平裂によって上葉・中葉・下葉の3葉に分けられる.両肺の肺尖は頸の基部に入りこんでいる.

Left Lung

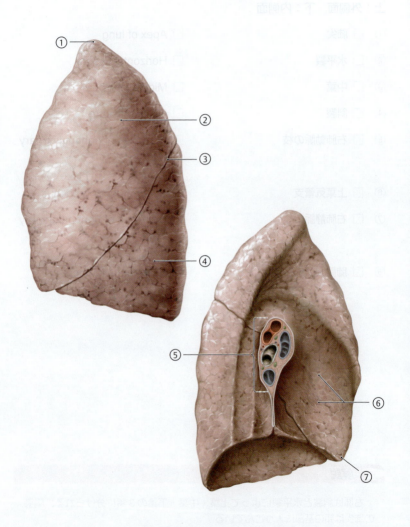

左肺

上:外側面,下:内側面

① □ 肺尖 　　　　　　　□ Apex of lung
② □ 上葉 　　　　　　　□ Superior lobe
③ □ 斜裂 　　　　　　　□ Oblique fissure
④ □ 下葉 　　　　　　　□ Inferior lobe
⑤ □ 肺門 　　　　　　　□ Hilum of lung
⑥ □ 心圧痕 　　　　　　□ Cardiac impression
⑦ □ 小舌 　　　　　　　□ Lingula

解説

　左肺は斜裂によって上葉と下葉に分けられる.肺門は気管支や神経・脈管が肺に出入りする部位.

Trachea

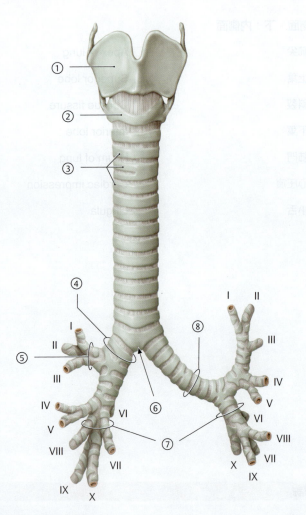

気管竜骨とは何か？

気管

前面

① □ 甲状軟骨 — □ Thyroid cartilage
② □ 輪状軟骨 — □ Cricoid cartilage
③ □ 気管軟骨 — □ Tracheal cartilages
④ □ 右主気管支 — □ Right main bronchus
⑤ □ 右上葉気管支 — □ Right superior lobar bronchus
⑥ □ 気管分岐部 — □ Tracheal bifurcation
⑦ □ 右・左下葉気管支 — □ Right / left inferior lobar bronchi
⑧ □ 左主気管支 — □ Left main bronchus

A 気管竜骨は気管最下部の分岐部にあり，左主気管支と右主気管支を分ける．

Divisions of the Bronchial Tree

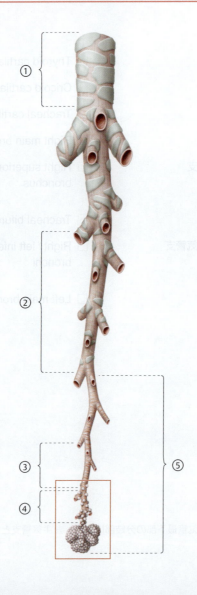

胸部 185

気管支樹の区分

① □ 区域気管支　　　　　　　□ Segmental bronchus
② □ 小さい亜区域気管支　　　□ Small subsegmental bronchus
③ □ 終末細気管支　　　　　　□ Terminal bronchiole
④ □ 呼吸細気管支　　　　　　□ Respiratory bronchiole
⑤ □ 細気管支（軟骨がない）　□ Bronchiole (cartilage-free wall)

解説

気管支樹の伝導部は気管分岐部から終末細気管支に及び，呼吸部は呼吸細気管支，肺胞管，肺胞嚢，肺胞を含む．

Respiratory Portion of the Bronchial Tree

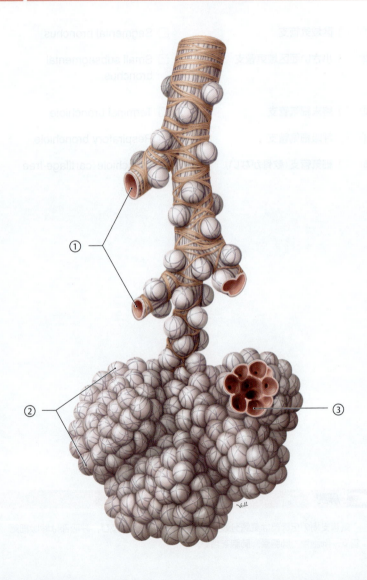

気管支樹の呼吸部

① ☐ 呼吸細気管支　　☐ Respiratory bronchioles
② ☐ 肺胞嚢　　　　　☐ Alveolar sac
③ ☐ 肺胞　　　　　　☐ Alveolus

臨床

気管支レベルでの呼吸器不全の最も一般的な原因は喘息である．肺胞レベルでの呼吸不全は拡散距離の増大，低換気（肺気腫），液体浸潤（肺炎など）から起こる．

Pulmonary Arteries & Veins

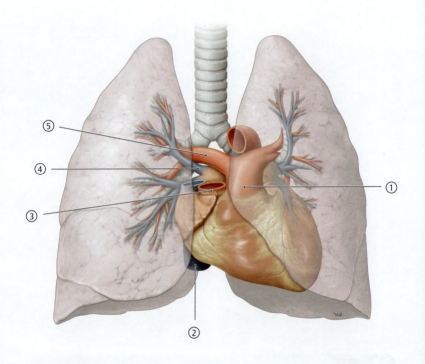

肺動脈と肺静脈

前面

① □ 肺動脈幹　　　　　□ Pulmonary trunk
② □ 下大静脈　　　　　□ Inferior vena cava
③ □ 上行大動脈　　　　□ Ascending aorta
④ □ 右上肺静脈　　　　□ Superior right pulmonary vein
⑤ □ 右肺動脈　　　　　□ Right pulmonary artery

 解説

　肺動脈幹は右心室から起こり，両肺への左右の肺動脈に分かれる．肺静脈は左右それぞれ2本ずつ両側から左心房に注ぐ．肺動脈は気管支樹に沿って追随しながら分岐していくが，肺静脈は肺小葉の辺縁部にあり，気管支樹に随伴しない．

Lymph Nodes of the Pleural Cavity

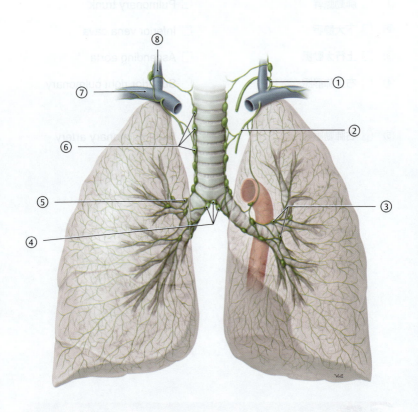

各肺のリンパ流路はどのようなものか？

胸膜腔のリンパ節

前面

① □ 胸管　　　　　　　　　□ Thoracic duct
② □ 左気管支縦隔リンパ本幹　□ Left bronchomediastinal trunk
③ □ 気管支肺リンパ節　　　　□ Bronchopulmonary node
④ □ 下気管気管支リンパ節　　□ Inferior tracheobronchial node
⑤ □ 上気管気管支リンパ節　　□ Superior tracheobronchial node
⑥ □ 気管傍リンパ節　　　　　□ Paratracheal node
⑦ □ 右鎖骨下静脈　　　　　　□ Right subclavian vein
⑧ □ 右内頸静脈　　　　　　　□ Right internal jugular vein

A 右肺と左肺の下半分は右側の気管気管支リンパ節に流入する．左側の気管気管支リンパ節に流入するのは左肺の上葉だけである．

Surface Anatomy

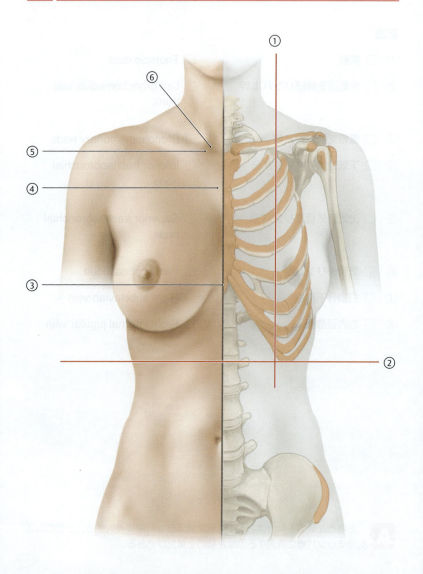

胸部の体表解剖

胸部の触知可能構造，前面

① □ 鎖骨中線　　　　　□ Midclavicular line（MCL）

② □ 肋骨下平面　　　　□ Subcostal plane

③ □ 剣状突起　　　　　□ Xiphoid process

④ □ 胸骨角　　　　　　□ Sternal angle of sternum

⑤ □ 鎖骨の胸骨端　　　□ Sternal end clavicle

⑥ □ 頸切痕　　　　　　□ Jugular notch

腹部・骨盤部 Abdomen & Pelvis

寛骨 196
下肢帯 198
骨盤部の靱帯 1, 2 200
腹壁の筋の概観 1-3 204
腹壁の筋 1-5 210
鼡径部 1, 2 220
骨盤底の筋の概観 1-3 224
骨盤底の筋 1-3 230
腹腔・骨盤腔 236
腹膜腔 238
網嚢 240
腸間膜と臓器 242
腹膜腔の後壁 244
男性骨盤部の内容 246
女性骨盤部の内容 248
腹部の水平断面 250
原位置の胃 252
十二指腸 254
大腸 256
原位置の直腸 258
直腸と肛門管 260
肝臓の表面 1, 2 262
肝外胆管 266
原位置の胆路 268
膵臓 270
原位置の腎臓と尿管 272
女性の膀胱と尿道 274
膀胱三角 276

子宮と卵管 1, 2 278
女性の外生殖器 282
女性の勃起組織 284
女性会陰の神経・血管 286
陰茎の横断面 288
陰茎 290
精巣と精巣上体 292
精巣の被膜 294
男性の付属生殖腺 296
原位置の前立腺 298
男性会陰の神経・血管 300
腹大動脈 302
腎動脈 304
腹腔動脈 1, 2 306
上腸間膜動脈 310
下腸間膜動脈 312
下大静脈の支脈 314
腎動脈・静脈 316
門脈の分布 318
原位置の門脈 320
女性骨盤部の血管 322
直腸の血管 324
男性生殖器の血管 326
壁側リンパ節 328
自律神経叢 330
女性骨盤部の神経支配 332
男性骨盤部の神経支配 334
腹部・骨盤部の体表解剖 336

Hip Bone

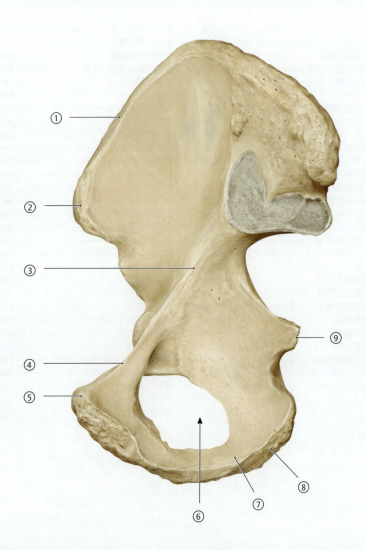

寛骨

内側面

① ☐ 腸骨稜 ☐ Iliac crest
② ☐ 上前腸骨棘 ☐ Anterior superior iliac spine
③ ☐ 弓状線 ☐ Arcuate line
④ ☐ 恥骨筋線 ☐ Pectineal line
⑤ ☐ 恥骨結節 ☐ Pubic tubercle
⑥ ☐ 閉鎖孔 ☐ Obturator foramen
⑦ ☐ 坐骨枝 ☐ Ischial ramus
⑧ ☐ 坐骨結節 ☐ Ischial tuberosity
⑨ ☐ 坐骨棘 ☐ Ischial spine

Pelvic Girdle

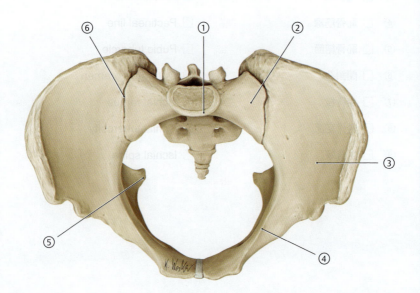

Q 骨盤上口の境界をなすのは何か？

下肢帯

女性骨盤部（Female pelvis），上面

① □ 岬角　　　　　　□ Promontory
② □ 仙骨翼　　　　　□ Ala of sacrum
③ □ 腸骨窩　　　　　□ Iliac fossa
④ □ 恥骨櫛　　　　　□ Pecten pubis
⑤ □ 坐骨棘　　　　　□ Ischial spine
⑥ □ 仙腸関節　　　　□ Sacro-iliac joint

A 骨盤上口は恥骨結合の上縁，恥骨稜，恥骨櫛，腸骨の弓状線，仙骨翼の前縁，仙骨の岬角からなる．

Pelvic Ligaments I

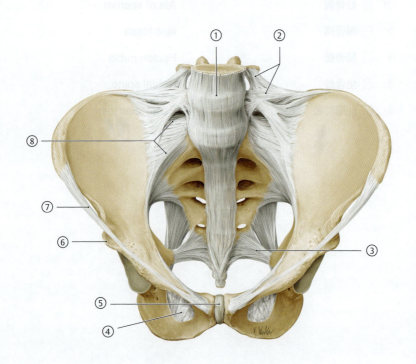

骨盤部の靱帯 1

男性骨盤部（Male pelvis），前上面

① □ 前縦靱帯　　　　　□ Anterior longitudinal ligament
② □ 腸腰靱帯　　　　　□ Iliolumbar ligament
③ □ 仙棘靱帯　　　　　□ Sacrospinous ligament
④ □ 閉鎖膜　　　　　　□ Obturator membrane
⑤ □ 恥骨結合　　　　　□ Pubic symphysis
⑥ □ 下前腸骨棘　　　　□ Anterior inferior iliac spine
⑦ □ 鼠径靱帯　　　　　□ Inguinal ligament
⑧ □ 前仙腸靱帯　　　　□ Anterior sacro-iliac ligaments

Pelvic Ligaments II

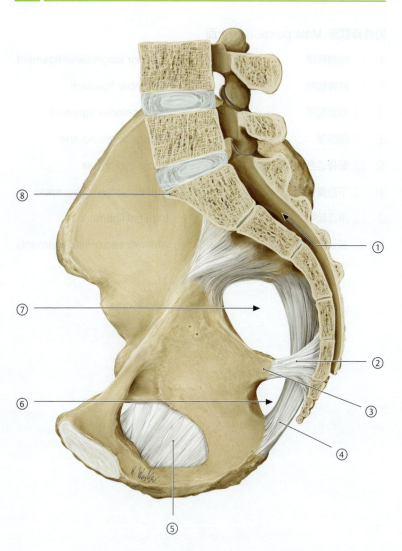

骨盤部の靱帯 2

骨盤部の右半分，内側面

① □ 仙骨管　　　　　　　□ Sacral canal
② □ 仙棘靱帯　　　　　　□ Sacrospinous ligament
③ □ 坐骨棘　　　　　　　□ Ischial spine
④ □ 仙結節靱帯　　　　　□ Sacrotuberous ligament
⑤ □ 閉鎖膜　　　　　　　□ Obturator membrane
⑥ □ 小坐骨孔　　　　　　□ Lesser sciatic foramen
⑦ □ 大坐骨孔　　　　　　□ Greater sciatic foramen
⑧ □ 岬角　　　　　　　　□ Promontory

Abdominal Wall Muscles I

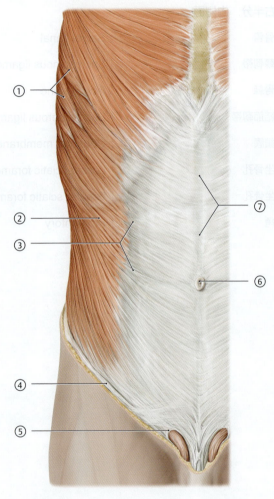

Q 白線とは何か？

腹壁の筋の概観 1

浅層の筋（Superficial muscles），前面

① □ 前鋸筋　　　　　　□ Serratus anterior
② □ 外腹斜筋　　　　　□ External oblique
③ □ 外腹斜筋腱膜　　　□ External oblique aponeurosis
④ □ 鼠径靱帯　　　　　□ Inguinal ligament
⑤ □ 浅鼠径輪　　　　　□ Superficial inguinal ring
⑥ □ 臍　　　　　　　　□ Umbilicus
⑦ □ 白線　　　　　　　□ Linea alba

A 　白線は正中線上を剣状突起から恥骨まで伸びる．白線は左右の前側腹壁にある筋肉の腱膜の線維が重なり合ってできる比較的血管の少ない面であり，しばしば外科手術において切開される．

Abdominal Wall Muscles II

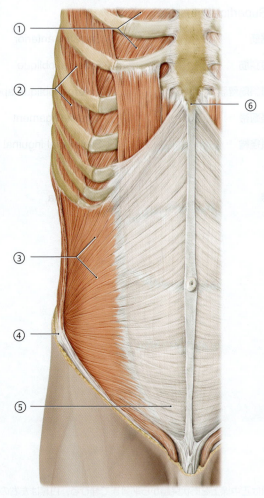

①
②
③
④
⑤
⑥

Q 前側腹壁の支配神経は何か？

腹壁の筋の概観 2

中層の筋（Intermediate muscles），前面

① □ 内肋間筋　　　　　□ Internal intercostal muscles
② □ 外肋間筋　　　　　□ External intercostal muscles
③ □ 内腹斜筋　　　　　□ Internal oblique
④ □ 上前腸骨棘　　　　□ Anterior superior iliac spine
⑤ □ 腹直筋鞘の前葉　　□ Anterior layer of rectus sheath
⑥ □ 剣状突起　　　　　□ Xiphoid process

A 前側腹壁の筋肉（外腹斜筋，内腹斜筋，腹横筋）は T7-T12 の肋間神経によって支配される．内腹斜筋と腹横筋は腸骨下腹神経と腸骨鼡径神経にも支配される．デルマトームの指標として，T10 が臍を支配することが用いられる．

Abdominal Wall Muscles III

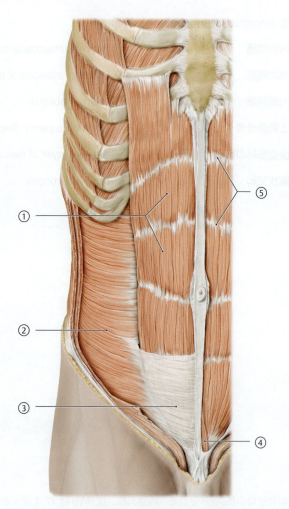

Q 弓状線より下の部分の腹直筋鞘の前葉と後葉を構成するのは何か？

腹壁の筋の概観 3

深層の筋（Deep muscles），前面

① □ 腹直筋　　　　　　　　　□ Rectus abdominis

② □ 腹横筋　　　　　　　　　□ Transversus abdominis

③ □ 腹横筋の腱膜　　　　　　□ Transversus abdominis
　　（腹直筋鞘の前葉）　　　　　aponeurosis（anterior layer of
　　　　　　　　　　　　　　　　rectus sheath）

④ □ 錐体筋　　　　　　　　　□ Pyramidalis

⑤ □ 腱画　　　　　　　　　　□ Tendinous intersections

A 弓状線より下では，腹壁筋の腱膜は腹直筋の前面に集まり，腹直筋鞘の前葉を構成する．後葉は横筋筋膜と壁側筋膜からのみなる．

System of the Abdominal Wall Muscles I

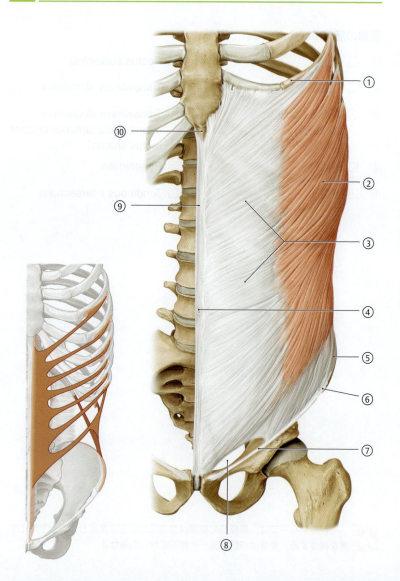

腹壁の筋 1

前外側腹壁筋：外腹斜筋

① □ 第5肋骨　　　　　　　　　　□ 5th rib
② □ 外腹斜筋　　　　　　　　　　□ **External oblique**
③ □ 外腹斜筋腱膜　　　　　　　　□ External oblique aponeurosis
④ □ 臍輪　　　　　　　　　　　　□ Umbilical ring
⑤ □ 腸骨稜の外唇　　　　　　　　□ Outer lip of iliac crest
⑥ □ 上前腸骨棘　　　　　　　　　□ Anterior superior iliac spine
⑦ □ 鼡径靱帯　　　　　　　　　　□ Inguinal ligament
⑧ □ 浅鼡径輪　　　　　　　　　　□ Superficial inguinal ring
⑨ □ 白線　　　　　　　　　　　　□ Linea alba
⑩ □ 剣状突起　　　　　　　　　　□ Xiphoid process

筋	起始	停止	作用	神経支配
外腹斜筋	第5-12肋骨（外側面）	・腸骨稜（外唇） ・腹直筋鞘の前葉 ・白線	・片側：体幹を同側に曲げる，体幹を反対側に回旋させる ・両側：体幹の屈曲，骨盤の固定，腹圧を高める，呼出	肋間神経(T7-T11)，肋下神経(T12)

System of the Abdominal Wall Muscles II

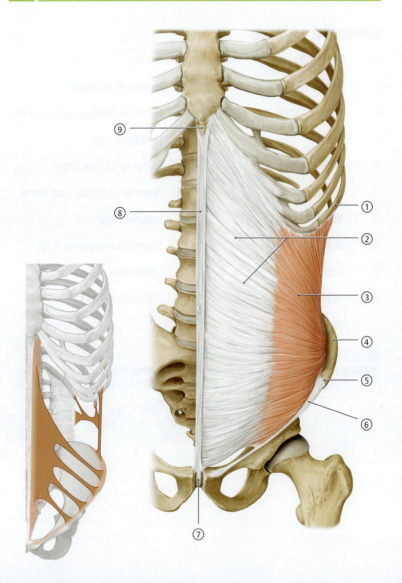

腹壁の筋 2

前外側腹壁筋：内腹斜筋

① □ 第10肋骨　　　　　□ 10th rib
② □ 内腹斜筋腱膜　　　□ Internal oblique aponeurosis
③ □ 内腹斜筋　　　　　□ **Internal oblique**
④ □ 腸骨稜，中間線　　□ Intermediate zone of iliac crest
⑤ □ 上前腸骨棘　　　　□ Anterior superior iliac spine
⑥ □ 鼠径靱帯　　　　　□ Inguinal ligament
⑦ □ 恥骨結合　　　　　□ Pubic symphysis
⑧ □ 白線　　　　　　　□ Linea alba
⑨ □ 剣状突起　　　　　□ Xiphoid process

筋	起始	停止	作用	神経支配
内腹斜筋	・胸腰筋膜（深層） ・腸骨稜（中間線） ・上前腸骨棘 ・鼠径靱帯（外側半）	・第10-12肋骨（下縁） ・腹直筋鞘（前葉・後葉） ・白線 ・精巣挙筋に移行	・片側：体幹を同側に曲げる，体幹を同側に回旋させる ・両側：体幹の屈曲，骨盤の固定，腹圧を高める，呼出	・肋間神経（T8-T11），肋下神経（T12），腸骨下腹神経，腸骨鼠径神経 ・精巣挙筋（陰部大腿神経の陰部枝）

System of the Abdominal Wall Muscles III

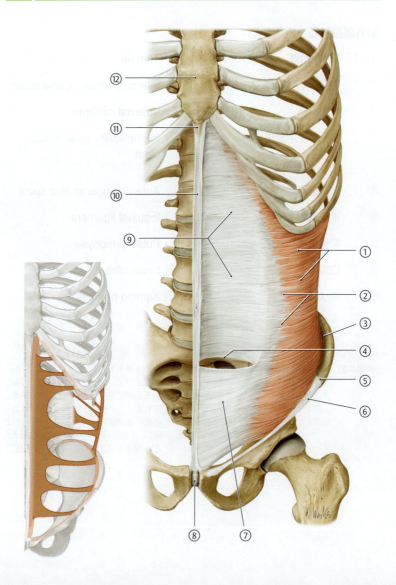

腹部・骨盤部　**215**

腹壁の筋 3

前外側腹壁筋：腹横筋

① ☐ 腹横筋　　　　　　　　　　☐ **Transversus abdominis**
② ☐ 半月線　　　　　　　　　　☐ Semilunar line
③ ☐ 腸骨稜の内唇　　　　　　　☐ Inner lip of iliac crest
④ ☐ 弓状線　　　　　　　　　　☐ Arcuate line
⑤ ☐ 上前腸骨棘　　　　　　　　☐ Anterior superior iliac spine
⑥ ☐ 鼡径靱帯　　　　　　　　　☐ Inguinal ligament
⑦ ☐ 腹直筋鞘の前葉　　　　　　☐ Anterior layer of rectus sheath
⑧ ☐ 恥骨結合　　　　　　　　　☐ Pubic symphysis
⑨ ☐ 腹横筋腱膜（＝腹直筋鞘の後葉）　☐ Transversus abdominis aponeurosis（＝ posterior layer of rectus sheath）
⑩ ☐ 白線　　　　　　　　　　　☐ Linea alba
⑪ ☐ 剣状突起　　　　　　　　　☐ Xiphoid process
⑫ ☐ 胸骨　　　　　　　　　　　☐ Sternum

筋	起始	停止	作用	神経支配
腹横筋	・第 7-12 肋軟骨（内側面） ・胸腰筋膜（深層） ・腸骨稜（内唇） ・上前腸骨棘	・腹直筋鞘（後葉） ・白線	・片側：体幹を同側に回旋させる ・両側：腹圧を高める，呼出	・肋間神経（T7-T11），肋下神経（T12） ・腸骨下腹神経，腸骨鼡径神経

System of the Abdominal Wall Muscles IV

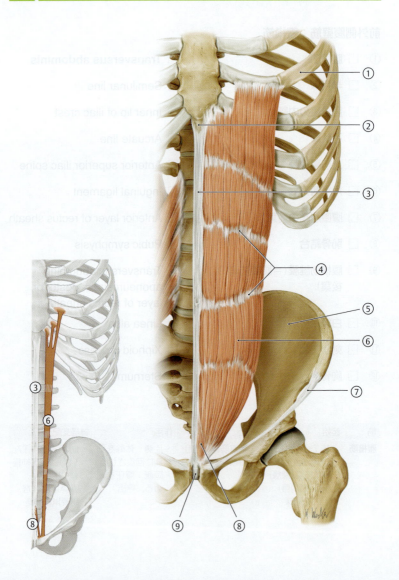

腹壁の筋 4

前腹壁筋：腹直筋と錐体筋

① ☐ 第 5 肋骨　　　　　　　　☐ 5th rib

② ☐ 剣状突起　　　　　　　　☐ Xiphoid process

③ ☐ 白線　　　　　　　　　　☐ Linea alba

④ ☐ 腱画　　　　　　　　　　☐ Tendinous intersections

⑤ ☐ 腸骨窩　　　　　　　　　☐ Iliac fossa

⑥ ☐ 腹直筋　　　　　　　　　☐ **Rectus abdominis**

⑦ ☐ 鼡径靱帯　　　　　　　　☐ Inguinal ligament

⑧ ☐ 錐体筋　　　　　　　　　☐ **Pyramidalis**

⑨ ☐ 恥骨結合　　　　　　　　☐ Pubic symphysis

筋	起始	停止	作用	神経支配
腹直筋	・第 5-7 肋軟骨 ・胸骨剣状突起	恥骨（恥骨結節と恥骨結合の間）	・腹部の屈曲 ・骨盤の固定 ・腹圧を高める ・呼出	肋間神経（T5-T11），肋下神経（T12）
錐体筋	恥骨（腹直筋の前方）	白線	白線の緊張	肋下神経（T12）

System of the Abdominal Wall Muscles V

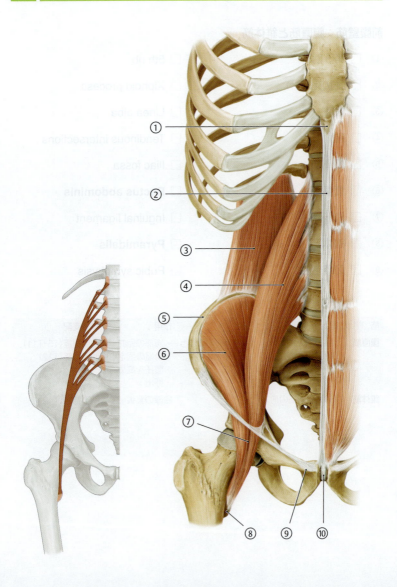

腹壁の筋 5

後腹壁筋：腰方形筋と大腰筋

① □ 剣状突起　　　　□ Xiphoid process
② □ 白線　　　　　　□ Linea alba
③ □ **腰方形筋**　　　□ **Quadratus lumborum**
④ □ **大腰筋**　　　　□ **Psoas major**
⑤ □ 腸骨稜　　　　　□ Iliac crest
⑥ □ 腸骨筋　　　　　□ Iliacus
⑦ □ 腸腰筋　　　　　□ Iliopsoas
⑧ □ 小転子　　　　　□ Lesser trochanter
⑨ □ 恥骨結節　　　　□ Pubic tubercle
⑩ □ 恥骨結合　　　　□ Pubic symphysis

筋	起始	停止	作用	神経支配
腰方形筋	腸骨稜の内唇	・第12肋骨 ・L1-L4 （肋骨突起）	・片側：体幹を同側に曲げる ・両側：腹圧を高める，呼出	肋下神経(T12)，L1-L4
大腰筋	・浅層：T12-L4の椎体側面とそれらの間の椎間円板の側面 ・深層：L1-L5（肋骨突起）	腸骨筋と合体して腸腰筋*となり，大腿骨の小転子に停止	・片側：(大腿骨固定時)体幹の同側への側屈 ・両側：体幹を仰臥位から起こす	・大腿神経(L2-L4) ・腰神経叢からの直接の枝

*大腰筋は局所解剖学的に後腹壁筋に属する．大腰筋は，腸骨筋と同様に機能面で大腿の筋に属する(pp.524, 525を参照)．

Inguinal Region I

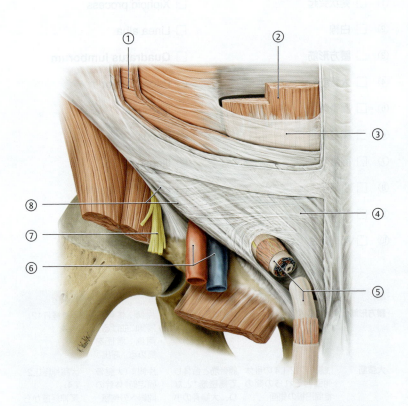

Q 鼠径管の経路を説明せよ．

鼠径部 1

右側，前面

① □ 内腹斜筋　　　　□ Internal oblique
② □ 腹直筋　　　　　□ Rectus abdominis
③ □ 腹直筋鞘の前葉　□ Anterior layer of rectus sheath
④ □ 外腹斜筋腱膜　　□ External oblique aponeurosis
⑤ □ 精索　　　　　　□ Spermatic cord
⑥ □ 大腿動脈・静脈　□ Femoral artery and vein
⑦ □ 大腿神経　　　　□ Femoral nerve
⑧ □ 鼠径靱帯　　　　□ Inguinal ligament

A 鼠径管は前腹壁の下部を斜めに貫通し，最深層外側の深鼠径輪から始まる．深鼠径輪は鼠径靱帯の中点のやや外側にあり，鼠径管の最浅層は内側で終わり，恥骨結節の外側で浅鼠径輪が開口する．

Inguinal Region II

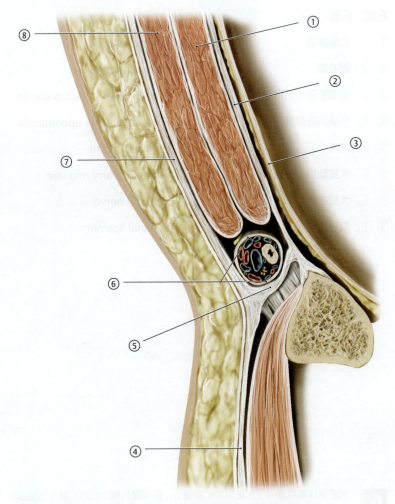

 精索に含まれるのは何か？

鼠径部 2

矢状断面

① □ 腹横筋　　　　　□ Transversus abdominis
② □ 横筋筋膜　　　　□ Transversalis fascia
③ □ 壁側腹膜　　　　□ Parietal peritoneum
④ □ 大腿筋膜　　　　□ Fascia lata
⑤ □ 鼠径靭帯　　　　□ Inguinal ligament
⑥ □ 精索　　　　　　□ Spermatic cord
⑦ □ 外腹斜筋腱膜　　□ External oblique aponeurosis
⑧ □ 内腹斜筋　　　　□ Internal oblique

A 精索には，精管，精巣動脈，蔓状静脈叢，自律神経，リンパ管，鞘状突起の遺残が含まれる．

Pelvic Floor Muscles I

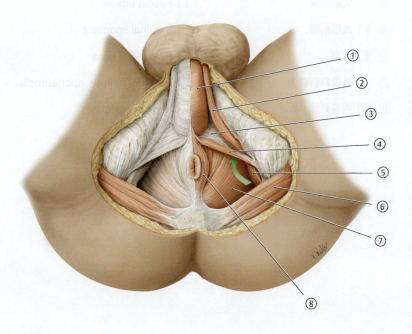

骨盤底の筋の概観 1

男性の骨盤部，切石位

① □ 球海綿体筋　　　　　□ Bulbospongiosus

② □ 坐骨海綿体筋　　　　□ Ischiocavernosus

③ □ 下尿生殖隔膜筋膜（会陰膜）　□ Perineal membrane

④ □ 浅会陰横筋　　　　　□ Superficial transverse perineal muscle

⑤ □ 内閉鎖筋　　　　　　□ Obturator internus

⑥ □ 大殿筋　　　　　　　□ Gluteus maximus

⑦ □ 肛門挙筋　　　　　　□ Levator ani

⑧ □ 外肛門括約筋　　　　□ External anal sphincter

解説

男女を問わず会陰の左右の境界をなすのは，恥骨結合，坐骨恥骨枝，坐骨結節，仙結節靱帯，尾骨である．

Pelvic Floor Muscles II

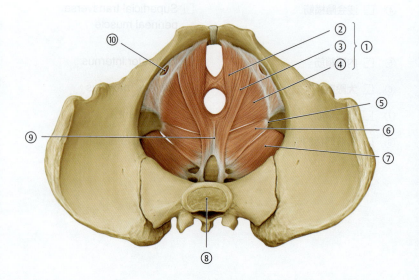

Q 骨盤隔膜をなす筋肉は何か？

骨盤底の筋の概観 2

女性の骨盤部，上面

① □ 肛門挙筋　　　　　□ Levator ani
② □ 恥骨直腸筋　　　　□ Puborectalis
③ □ 恥骨尾骨筋　　　　□ Pubococcygeus
④ □ 腸骨尾骨筋　　　　□ Iliococcygeus
⑤ □ 坐骨棘　　　　　　□ Ischial spine
⑥ □ 尾骨筋　　　　　　□ Coccygeus
⑦ □ 梨状筋　　　　　　□ Piriformis
⑧ □ 仙骨　　　　　　　□ Sacrum
⑨ □ 肛門尾骨靱帯　　　□ Anococcygeal ligament
⑩ □ 閉鎖管　　　　　　□ Obturator canal

A 肛門挙筋(恥骨直腸筋, 恥骨尾骨筋, 腸骨尾骨筋)と尾骨筋が骨盤隔膜として知られる骨盤底をなしている.

Pelvic Floor Muscles III

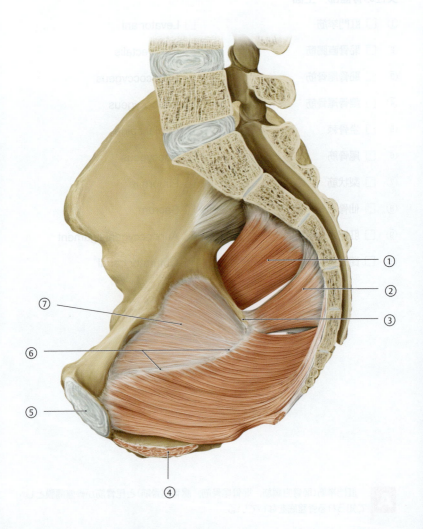

骨盤底の筋の概観 3

女性の骨盤部の右半分，内側面

① □ 梨状筋　　　　　□ Piriformis
② □ 尾骨筋　　　　　□ Coccygeus
③ □ 坐骨棘　　　　　□ Ischial spine
④ □ 深会陰横筋　　　□ Deep transverse perineal muscle
⑤ □ 恥骨結合　　　　□ Pubic symphysis
⑥ □ 肛門挙筋腱弓　　□ Tendinous arch of levator ani
⑦ □ 内閉鎖筋筋膜　　□ Obturator internus fascia

System of the Pelvic Floor Muscles I

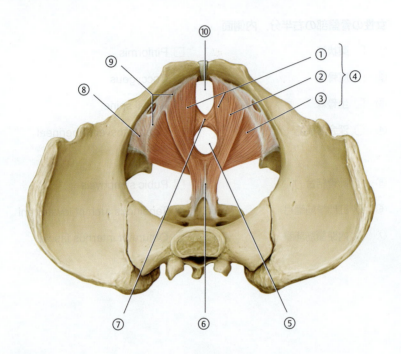

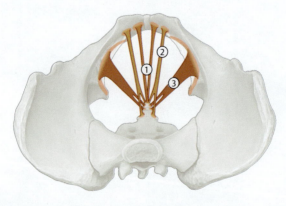

骨盤底の筋 1

骨盤隔膜：肛門挙筋，女性の骨盤部．上方から見たところ．

① □ 恥骨直腸筋　　　　　□ **Puborectalis**
② □ 恥骨尾骨筋　　　　　□ **Pubococcygeus**
③ □ 腸骨尾骨筋　　　　　□ **Iliococcygeus**
④ □ 肛門挙筋　　　　　　□ **Levator ani**
⑤ □ 肛門裂孔　　　　　　□ Anal aperture
⑥ □ 腸骨尾骨筋縫線　　　□ Iliococcygeal raphe
⑦ □ 直腸前線維　　　　　□ Prerectal fibers
⑧ □ 内閉鎖筋　　　　　　□ Obturator internus
⑨ □ 肛門挙筋腱弓　　　　□ Tendinous arch of levator ani
⑩ □ 尿生殖裂孔　　　　　□ Urogenital hiatus

筋	起始	停止	作用	神経支配
肛門挙筋（恥骨直腸筋）	恥骨結合の両側の恥骨上肢	肛門直腸移行部の周囲を係蹄状に，外肛門括約筋の深部と絡み合っている	骨盤内臓の支持	陰部神経（S2-S4）
肛門挙筋（恥骨尾骨筋）	恥骨（恥骨直腸筋の起始の外側）	尾骨，肛門尾骨靱帯		
肛門挙筋（腸骨尾骨筋）	内閉鎖筋筋膜の腱様弓（肛門挙筋腱弓）	尾骨，腸骨尾骨筋縫線		

System of the Pelvic Floor Muscles II

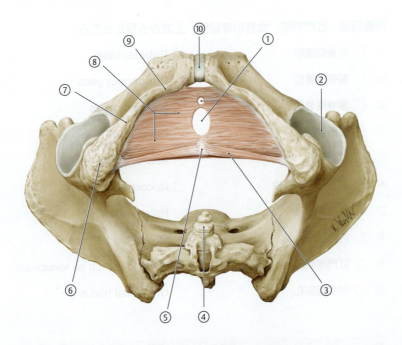
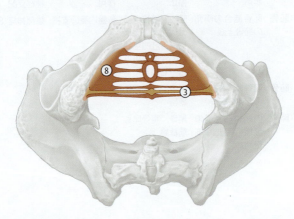

骨盤底の筋 2

尿生殖隔膜：深・浅会陰横筋，女性の骨盤部．下方から見たところ

① □ 尿生殖裂孔　　　　　　　　□ Urogenital hiatus

② □ 寛骨臼　　　　　　　　　　□ Acetabulum

③ □ 浅会陰横筋　　　　　　　　□ **Superficial transverse perineal muscle**

④ □ 尾骨　　　　　　　　　　　□ Coccyx

⑤ □ 会陰腱中心　　　　　　　　□ Perineal body

⑥ □ 坐骨結節　　　　　　　　　□ Ischial tuberosity

⑦ □ 坐骨枝　　　　　　　　　　□ Ramus of ischium

⑧ □ 深会陰横筋　　　　　　　　□ **Deep transverse perineal muscle**

⑨ □ 恥骨下肢　　　　　　　　　□ Inferior pubic ramus

⑩ □ 恥骨結合　　　　　　　　　□ Pubic symphysis

筋	起始	停止	作用	神経支配
深会陰横筋	恥骨下肢，坐骨枝	・腟壁 ・女性・男性それぞれの尿道の壁 ・会陰腱中心	・骨盤内臓の支持 ・尿道を閉める	陰部神経 (S2-S4)
浅会陰横筋	坐骨枝	会陰腱中心		

System of the Pelvic Floor Muscles III

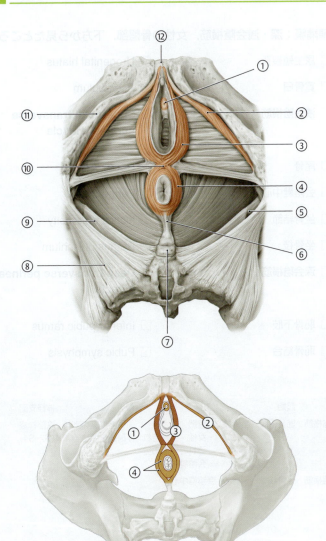

骨盤底の筋 3

括約筋と勃起筋：外肛門括約筋，外尿道括約筋，球海綿体筋，坐骨海綿体筋，女性の骨盤部，下方から見たところ

① ☐ 外尿道括約筋　　　☐ External urethral sphincter
② ☐ 坐骨海綿体筋　　　☐ Ischiocavernosus
③ ☐ 球海綿体筋　　　　☐ Bulbospongiosus
④ ☐ 外肛門括約筋　　　☐ External anal sphincter
⑤ ☐ 坐骨棘　　　　　　☐ Ischial spine
⑥ ☐ 肛門尾骨靱帯　　　☐ Anococcygeal ligament
⑦ ☐ 尾骨　　　　　　　☐ Coccyx
⑧ ☐ 仙結節靱帯　　　　☐ Sacrotuberous ligament
⑨ ☐ 仙棘靱帯　　　　　☐ Sacrospinous ligament
⑩ ☐ 会陰腱中心　　　　☐ Perineal body
⑪ ☐ 恥骨下肢　　　　　☐ Inferior pubic ramus
⑫ ☐ 恥骨結合　　　　　☐ Pubic symphysis

筋	起始	停止	作用	神経支配
外肛門括約筋，皮下部，表面部および深部	肛門を取り囲む（会陰体より肛門尾骨靱帯まで後方に走る）		肛門を閉める	陰部神経 (S2-S4)
外尿道括約筋	深会陰横筋から分束し，尿道を取り囲む（pp.284, 285を参照）		尿道を閉める	
球海綿体筋	会陰腱中心から前方へ，女性では陰核に，男性では陰茎縫線に至る．		・女性：大前庭腺を収縮 ・男性：陰茎海綿体を包む	
坐骨海綿体筋	坐骨枝	陰核脚または陰茎脚	陰核海綿体あるいは陰茎海綿体に血液を押し込める	

Abdominopelvic Cavity

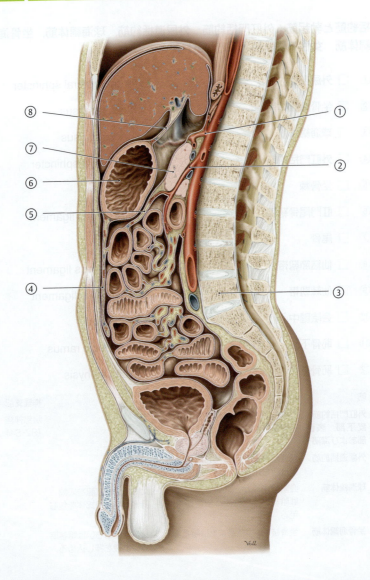

腹腔・骨盤腔

正中矢状断面，左側面

① □ 腹腔動脈　　　　　　□ Celiac trunk
② □ 上腸間膜動脈　　　　□ Superior mesenteric artery
③ □ 第5腰椎　　　　　　□ L5 vertebra
④ □ 大網　　　　　　　　□ Greater omentum
⑤ □ 横行結腸間膜　　　　□ Transverse mesocolon
⑥ □ 胃　　　　　　　　　□ Stomach
⑦ □ 膵臓　　　　　　　　□ Pancreas
⑧ □ 肝胃間膜（小網）　　□ Hepatogastric ligament

解説

腹膜内器官は臓側腹膜に包まれ，血管と神経を腸間膜を通して受け取る．腹膜後器官は後腹壁に位置し，前面だけが臓側腹膜に覆われる．

Greater Sac (Peritoneal Cavity)

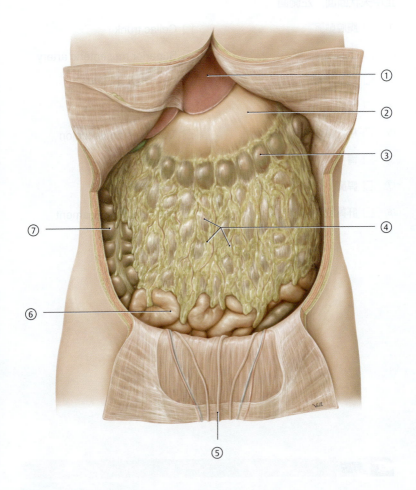

Q 大網とは何か？

腹膜腔

前面

① □ 肝臓, 左葉　　　　　　　　□ Liver, left lobe
② □ 胃　　　　　　　　　　　　□ Stomach
③ □ 横行結腸　　　　　　　　　□ Transverse colon
④ □ 大網　　　　　　　　　　　□ Greater omentum
⑤ □ 正中臍ヒダ（中に閉鎖した　□ Median umbilical fold
　　　尿膜管が走る）　　　　　　　　（with obliterated urachus）
⑥ □ 回腸　　　　　　　　　　　□ Ileum
⑦ □ 上行結腸　　　　　　　　　□ Ascending colon

大網は胃の大弯から垂れ下がり, 横行結腸と小腸の前面を覆っているエプロン状の4層の腹膜のヒダである. 横行結腸と小腸の前面で折れ返り, 横行結腸間膜より上で後腹壁に付着する.

Omental Bursa

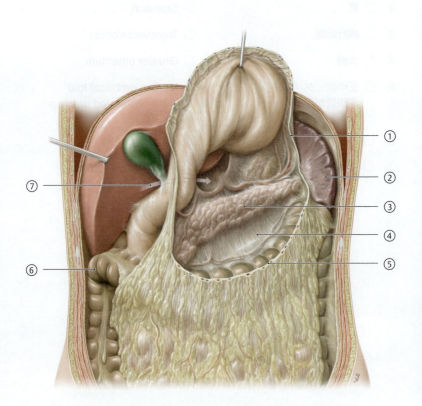

網囊

前面

① ☐ 胃脾間膜　　　　　☐ Gastrosplenic ligament
② ☐ 脾臟　　　　　　　☐ Spleen
③ ☐ 膵臟　　　　　　　☐ Pancreas
④ ☐ 橫行結腸間膜　　　☐ Transverse mesocolon
⑤ ☐ 胃結腸間膜　　　　☐ Gastrocolic ligament
⑥ ☐ 右結腸曲　　　　　☐ Right colic flexure
⑦ ☐ 網囊孔　　　　　　☐ Omental foramen

Mesenteries & Organs

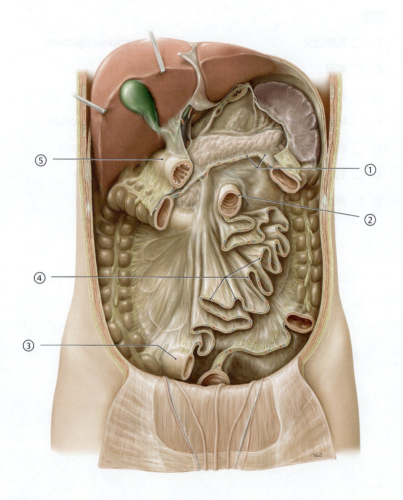

①
②
③
④
⑤

Q 小腸と大腸のどの部分に間膜が付着するか？

腸間膜と臓器

前面

① ☐ 横行結腸間膜，根 ☐ Transverse mesocolon, root
② ☐ 十二指腸空腸曲 ☐ Duodenojejunal flexure
③ ☐ 回腸 ☐ Ileum
④ ☐ 腸間膜（断端） ☐ Mesentery（cut）
⑤ ☐ 十二指腸の上部 ☐ Superior part of duodenum

　小腸の空腸と回腸，大腸の横行結腸とS状結腸は間膜によって，吊り下げられている．

Posterior Wall of the Peritoneal Cavity

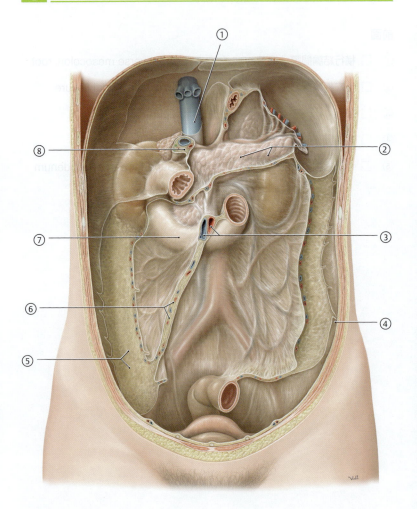

Q 結腸の右下半領域の境界をなすもののうち，排液を制限するのはどれか？

腹膜腔の後壁

前面

① □ 下大静脈　　　　　　　　　□ Inferior vena cava

② □ 膵臓（膵体，膵尾）　　　　□ Pancreas, body and tail

③ □ 上腸間膜動脈・静脈　　　　□ Superior mesenteric artery and vein

④ □ 結腸傍溝　　　　　　　　　□ Paracolic gutter

⑤ □ 上行結腸（付着部）　　　　□ Ascending colon (site of attachment)

⑥ □ 腸間膜根　　　　　　　　　□ Root of mesentery

⑦ □ 十二指腸の水平部　　　　　□ Horizontal part of duodenum

⑧ □ 肝十二指腸間膜（門脈，固有肝動脈，総胆管が入っている）　□ Hepatoduodenal ligament (with hepatic portal vein, hepatic artery proper, and bile duct)

結腸の右下半領域は後腹壁上の三角形の部分であり，横行結腸間膜，腸間膜根，上行結腸が境界をなしている．液体の移動はこの境界によって制限されるが，腹膜腔においては結腸傍溝に沿って下へと移動して骨盤に至ることが可能である．

Contents of the Male Pelvis

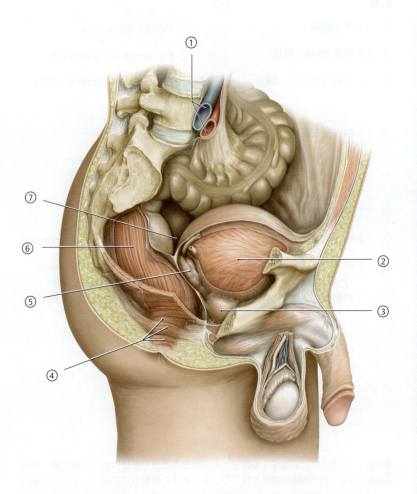

男性骨盤部の内容

傍矢状断面, 右側面

① □ 右総腸骨動脈・静脈　　□ Right common iliac artery and vein
② □ 膀胱　　□ Urinary bladder
③ □ 前立腺　　□ Prostate
④ □ 外肛門括約筋　　□ External anal sphincter
⑤ □ 右の精嚢　　□ Right seminal gland
⑥ □ 直腸　　□ Rectum
⑦ □ 直腸膀胱窩　　□ Rectovesical pouch

Contents of the Female Pelvis

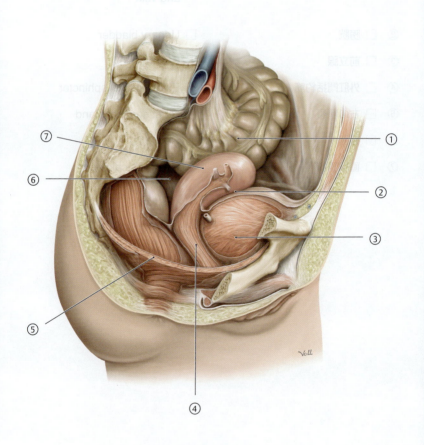

女性骨盤部の内容

傍矢状断面，右側面

① □ S状結腸　　　　　□ Sigmoid colon
② □ 膀胱子宮窩　　　　□ Vesico-uterine pouch
③ □ 膀胱　　　　　　　□ Urinary bladder
④ □ 腟　　　　　　　　□ Vagina
⑤ □ 肛門挙筋　　　　　□ Levator ani
⑥ □ 直腸子宮窩　　　　□ Recto-uterine pouch
⑦ □ 子宮　　　　　　　□ Uterus

Transverse Section of the Abdomen

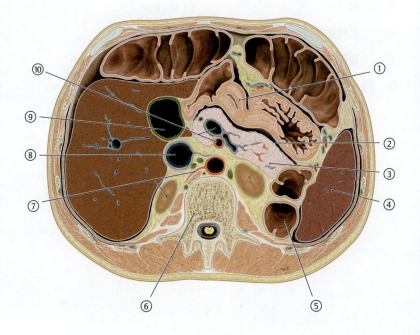

腹部の水平断面

下面

① □ 胃の幽門部　　　　　□ Pyloric part of stomach
② □ 網嚢　　　　　　　　□ Omental bursa
③ □ 膵臓　　　　　　　　□ Pancreas
④ □ 脾臓　　　　　　　　□ Spleen
⑤ □ 下行結腸　　　　　　□ Descending colon
⑥ □ 第1腰椎　　　　　　□ L1 vertebra
⑦ □ 腎臓(右腎動脈)　　　□ Kidney (with right renal artery)
⑧ □ 下大静脈　　　　　　□ Inferior vena cava
⑨ □ 胆嚢　　　　　　　　□ Gallbladder
⑩ □ 上腸間膜動脈・静脈　□ Superior mesenteric artery and vein

Stomach in situ

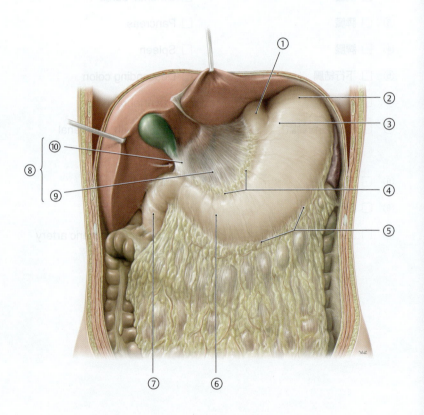

原位置の胃

前面

① □ 食道　　　　　　　□ Esophagus
② □ 胃底　　　　　　　□ Fundus of stomach
③ □ 噴門　　　　　　　□ Cardia
④ □ 小弯　　　　　　　□ Lesser curvature
⑤ □ 大弯　　　　　　　□ Greater curvature
⑥ □ 幽門洞　　　　　　□ Pyloric antrum
⑦ □ 十二指腸　　　　　□ Duodenum
⑧ □ 小網　　　　　　　□ Lesser omentum
⑨ □ 肝胃間膜　　　　　□ Hepatogastric ligament
⑩ □ 肝十二指腸間膜　　□ Hepatoduodenal ligament

臨床

よく知られた胃の疾患である胃炎と胃潰瘍は，胃酸産生過多と関連し，アルコールやアスピリンなどの薬物，細菌のヘリコバクター・ピロリが原因となる．食欲減退，胃痛が症状として現れるが，出血があった場合には，黒色便や吐瀉物中に暗褐色の物質が見られることもある．胃炎は胃壁の内側面に限られるが，胃潰瘍は胃壁に及ぶ．

Duodenum

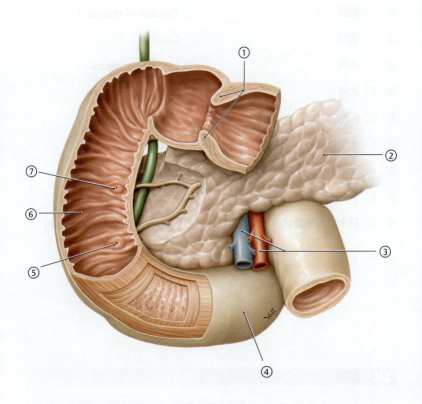

Q 十二指腸を支える靱帯は何か？

十二指腸

前面

① □ 幽門括約筋　　　　　□ Pyloric sphincter
② □ 膵臓　　　　　　　　□ Pancreas
③ □ 上腸間膜動脈・静脈　□ Superior mesenteric artery and vein
④ □ 十二指腸の水平部　　□ Horizontal part of duodenum
⑤ □ 大十二指腸乳頭　　　□ Major duodenal papilla
⑥ □ 十二指腸の下行部　　□ Descending part of duodenum
⑦ □ 小十二指腸乳頭　　　□ Minor duodenal papilla

A 　トライツ靱帯は線維筋性のヒモであり，十二指腸空腸曲において十二指腸を横隔膜右脚から吊り下げる．

Large Intestine

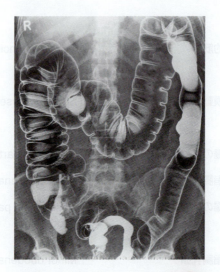

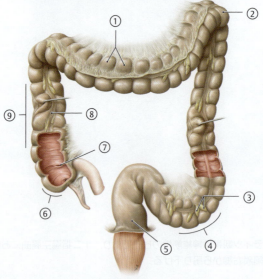

大腸

前面

① ☐ 結腸膨起 ☐ Haustra of colon
② ☐ 左結腸曲 ☐ Left colic flexure
③ ☐ 腹膜垂 ☐ Omental appendices
④ ☐ S状結腸 ☐ Sigmoid colon
⑤ ☐ 直腸（腹膜反転部） ☐ Rectum (with peritoneal reflection)
⑥ ☐ 盲腸 ☐ Cecum
⑦ ☐ 回腸口 ☐ Ileocecal orifice
⑧ ☐ 自由ヒモ ☐ Taeniae coli
⑨ ☐ 上行結腸 ☐ Ascending colon

 解説

　発生学的には，大腸は腹膜内器官として発生するが，腸の回転に伴って上行結腸と下行結腸は後腹壁に固定されて間膜を失う．腎臓などの一次性腹膜後器官は後腹壁の壁側腹膜の後方で形成されるので，間膜と結合することはない．

Rectum in situ

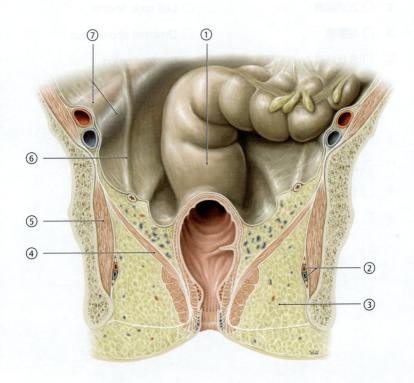

Q S状結腸と直腸の移行部には何があるか？

原位置の直腸

冠状断面，女性骨盤部の前面

① □ 直腸　　　　　　　　　　□ Rectum
② □ 内陰部動脈・静脈　　　　□ Internal pudendal artery and vein
③ □ 坐骨肛門窩（坐骨直腸窩）　□ Ischio-anal fossa
④ □ 肛門挙筋　　　　　　　　□ Levator ani
⑤ □ 内閉鎖筋　　　　　　　　□ Obturator internus
⑥ □ 尿管　　　　　　　　　　□ Ureter
⑦ □ 外腸骨動脈・静脈　　　　□ External iliac artery and vein

　直腸とS状結腸の移行部はほぼS3の高さであり，S状結腸間膜と結腸ヒモの終端が見られる．

Rectum & Anal Canal

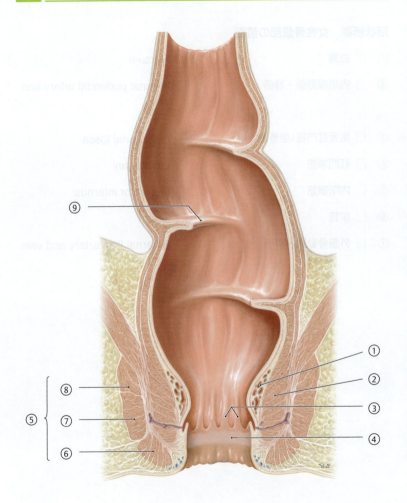

直腸と肛門管

冠状断面, 前面

① □ 直腸静脈叢　　　　　□ Rectal venous plexus
② □ 内肛門括約筋　　　　□ Internal anal sphincter
③ □ 肛門柱　　　　　　　□ Anal columns
④ □ 肛門櫛（白帯）　　　□ Anal pecten (white zone)
⑤ □ 外肛門括約筋　　　　□ External anal sphincter
⑥ □ 皮下部　　　　　　　□ Subcutaneous part
⑦ □ 浅部　　　　　　　　□ Superficial part
⑧ □ 深部　　　　　　　　□ Deep part
⑨ □ 中直腸横ヒダ　　　　□ Middle transverse rectal fold

Surfaces of the Liver I

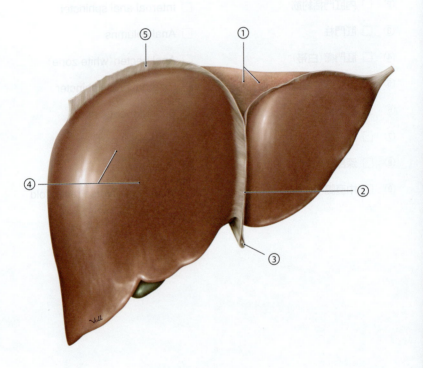

Q 肝臓の無漿膜野はどこか？

肝臓の表面 1

前面

① ☐ 無漿膜野（横隔面） ☐ Bare area (diaphragmatic surface of liver)

② ☐ 肝鎌状間膜 ☐ Falciform ligament

③ ☐ 肝円索（痕跡化した臍静脈を含む） ☐ Round ligament of liver (contains obliterated umbilical vein)

④ ☐ 肝臓の右葉，横隔面 ☐ Right lobe, diaphragmatic surface

⑤ ☐ 肝冠状間膜 ☐ Coronary ligament

肝臓の上面と後面は腹膜に覆われない無漿膜野であり，横隔膜の下面に直接接している．無漿膜野の境界をなすのは，肝冠状間膜と三角間膜の折れ返り部分である．

Surfaces of the Liver II

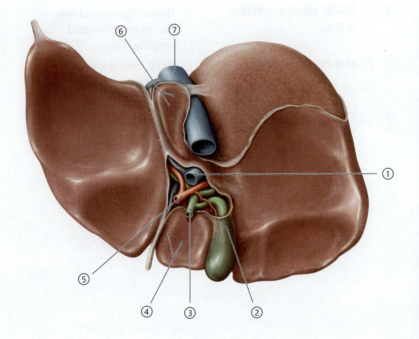

肝臓の表面 2

下面

① □ 門脈 □ Hepatic portal vein
② □ 胆嚢 □ Gallbladder
③ □ 総胆管 □ Bile duct
④ □ 方形葉 □ Quadrate lobe
⑤ □ 固有肝動脈 □ Hepatic artery proper
⑥ □ 尾状葉 □ Caudate lobe
⑦ □ 下大静脈 □ Inferior vena cava

Extrahepatic Bile Ducts

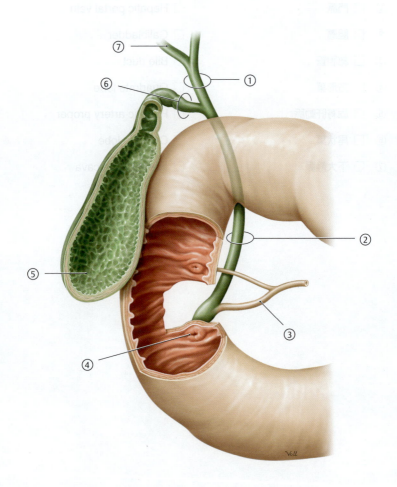

肝外胆管

前面

① □ 総肝管　　　　　□ Common hepatic duct
② □ 総胆管　　　　　□ Bile duct
③ □ 膵管　　　　　　□ Pancreatic duct
④ □ 大十二指腸乳頭　□ Major duodenal papilla
⑤ □ 胆嚢底　　　　　□ Fundus of gallbladder
⑥ □ 胆嚢管　　　　　□ Cystic duct
⑦ □ 右肝管　　　　　□ Right hepatic duct

臨床

胆汁が胆嚢で貯蔵・濃縮される間に，コレステロールなどの物質は結晶化し胆石となる．胆石が胆管に移動すると激しい痛み（疝痛）を起こす．胆石は十二指腸乳頭で膵管の閉塞を起こすことがあり，死に至らしめるような重度の急性膵炎を起こす．

Biliary Tract in situ

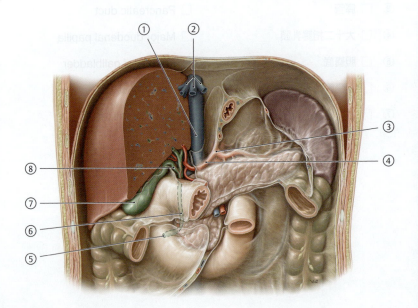

Q 肝十二指腸間膜内にある構造は何か？

原位置の胆路

前面

① □ 下大静脈　　　　　　　　　□ Inferior vena cava

② □ 肝静脈　　　　　　　　　　□ Hepatic veins

③ □ 腹腔動脈　　　　　　　　　□ Celiac trunk

④ □ 総肝動脈　　　　　　　　　□ Common hepatic artery

⑤ □ 胆膵管膨大部(大十二指腸乳頭へ開口)　□ Hepatopancreatic duct (opening on major duodenal papilla)

⑥ □ 総胆管　　　　　　　　　　□ Bile duct

⑦ □ 胆嚢　　　　　　　　　　　□ Gallbladder

⑧ □ 胆嚢管　　　　　　　　　　□ Cystic duct

A 総胆管，肝動脈，門脈が肝十二指腸間膜内を通る．

Pancreas

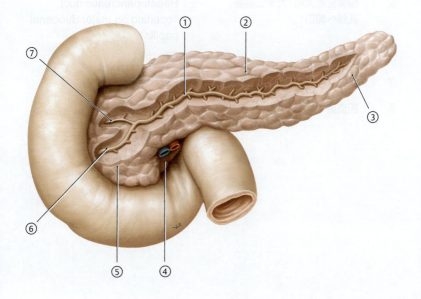

膵臓

前面

① □ 膵管　　　　　　　　　　□ Pancreatic duct

② □ 膵体　　　　　　　　　　□ Body of pancreas

③ □ 膵尾　　　　　　　　　　□ Tail of pancreas

④ □ 膵臓（鈎状突起）　　　　□ Uncinate process of pancreas

⑤ □ 膵頭　　　　　　　　　　□ Head of pancreas

⑥ □ 膵管（腹側膵芽から由来）　□ Pancreatic duct (from the ventral pancreatic bud)

⑦ □ 副膵管（背側膵芽から由来）□ Accessory pancreatic duct (from the dorsal pancreatic bud)

解説

　膵管は胎生期の腹側膵と背側膵から生じる．膵管の近位部は腹側膵に由来し，大十二指腸乳頭で十二指腸に開口する．残りの背側膵から起こった部分は副膵管であり，大十二指腸乳頭の近傍で十二指腸に開口する．膵管の走行には変異が多い．

Kidneys & Ureters in situ

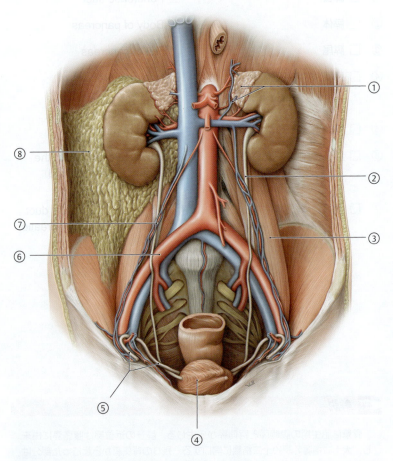

尿管の狭窄が起こりやすい部位はどこか？

原位置の腎臓と尿管

男性腹部，前面

① □ 左の副腎，左副腎静脈　　□ Left suprarenal gland and vein

② □ 尿管の腹部　　□ Abdominal part of ureter

③ □ 大腰筋　　□ Psoas major

④ □ 膀胱　　□ Urinary bladder

⑤ □ 右の精管　　□ Right ductus deferens

⑥ □ 右総腸骨動脈　　□ Right common iliac artery

⑦ □ 右精巣/卵巣動脈・静脈　　□ Right ovarian / testicular artery and vein

⑧ □ 脂肪被膜　　□ Perirenal fat capsule

　尿管は次の3ヵ所で狭窄を起こしやすい．腎盂が狭くなって尿管になる部位（腎盂尿管移行部），総腸骨動静脈の遠位端で骨盤上口と交差する部位，膀胱を貫通する部位．

Female Urinary Bladder & Urethra

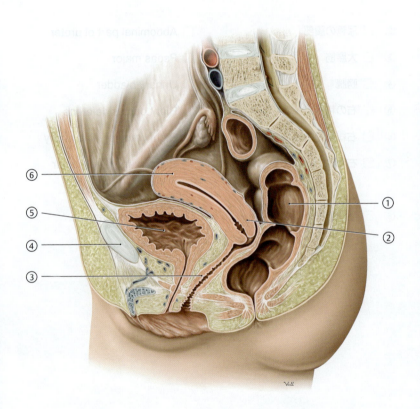

女性の膀胱と尿道

正中矢状断面，左側面

① ☐ 直腸　　　　　☐ Rectum
② ☐ 子宮頸　　　　☐ Cervix of uterus
③ ☐ 腟　　　　　　☐ Vagina
④ ☐ 恥骨結合　　　☐ Pubic symphysis
⑤ ☐ 膀胱　　　　　☐ Urinary bladder
⑥ ☐ 子宮底　　　　☐ Fundus of uterus

Trigone of the Bladder

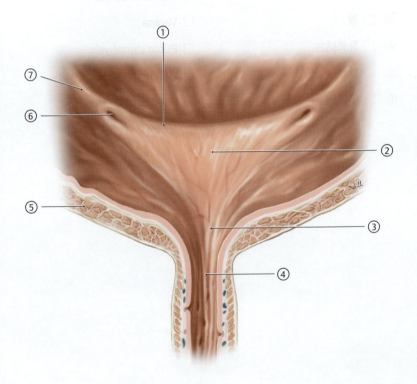

膀胱三角

冠状断面, 前面

① □ 尿管間ヒダ　　　　□ Interureteral fold
② □ 膀胱三角　　　　　□ Trigone of bladder
③ □ 膀胱頸　　　　　　□ Neck of bladder
④ □ 尿道　　　　　　　□ Urethra
⑤ □ 筋層(＝排尿筋)　　□ Muscularis(＝ detrusor)
⑥ □ 尿管口　　　　　　□ Ureteric orifice
⑦ □ 右の尿管, 壁内部　□ Right ureter, intramural part

Uterus & Uterine Tube I

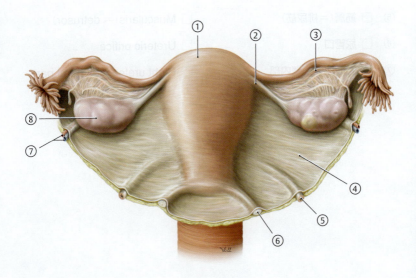

子宮と卵管 1

後上面

① ☐ 子宮底 — ☐ Fundus of uterus

② ☐ 固有卵巣索 — ☐ Ligament of ovary

③ ☐ 卵管間膜(中を子宮動脈・静脈の卵管枝が走る) — ☐ Mesosalpinx (with tubal branches of uterine artery and vein)

④ ☐ 子宮間膜 — ☐ Mesometrium

⑤ ☐ 右の尿管 — ☐ Right ureter

⑥ ☐ 直腸子宮靱帯(直腸子宮ヒダの中を走る) — ☐ Uterosacral ligament (in uterosacral fold)

⑦ ☐ 卵巣動脈・静脈(卵巣提靱帯の中を走る) — ☐ Ovarian artery and vein (in suspensory ligament of ovary)

⑧ ☐ 左の卵巣 — ☐ Left ovary

臨床

通常，卵子は受精後に子宮腔の壁に着床するが，他の場所(卵管や場合によっては腹膜腔)に着床することもある．最も一般的な異所性妊娠である卵管妊娠では卵管壁が破裂し，腹膜腔内に出血することで生命の危機に陥る可能性がある．卵管妊娠の多くは炎症の後に卵管粘膜に癒着が生じることにより起こる．

Uterus & Uterine Tube II

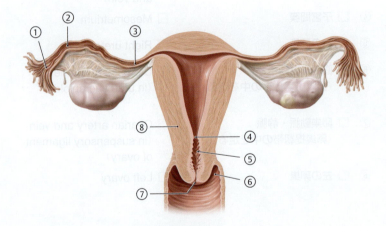

受精が起こるのは通常は女性生殖路のどこか？

子宮と卵管 2

冠状断面，子宮を垂直に示し，後方から見たところ

① □ 卵管漏斗　　　　　　　　　□ Infundibulum
② □ 卵管膨大部　　　　　　　　□ Ampulla
③ □ 卵管峡部　　　　　　　　　□ Isthmus of uterine tube
④ □ 内子宮口（子宮峡部の）　　□ Internal os（at uterine isthmus）
⑤ □ 子宮頸管　　　　　　　　　□ Cervical canal
⑥ □ 腟円蓋の外側部　　　　　　□ Lateral part of vaginal fornix
⑦ □ 外子宮口　　　　　　　　　□ External os
⑧ □ 子宮筋層　　　　　　　　　□ Myometrium

卵子と精子の受精は，通常は卵管漏斗か卵管膨大部で起こる．

Female External Genitalia

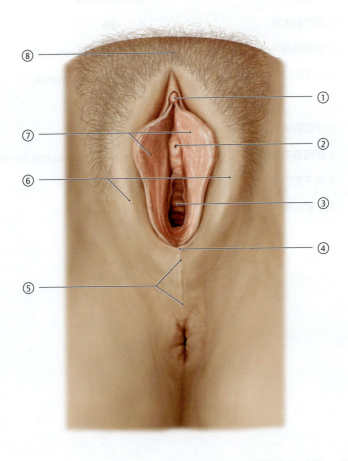

女性の外生殖器

切石位

① □ 陰核　　　　　　□ Clitoris

② □ 外尿道口　　　　□ External urethral orifice

③ □ 腟口　　　　　　□ Vaginal orifice

④ □ 後陰唇交連　　　□ Posterior labial commissure

⑤ □ 会陰縫線　　　　□ Perineal raphe

⑥ □ 大陰唇　　　　　□ Labia majora

⑦ □ 小陰唇　　　　　□ Labia minora

⑧ □ 恥丘　　　　　　□ Mons pubis

Female Erectile Muscles & Tissue

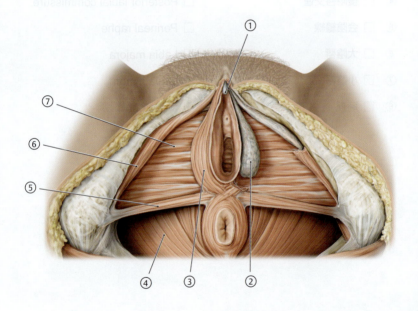

女性の勃起組織

切石位

① □ 陰核亀頭　　　　　□ Glans of clitoris

② □ 前庭球　　　　　　□ Bulb of vestibule

③ □ 球海綿体筋　　　　□ Bulbospongiosus

④ □ 肛門挙筋　　　　　□ Levator ani

⑤ □ 浅会陰横筋　　　　□ Superficial transverse perineal muscle

⑥ □ 坐骨海綿体筋　　　□ Ischiocavernosus

⑦ □ 深会陰横筋　　　　□ Deep transverse perineal muscle

> **臨床**
>
> 会陰切開術は分娩の娩出期に産道を拡大する産科的手技である．この手技は一般には，娩出期の低酸素症を防ぎ娩出を早めるために用いられる．そのほか，会陰の皮膚が白色になった場合（血流の低下を表す）は，会陰裂傷の危険が切迫しており，会陰切開術がしばしば行われる．側切開が切開の幅を最も広くとれるが，回復は難しくなる．

Neurovasculature of the Female Perineum

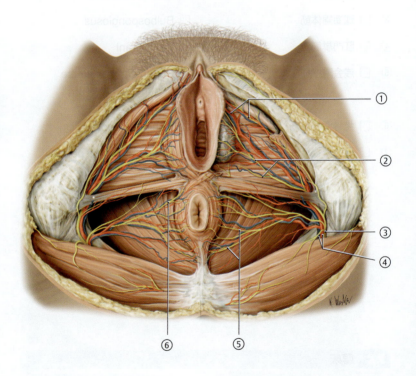

Q 陰部神経の起始と走行は？

女性会陰の神経・血管

切石位

① □ 陰核背動脈・神経 □ Dorsal artery of clitoris, dorsal nerve of clitoris

② □ 後陰唇神経（陰部神経の枝） □ Posterior labial nerves (branches of pudendal nerve)

③ □ 陰部神経 □ Pudendal nerve

④ □ 内陰部動脈・静脈 □ Internal pudendal artery and vein

⑤ □ 下直腸神経 □ Inferior rectal nerves

⑥ □ 会陰神経 □ Perineal nerves

 陰部神経はS2-S4の前枝から仙骨神経叢の一枝として起こり，大坐骨孔から骨盤外に出て，仙棘靱帯の後方を通り，小坐骨孔から会陰へ至る．陰部神経の枝は肛門三角と尿生殖三角の各構造に分布する．

Cross Section of the Penis

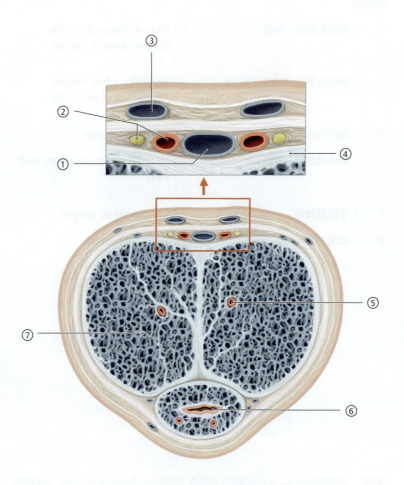

陰茎の横断面

陰茎体での横断面

① □ 深陰茎背静脈 □ Deep dorsal vein of penis
② □ 陰茎背動脈・神経 □ Dorsal artery of penis, dorsal nerve of penis
③ □ 浅陰茎背静脈 □ Superficial dorsal vein of penis
④ □ 陰茎海綿体白膜 □ Tunica albuginea of corpus cavernosum
⑤ □ 陰茎深動脈 □ Deep artery of penis
⑥ □ 尿道の海綿体部 □ Spongy urethra
⑦ □ 陰茎海綿体 □ Corpus cavernosum penis

Penis

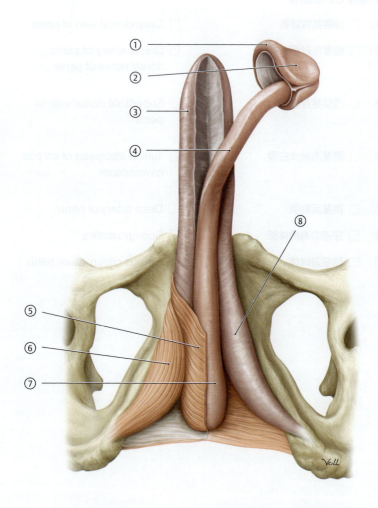

陰茎

下面

① □ 亀頭冠 □ Corona of glans
② □ 陰茎亀頭 □ Glans penis
③ □ 陰茎海綿体 □ Corpus cavernosum penis
④ □ 尿道海綿体 □ Corpus spongiosum penis
⑤ □ 球海綿体筋 □ Bulbospongiosus
⑥ □ 坐骨海綿体筋 □ Ischiocavernosus
⑦ □ 尿道球 □ Bulb of penis
⑧ □ 陰茎脚 □ Crus of penis

Testis & Epididymis

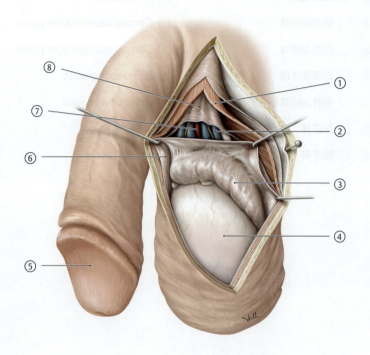

Q 精巣上体とは何か？

精巣と精巣上体

左外側面

① □ 精巣挙筋，精巣挙筋膜　　□ Cremaster and cremasteric (cremaster) fascia

② □ 蔓状静脈叢（精巣静脈）　　□ Pampiniform plexus (testicular veins)

③ □ 精巣上体の体　　□ Body of epididymis

④ □ 精巣と精巣鞘膜の臓側板　　□ Testis with visceral layer of tunica vaginalis

⑤ □ 陰茎亀頭　　□ Glans penis

⑥ □ 精巣鞘膜の壁側板　　□ Parietal layer of tunica vaginalis

⑦ □ 精巣動脈　　□ Testicular artery

⑧ □ 内精筋膜　　□ Internal spermatic fascia

A 　精巣上体は大きく曲がりくねった管であり，精巣から未成熟な精子を受け取って貯蔵する．尾部は精管につながる．

Coverings of the Testis

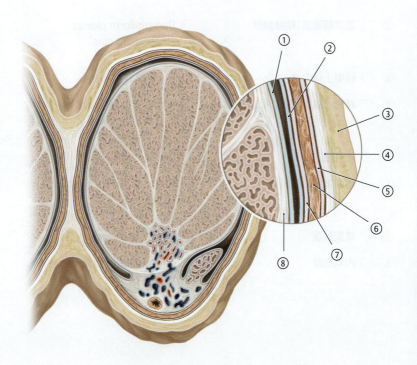

Q 腹壁を構成する層のうち，精索と精巣の被膜に関与しないのはどれか？

精巣の被膜

横断面，上面

① ☐ 精巣鞘膜の臓側板　　☐ Visceral layer of tunica vaginalis

② ☐ 精巣鞘膜の壁側板　　☐ Parietal layer of tunica vaginalis

③ ☐ 陰嚢の皮膚　　☐ Scrotal skin

④ ☐ 肉様膜　　☐ Dartos fascia

⑤ ☐ 外精筋膜　　☐ External spermatic fascia

⑥ ☐ 精巣挙筋, 精巣挙筋膜　　☐ Cremaster and cremasteric (cremaster) fascia

⑦ ☐ 内精筋膜　　☐ Internal spermatic fascia

⑧ ☐ 白膜　　☐ Tunica albuginea

A 腹横筋は精索と精巣の被膜に関与しない．

Male Accessory Sex Glands

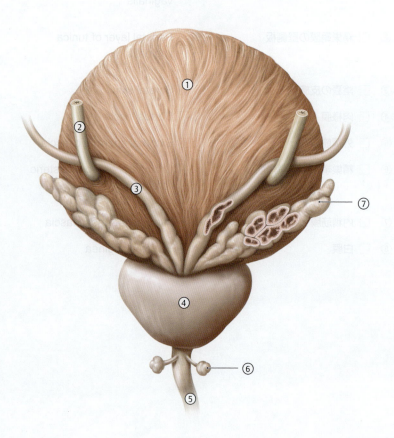

男性の付属生殖腺

後面

① □ 膀胱 □ Urinary bladder
② □ 尿管の骨盤部 □ Pelvic part of ureter
③ □ 精管 □ Ductus deferens
④ □ 前立腺 □ Prostate
⑤ □ 尿道 □ Urethra
⑥ □ 尿道球腺 □ Bulbo-urethral gland
⑦ □ 精嚢 □ Seminal gland

Prostate in situ

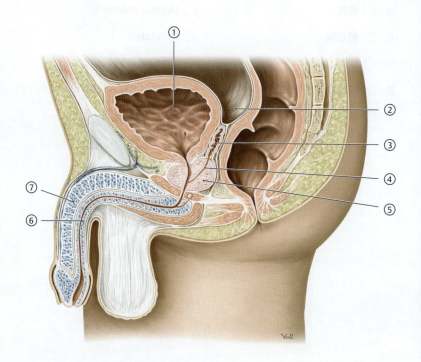

原位置の前立腺

矢状断，左外側面

① □ 膀胱，体　　　　　　□ Body of bladder
② □ 直腸膀胱窩　　　　　□ Rectovesical pouch
③ □ 精嚢　　　　　　　　□ Seminal gland
④ □ 射精管　　　　　　　□ Ejaculatory duct
⑤ □ 前立腺　　　　　　　□ Prostate
⑥ □ 尿道の海綿体部　　　□ Spongy urethra
⑦ □ 陰茎海綿体　　　　　□ Corpus cavernosum penis

臨床

　前立腺癌は，高齢の男性において最もよく見られる悪性腫瘍の1つで，前立腺の辺縁領域の被膜下に増殖する．良性の前立腺肥大が中心領域で生じるのとは対照的に，前立腺癌は早期では尿路を閉塞しない．辺縁領域にある腫瘍は，直腸内診によって直腸の前壁を介して硬い塊として触知される．

Neurovasculature of the Male Perineum

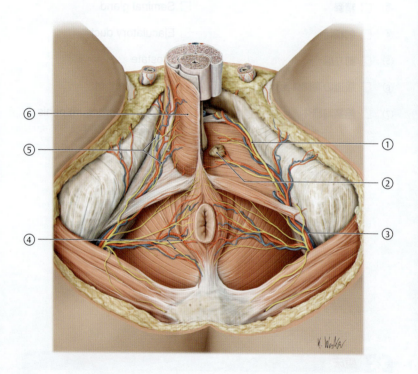

男性会陰の神経・血管

切石位

① □ 陰茎背神経　　　　　□ Dorsal nerve of penis

② □ 尿道球腺　　　　　　□ Bulbo-urethral gland

③ □ 内陰部動脈・静脈　　□ Internal pudendal artery and vein

④ □ 下直腸神経　　　　　□ Inferior rectal nerves

⑤ □ 後陰嚢神経　　　　　□ Posterior scrotal nerves

⑥ □ 球海綿体筋　　　　　□ Bulbospongiosus

Abdominal Aorta

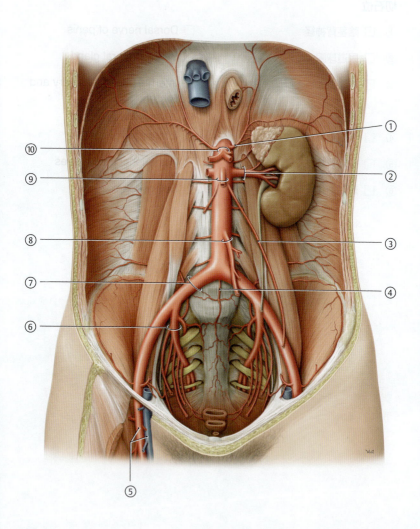

腹大動脈

女性の腹部，前面

① ☐ 左下横隔動脈　　　　　☐ Left inferior phrenic artery
② ☐ 左腎動脈　　　　　　　☐ Left renal artery
③ ☐ 左卵巣動脈（男性の場合は　☐ Left ovarian artery（testicular
　　　精巣動脈）　　　　　　　　artery in males）
④ ☐ 正中仙骨動脈　　　　　☐ Median sacral artery
⑤ ☐ 大腿動脈・静脈　　　　☐ Femoral artery and vein
⑥ ☐ 右内腸骨動脈　　　　　☐ Right internal iliac artery
⑦ ☐ 右総腸骨動脈　　　　　☐ Right common iliac artery
⑧ ☐ 下腸間膜動脈　　　　　☐ Inferior mesenteric artery
⑨ ☐ 上腸間膜動脈　　　　　☐ Superior mesenteric artery
⑩ ☐ 腹腔動脈　　　　　　　☐ Celiac trunk

解説

　腹大動脈は胸大動脈の延長であり，T12の高さで腹部に入り，L4の高さで二分岐して総腸骨動脈になる．

Renal Arteries

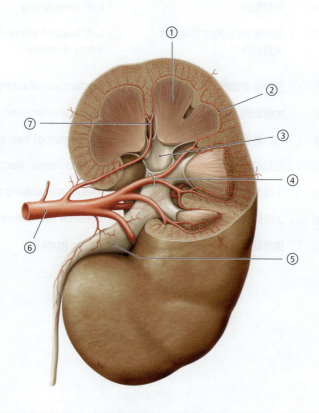

腎動脈

左の腎臓，前面

① □ 腎錐体　　　　　　　　　　□ Renal pyramid

② □ 弓状動脈〔腎錐体の錐体底に〕　□ Arcuate artery (at base of renal pyramids)

③ □ 大腎杯　　　　　　　　　　□ Major calyces

④ □ 上前区動脈　　　　　　　　□ Anterior superior segmental artery

⑤ □ 左の尿管〔腎盂（腎盤）からの起始部〕　□ Left ureter (origin from renal pelvis)

⑥ □ 左腎動脈（本幹）　　　　　　□ Left renal artery (main trunk)

⑦ □ 葉間動脈（腎錐体の間）　　　□ Interlobar artery (between the medullary pyramids)

臨床

腎臓は血圧を感知して制御する重要な器官である．腎動脈の狭窄によって腎臓の血流量が減少すると，アンギオテンシノゲンを開裂させてアンギオテンシンⅠを遊離させるホルモンであるレニンの分泌が促進される．さらに，開裂することで血管収縮を促進して血圧を高めるアンギオテンシンⅡが生じる．腎性高血圧症は高血圧症の診断において除外されるか，確定される必要がある．

Celiac Trunk I

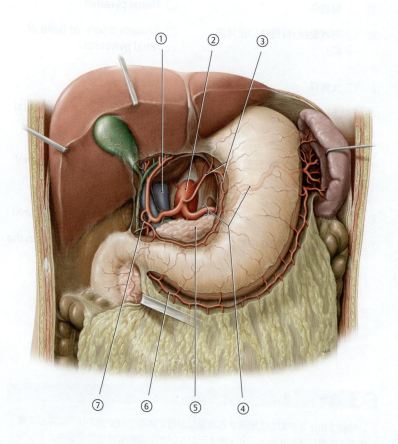

Q 腹腔動脈は前腸に血液を供給する．ここに含まれる構造は何か？

腹腔動脈 1

前面

① ☐ 下大静脈　　　　　　☐ Inferior vena cava
② ☐ 腹大動脈　　　　　　☐ Abdominal aorta
③ ☐ 左胃動脈　　　　　　☐ Left gastric artery
④ ☐ 脾動脈　　　　　　　☐ Splenic artery
⑤ ☐ 膵臓　　　　　　　　☐ Pancreas
⑥ ☐ 右胃大網動脈　　　　☐ Right gastro-omental artery
⑦ ☐ 右胃動脈　　　　　　☐ Right gastric artery

　腹腔動脈はT12の高さで腹大動脈から起こり，前腸の諸構造に分布する．腹腔動脈から枝を受けるものには，食道の遠位半，胃，十二指腸の近位半，肝臓，胆嚢，膵臓の上部がある．脾臓は前腸に含まれないが，腹腔動脈から枝を受ける．

Celiac Trunk II

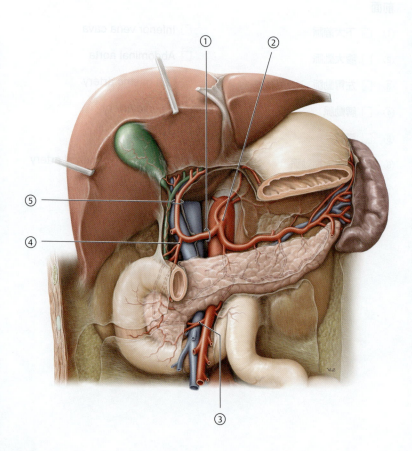

Q 膵十二指腸動脈弧はどの動脈から生じるか？

腹腔動脈 2

前面

① □ 総肝動脈 □ Common hepatic artery
② □ 腹腔動脈 □ Celiac trunk
③ □ 下膵十二指腸動脈 □ Inferior pancreaticoduodenal artery
④ □ 胃十二指腸動脈 □ Gastroduodenal artery
⑤ □ 固有肝動脈 □ Hepatic artery proper

膵十二指腸動脈弓は腹腔動脈と上腸間膜動脈の重要な吻合である．上膵十二指腸動脈は胃十二指腸動脈から起こり，下膵十二指腸動脈は上腸間膜動脈から起こる．上・下膵十二指腸動脈はともに前後に分かれ，膵頭内で吻合する．

Superior Mesenteric Artery

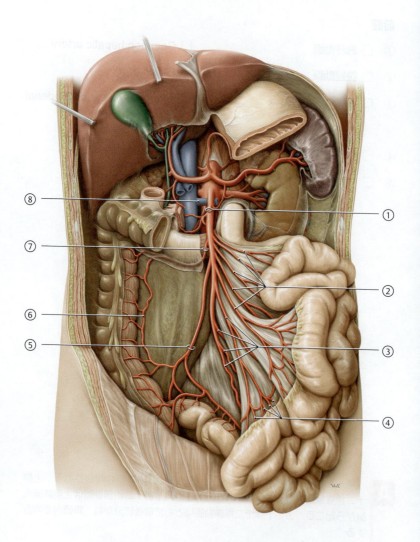

上腸間膜動脈

前面

① ☐ 中結腸動脈
② ☐ 空腸動脈
③ ☐ 回腸動脈
④ ☐ 直細動脈
⑤ ☐ 回結腸動脈
⑥ ☐ 結腸辺縁動脈
⑦ ☐ 右結腸動脈
⑧ ☐ 左腎静脈

☐ Middle colic artery
☐ Jejunal arteries
☐ Ileal arteries
☐ Vasa recta
☐ Ileocolic artery
☐ Marginal artery
☐ Right colic artery
☐ Left renal vein

解説

　上腸間膜動脈は中腸に分布し，そこには十二指腸の遠位部（膵臓の一部も含む），空腸，回腸，左結腸曲までの結腸が含まれる．結腸辺縁動脈は上腸間膜動脈の結腸枝を結び，下腸間膜動脈の枝と吻合する．

Inferior Mesenteric Artery

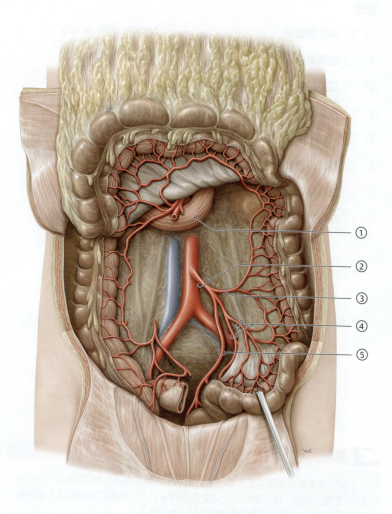

①
②
③
④
⑤

下腸間膜動脈

前面

① ☐ 十二指腸　　　　　　　　☐ Duodenum
② ☐ 下腸間膜動脈　　　　　　☐ Inferior mesenteric artery
③ ☐ 左結腸動脈　　　　　　　☐ Left colic artery
④ ☐ S状結腸動脈　　　　　　 ☐ Sigmoid arteries
⑤ ☐ 上直腸動脈　　　　　　　☐ Superior rectal artery

解説

　下腸間膜動脈は左結腸曲，下行結腸，S状結腸，および直腸の大部分に分布する．下腸間膜動脈は上腸間膜動脈とは結腸辺縁動脈において吻合し，骨盤内では直腸の動脈と上直腸動脈によって吻合する．

Tributaries of the Inferior Vena Cava

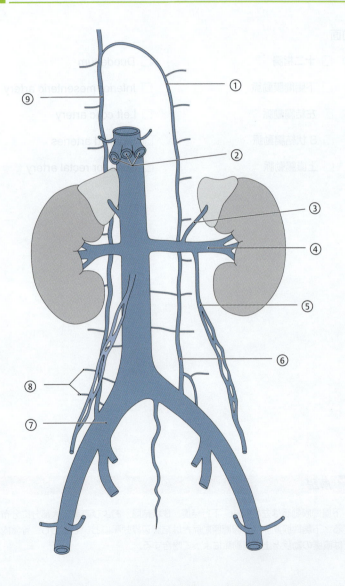

下大静脈の支脈

① □ 半奇静脈　　　　　□ Hemia-zygos vein
② □ 肝静脈　　　　　　□ Hepatic veins
③ □ 上副腎静脈　　　　□ Suprarenal vein
④ □ 腎静脈　　　　　　□ Renal vein
⑤ □ 精巣 / 卵巣静脈　　□ Testicular / ovarian vein
⑥ □ 上行腰静脈　　　　□ Ascending lumbar vein
⑦ □ 総腸骨静脈　　　　□ Common iliac vein
⑧ □ 腰静脈　　　　　　□ Lumbar veins
⑨ □ 奇静脈　　　　　　□ Azygos vein

Renal Arteries & Veins

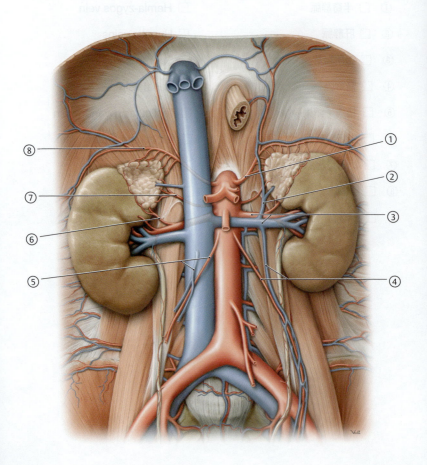

右腎静脈と左腎静脈の走行と枝を比較せよ.

腎動脈・静脈

前面

① ☐ 左下横隔動脈 ☐ Left inferior phrenic artery
② ☐ 左副腎静脈 ☐ Left suprarenal vein
③ ☐ 左腎動脈・静脈 ☐ Left renal artery and vein
④ ☐ 左精巣/卵巣動脈・静脈 ☐ Left testicular / ovarian artery and vein
⑤ ☐ 右精巣/卵巣動脈・静脈 ☐ Right testicular / ovarian artery and vein
⑥ ☐ 右下副腎動脈 ☐ Right inferior suprarenal artery
⑦ ☐ 右中副腎動脈 ☐ Right middle suprarenal artery
⑧ ☐ 右上副腎動脈 ☐ Right superior suprarenal artery

 左腎静脈には左副腎静脈と左精巣・卵巣静脈が注ぐが，右副腎静脈と右精巣・卵巣静脈は直接下大静脈に注ぐ．尿管から細い静脈が左右の腎静脈に注ぐ．

Portal Vein Distribution

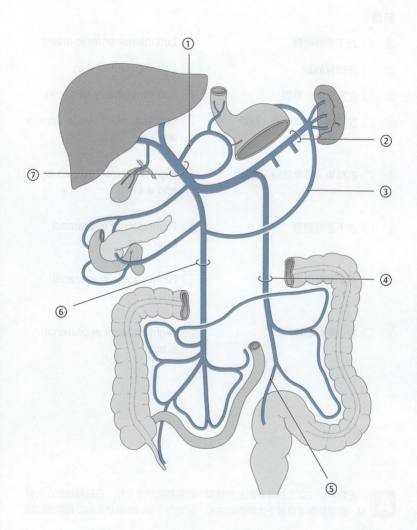

門脈の分布

① □ 左胃静脈と食道静脈　　□ Left gastric vein (with esophageal veins)

② □ 脾静脈　　□ Splenic vein

③ □ 左胃大網静脈　　□ Left gastro-omental vein

④ □ 下腸間膜静脈　　□ Inferior mesenteric vein

⑤ □ 上直腸静脈　　□ Superior rectal vein

⑥ □ 上腸間膜静脈　　□ Superior mesenteric vein

⑦ □ 門脈　　□ Hepatic portal vein

臨床

上腸間膜静脈が分布する部位の腫瘍は，門脈系を介して肝臓の毛細血管床に広がる(肝臓転移)．中直腸静脈と下直腸静脈が分布する部位の腫瘍は，下大静脈と右心を介して肺の毛細血管床に転移する(肺転移)．

Portal Vein in situ

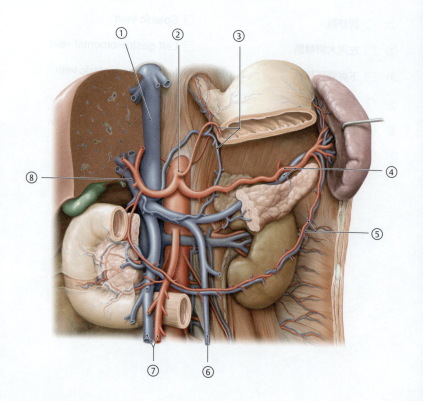

Q 門脈系が分布する腹部内臓は何か？

原位置の門脈

前面

① ☐ 下大静脈　　　　　　　☐ Inferior vena cava
② ☐ 腹腔動脈　　　　　　　☐ Celiac trunk
③ ☐ 左胃動脈・静脈　　　　☐ Left gastric artery and vein
④ ☐ 脾動脈・静脈　　　　　☐ Splenic artery and vein
⑤ ☐ 左胃大網動脈・静脈　　☐ Left gastro-omental artery and vein

⑥ ☐ 下腸間膜静脈　　　　　☐ Inferior mesenteric vein
⑦ ☐ 上腸間膜動脈・静脈　　☐ Superior mesenteric artery and vein

⑧ ☐ 門脈　　　　　　　　　☐ Hepatic portal vein

A 　門脈系は食道下部から直腸上部までの胃腸管，また胆囊，膵臓，脾臓に分布する．

Blood Vessels of the Female Pelvis

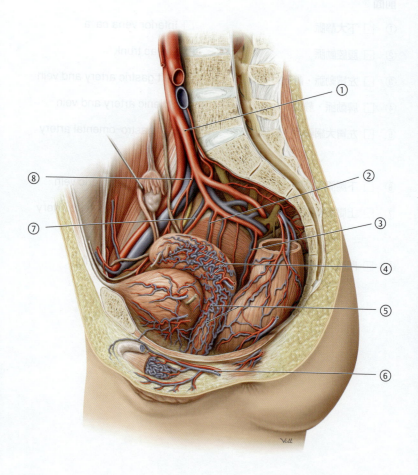

Q 外科手術において，脈管遮断の危険を恐れることなく内腸骨動脈を切断できるのはなぜか？

女性骨盤部の血管

骨盤部の右半分，左外側面

① □ 右内腸骨動脈　　　　　□ Right internal iliac artery
② □ 右子宮動脈・静脈　　　□ Right uterine artery and vein
③ □ 右中直腸動脈・静脈　　□ Right middle rectal artery and vein

④ □ 子宮静脈叢　　　　　　□ Uterine venous plexus
⑤ □ 腟静脈叢　　　　　　　□ Vaginal venous plexus
⑥ □ 左内陰部動脈・静脈　　□ Left internal pudendal artery and vein

⑦ □ 右閉鎖動脈・静脈　　　□ Right obturator artery and vein

⑧ □ 右臍動脈　　　　　　　□ Right umbilical artery

　内腸骨動脈は同側および対側の枝との間に多くの吻合がある．また，内腸骨動脈は外腸骨動脈，大腿動脈，下腸間膜動脈，卵巣動脈との間に側副路がある．

Blood Vessels of the Rectum

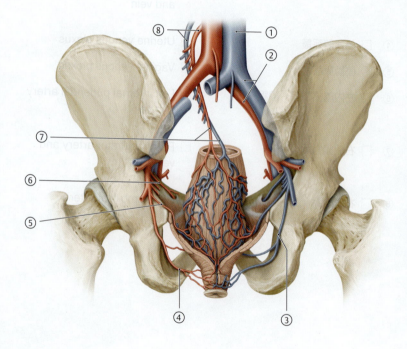

直腸の血管

後面

① □ 下大静脈　　　　　　　□ Inferior vena cava
② □ 右総腸骨動脈・静脈　　□ Right common iliac artery and vein
③ □ 右内陰部静脈　　　　　□ Right internal pudendal vein
④ □ 左下直腸動脈　　　　　□ Left inferior rectal artery
⑤ □ 左中直腸動脈　　　　　□ Left middle rectal artery
⑥ □ 左閉鎖動脈　　　　　　□ Left obturator artery
⑦ □ 上直腸動脈・静脈　　　□ Superior rectal artery and vein
⑧ □ 下腸間膜動脈・静脈　　□ Inferior mesenteric artery and vein

解説

主に直腸に分布するのは上直腸動脈である．中直腸動脈は上直腸動脈と下直腸動脈との間の吻合路となっている．

Blood Vessels of the Male Genitalia

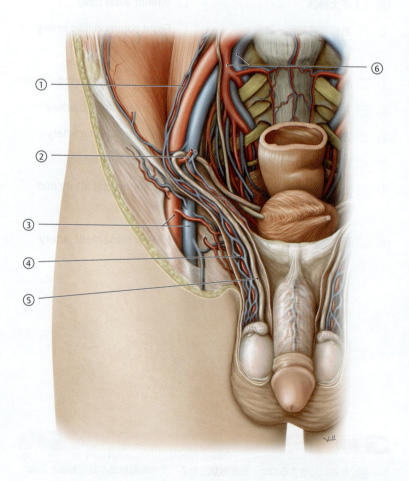

男性生殖器の血管

前面

① □ 精巣動脈・静脈 □ Testicular artery and vein
② □ 下腹壁動脈・静脈 □ Inferior epigastric artery and vein
③ □ 大腿動脈・静脈 □ Femoral artery and vein
④ □ 蔓状静脈叢（精巣静脈） □ Pampiniform plexus (testicular veins)
⑤ □ 右の精管 □ Right ductus deferens
⑥ □ 内腸骨動脈・静脈 □ Internal iliac artery and vein

Parietal Lymph Nodes

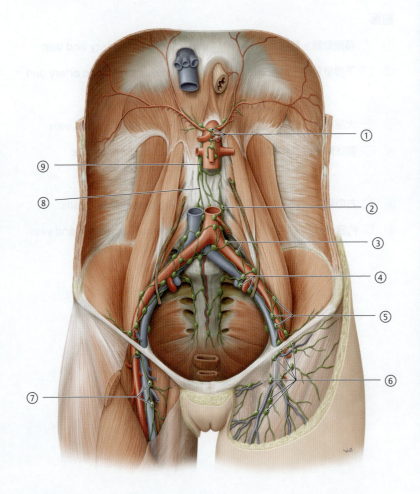

Q 腸のリンパ流路について簡単に説明せよ.

壁側リンパ節

前面

① □ 腹腔リンパ節　　　　　　　□ Celiac node

② □ 左外側大動脈リンパ節　　　□ Left lateral aortic node

③ □ 総腸骨リンパ節　　　　　　□ Common iliac node

④ □ 内腸骨リンパ節　　　　　　□ Internal iliac node

⑤ □ 外腸骨リンパ節　　　　　　□ External iliac node

⑥ □ 浅鼠径リンパ節　　　　　　□ Superficial inguinal node
　　（水平群と垂直群）　　　　　　（horizontal and vertical groups）

⑦ □ 深鼠径リンパ節　　　　　　□ Deep inguinal node

⑧ □ 右腰リンパ本幹　　　　　　□ Right lumbar trunk

⑨ □ 乳ビ槽　　　　　　　　　　□ Cisterna chyli

A 　腸のリンパ系は動脈の走行に従い，腹腔動脈・上腸間膜動脈・下腸間膜動脈周辺の大動脈前リンパ節を通過することになる．最終的には乳ビ槽に至り，そこから胸管へ入っていく．

Autonomic Plexuses

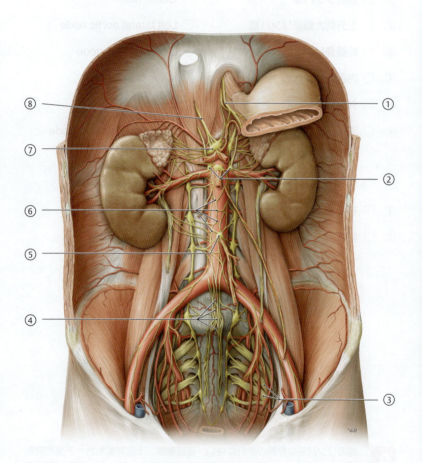

自律神経叢

男性腹部，前面

① □ 前迷走神経幹　□ Anterior vagal trunk
② □ 大動脈腎動脈神経節　□ Aorticorenal ganglia
③ □ 仙骨神経叢　□ Sacral plexus
④ □ 上下腹神経叢　□ Superior hypogastric plexus
⑤ □ 下腸間膜動脈神経節　□ Inferior mesenteric ganglion
⑥ □ 腸間膜動脈間神経叢　□ Intermesenteric plexus
⑦ □ 腹腔神経節　□ Celiac ganglion
⑧ □ 右大内臓神経　□ Right greater splanchnic nerve

Innervation of the Female Pelvis

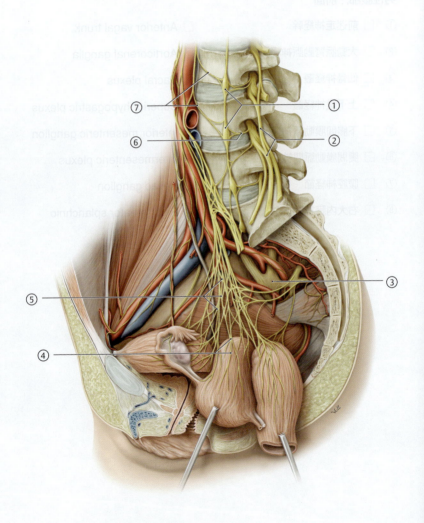

腹部・骨盤部 333

女性骨盤部の神経支配

右骨盤部，左外側面

① □ 交感神経幹，腰神経節　　□ Sympathetic trunk, lumbar ganglia

② □ 腰神経，前枝　　□ Lumbar nerves, anterior rami

③ □ 仙骨神経叢　　□ Sacral plexus

④ □ 右子宮腟神経叢　　□ Right uterovaginal plexus

⑤ □ 右下下腹神経叢　　□ Right inferior hypogastric plexus

⑥ □ 灰白交通枝　　□ Gray ramus communicans

⑦ □ 腰内臓神経　　□ Lumbar splanchnic nerve

Innervation of the Male Pelvis

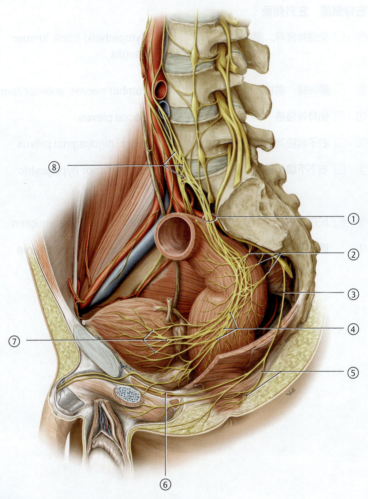

骨盤内臓の副交感神経系の起始はどこか？

男性骨盤部の神経支配

右骨盤部，左外側面

① ☐ 左下腹神経　　　　　☐ Left hypogastric nerve
② ☐ 骨盤内臓神経　　　　☐ Pelvic splanchnic nerves
③ ☐ 陰部神経　　　　　　☐ Pudendal nerve
④ ☐ 下直腸動脈神経叢　　☐ Inferior rectal plexus
⑤ ☐ 下直腸神経　　　　　☐ Inferior rectal nerves
⑥ ☐ 陰茎背神経　　　　　☐ Dorsal nerve of the penis
⑦ ☐ 膀胱神経叢　　　　　☐ Vesical plexus
⑧ ☐ 上下腹神経叢　　　　☐ Superior hypogastric plexus

　骨盤内臓神経は仙髄から起こり，仙骨神経を通って左右の下腹神経叢に至り，そこで骨盤神経叢を作る．

Surface Anatomy

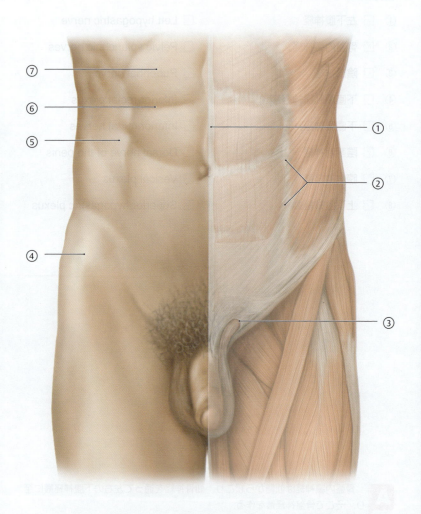

腹部・骨盤部の体表解剖

前面

① □ 白線　　　　　　　　□ Linea alba
② □ 半月線　　　　　　　□ Semilunar line
③ □ 浅鼠径輪　　　　　　□ Superficial inguinal ring
④ □ 上前腸骨棘　　　　　□ Anterior superior iliac spine (ASIS)
⑤ □ 外腹斜筋　　　　　　□ External oblique
⑥ □ 腱画　　　　　　　　□ Tendinous intersections
⑦ □ 腹直筋　　　　　　　□ Rectus abdominis

上肢 Upper Limb

上肢の骨格 ……………………………… *340*	手の筋 1-4 ……………………………… *434*
鎖骨 …………………………………………… *342*	手背 ……………………………………………… *442*
肩甲骨 1, 2 ………………………………… *344*	手の筋の区分 1-5 ……………………… *444*
上腕骨 1, 2 ………………………………… *348*	上肢の動脈 ………………………………… *454*
上肢帯の関節 ……………………………… *352*	上肢の皮静脈 ……………………………… *456*
胸鎖関節 …………………………………… *354*	腕神経叢の構造 …………………………… *458*
肩関節（肩甲上腕関節）1, 2 ………… *356*	腕神経叢の走行 …………………………… *460*
肩の冠状断面 ……………………………… *360*	腕神経叢からの神経 1-5 ……………… *462*
肩と上腕の筋（前面）1-4 …………… *362*	肩の後部における神経・血管 1, 2 …… *472*
肩と上腕の筋（後面）1-3 …………… *370*	腋窩の神経・血管 1-3 ………………… *476*
上肢帯の筋の区分 1-5 ………………… *376*	上腕の神経・血管 ………………………… *482*
肩関節の筋の区分 1-4 ………………… *386*	前腕の神経・血管 ………………………… *484*
上腕の筋の区分 1, 2 …………………… *394*	手根管 ………………………………………… *486*
橈骨と尺骨 ………………………………… *398*	浅掌動脈弓 ………………………………… *488*
肘関節 1, 2 ………………………………… *400*	深掌動脈弓 ………………………………… *490*
前腕の筋（前面）1-3 ………………… *404*	解剖学的嗅ぎタバコ入れ ……………… *492*
前腕の筋（後面）1, 2 ………………… *410*	手における感覚神経の分布 1, 2 …… *494*
前腕の筋の区分 1-7 …………………… *414*	上腕の横断面 ……………………………… *498*
手首と手の骨格 1, 2 …………………… *428*	前腕の横断面 ……………………………… *500*
手首と手の関節 …………………………… *432*	手の体表解剖 ……………………………… *502*

Bones of the Upper Limb

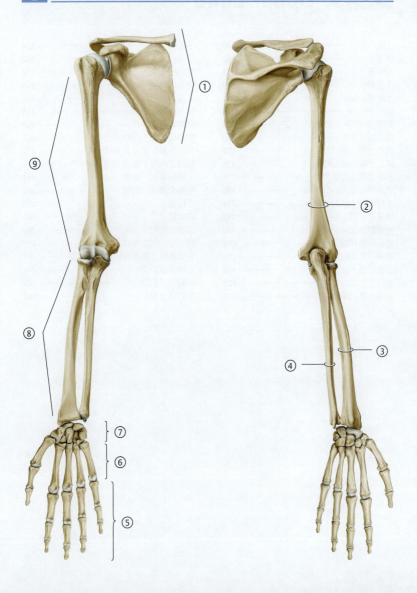

上肢の骨格

右上肢，左：前面，右：後面

① □ 上肢帯　　　　　　　□ Shoulder girdle

② □ 上腕骨　　　　　　　□ Humerus

③ □ 橈骨　　　　　　　　□ Radius

④ □ 尺骨　　　　　　　　□ Ulna

⑤ □ 指骨（指節骨）　　　□ Phalanges

⑥ □ 中手骨　　　　　　　□ Metacarpals

⑦ □ 手根骨　　　　　　　□ Carpal bones

⑧ □ 前腕　　　　　　　　□ Forearm

⑨ □ 上腕　　　　　　　　□ Arm

Clavicle

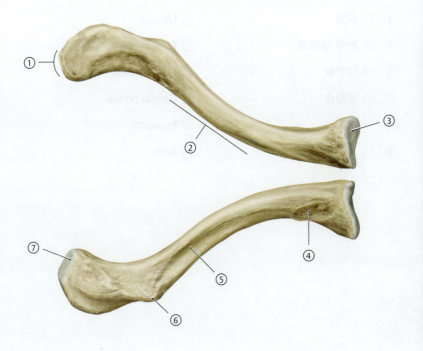

鎖骨

右鎖骨，上：上面，下：下面

① □ 肩峰端　　　　　□ Acromial end

② □ 鎖骨体　　　　　□ Shaft of clavicle

③ □ 胸骨関節面　　　□ Sternal articular surface

④ □ 肋鎖靱帯圧痕　　□ Impression for costoclavicular ligament

⑤ □ 鎖骨下筋溝　　　□ Groove for subclavius muscle

⑥ □ 円錐靱帯結節　　□ Conoid tubercle

⑦ □ 肩峰関節面　　　□ Acromial articular surface

 解説

　鎖骨はＳ字のような形をしており，全長（12〜15 cm）を体表から触知できる．鎖骨の内側端（胸骨端）は胸骨との間で胸鎖関節をなす．一方，外側端（肩峰端）は肩甲骨（肩峰）との間に肩鎖関節をなす．

Scapula I

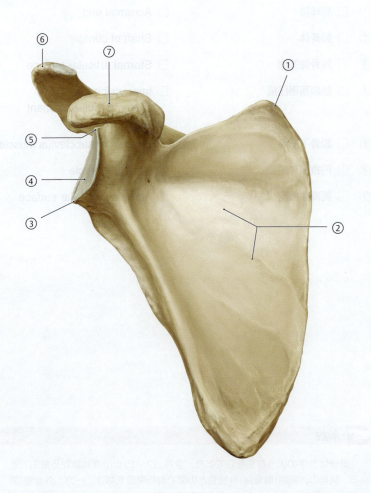

肩甲骨 1

右肩甲骨，前面

① □ 上角 □ Superior angle
② □ 肩甲下窩 □ Subscapular fossa
③ □ 関節下結節 □ Infraglenoid tubercle
④ □ 関節窩 □ Glenoid cavity
⑤ □ 関節上結節 □ Supraglenoid tubercle
⑥ □ 肩峰 □ Acromion
⑦ □ 烏口突起 □ Coracoid process

解説

解剖学的正位では，肩甲骨は第2肋骨から第7肋骨の間に位置する．

Scapula II

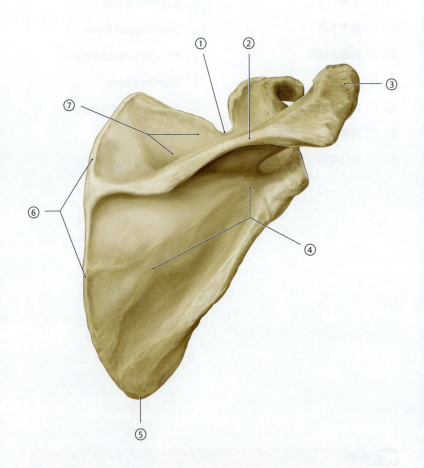

肩甲骨 2

右肩甲骨，後面

① □ 肩甲切痕　　　　　□ Scapular notch
② □ 肩甲棘　　　　　　□ Spine of scapular
③ □ 肩峰　　　　　　　□ Acromion
④ □ 棘下窩　　　　　　□ Infraspinous fossa
⑤ □ 下角　　　　　　　□ Inferior angle
⑥ □ 内側縁　　　　　　□ Medial border
⑦ □ 棘上窩　　　　　　□ Supraspinous fossa

臨床

上肩甲横靱帯の骨化により，肩甲切痕が骨性の孔（肩甲孔）となる場合がある．肩甲上神経は肩甲切痕を通過するので，上肩甲横靱帯の骨化に伴い，この神経が圧迫される場合がある．

Humerus I

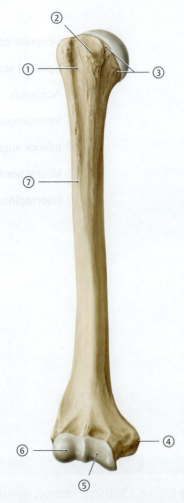

Q 上腕骨外科頸の骨折で損傷される場合がある神経・血管は何か？

上腕骨 1

右上腕骨，前面

① □ 結節間溝　　　　□ Intertubercular sulcus
② □ 小結節　　　　　□ Lesser tubercle
③ □ 解剖頸　　　　　□ Anatomical neck
④ □ 内側上顆　　　　□ Medial epicondyle
⑤ □ 上腕骨滑車　　　□ Trochlea
⑥ □ 上腕骨小頭　　　□ Capitellum
⑦ □ 三角筋粗面　　　□ Deltoid tuberosity

腋窩神経と前・後上腕回旋動脈が上腕骨外科頸の骨折で損傷される場合がある．

Humerus II

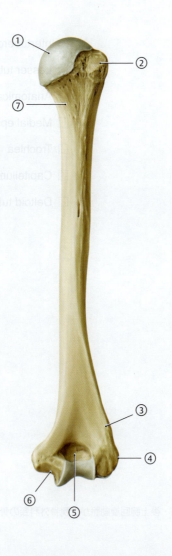

上腕骨 2

右上腕骨，後面

① ☐ 上腕骨頭　　　　　　　☐ Head of humerus
② ☐ 大結節　　　　　　　　☐ Greater tuberosity
③ ☐ 外側顆上稜　　　　　　☐ Lateral supracondylar ridge
④ ☐ 外側上顆　　　　　　　☐ Lateral epicondyle
⑤ ☐ 肘頭窩　　　　　　　　☐ Olecranon fossa
⑥ ☐ 尺骨神経溝　　　　　　☐ Ulnar groove (for ulnar nerve)
⑦ ☐ 外科頸　　　　　　　　☐ Surgical neck

Joints of the Shoulder Girdle

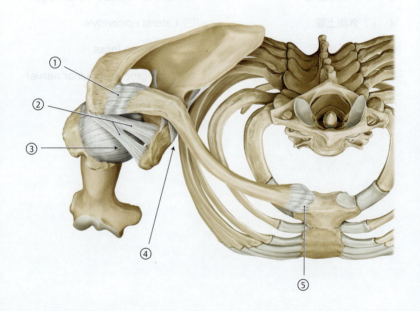

Q 上肢帯を体幹に連結する関節はどれか？

上肢帯の関節

右肩，上面

① ☐ 肩鎖関節（肩鎖靱帯） ☐ Acromioclavicular joint (with acromioclavicular ligament)

② ☐ 烏口肩峰靱帯 ☐ Coraco-acromial ligament

③ ☐ 肩関節（肩甲上腕関節） ☐ Glenohumeral joint

④ ☐ 肩甲胸郭関節 ☐ Scapulothoracic joint

⑤ ☐ 胸鎖関節（前胸鎖靱帯） ☐ Sternoclavicular joint (with anterior sternoclavicular ligament)

A 上肢帯の骨格は胸鎖関節のみによって体幹と連結する．肩甲骨は体幹の骨とは直接連結しない．上肢帯のすべての運動において，肩甲骨は胸郭の表面に存在する粗性結合組織（前鋸筋と肩甲下筋の間に形成される）の上を滑走する．肩甲骨とこの滑走面でできる連結を肩甲胸郭関節と呼ぶ場合がある．

Sternoclavicular Joint

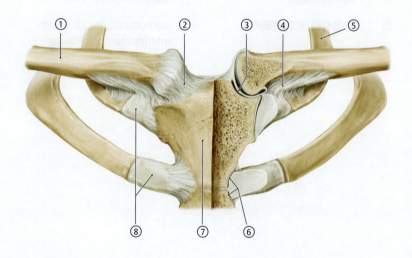

胸鎖関節

前面，左胸鎖関節の冠状断面が見えている

① □ 鎖骨　　　　　　　　　　□ Clavicle
② □ 前胸鎖靱帯　　　　　　　□ Anterior sternoclavicular ligament
③ □ 関節円板　　　　　　　　□ Articular disc
④ □ 肋鎖靱帯　　　　　　　　□ Costoclavicular ligament
⑤ □ 第1肋骨　　　　　　　　□ 1st rib
⑥ □ 胸肋関節　　　　　　　　□ Sternocostal joint
⑦ □ 胸骨柄　　　　　　　　　□ Manubrium of sternum
⑧ □ 肋軟骨　　　　　　　　　□ Costal cartilage

 解説

　線維軟骨でできた関節円板を介して，鎖骨の胸骨端と胸骨柄の関節面が密着する．

Shoulder Joint (Glenohumeral Joint) I

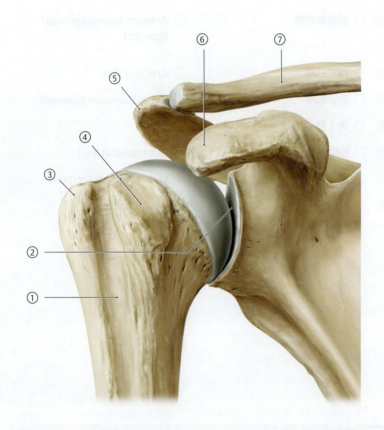

上肢 357

肩関節（肩甲上腕関節） 1

右肩，前面

① □ 結節間溝　　　　　　□ Intertubercular sulcus
② □ 関節窩　　　　　　　□ Glenoid cavity
③ □ 大結節　　　　　　　□ Greater tubercle
④ □ 小結節　　　　　　　□ Lesser tubercle
⑤ □ 肩峰　　　　　　　　□ Acromion
⑥ □ 烏口突起　　　　　　□ Coracoid process
⑦ □ 鎖骨　　　　　　　　□ Clavicle

Shoulder Joint (Glenohumeral Joint) II

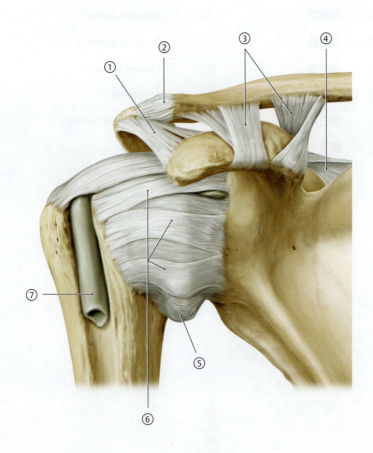

肩関節(肩甲上腕関節) 2

右肩,前面

① □ 烏口肩峰靭帯 　　　　　　□ Coracoacromial ligament

② □ 肩鎖靭帯 　　　　　　　　□ Acromioclavicular ligament

③ □ 烏口鎖骨靭帯 　　　　　　□ Coracoclavicular ligament

④ □ 上肩甲横靭帯 　　　　　　□ Superior transverse scapular ligament

⑤ □ 腋窩陥凹 　　　　　　　　□ Axillary recess

⑥ □ 関節包,関節上腕靭帯 　　□ Joint capsule, glenohumeral ligaments

⑦ □ 結節間滑液鞘 　　　　　　□ Intertubercular synovial sheath

Coronal Section of the Shoulder

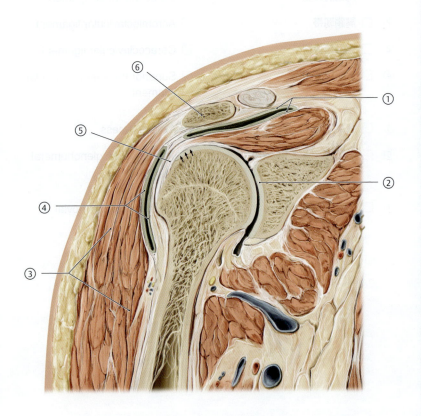

Q 棘上筋腱が断裂した場合，肩関節の運動にどのような影響が及ぶか？

肩の冠状断面

右肩，前面

① □ 肩峰下包　　　　　□ Subacromial bursa
② □ 肩甲骨の関節窩　　□ Glenoid cavity of scapula
③ □ 三角筋　　　　　　□ Deltoid
④ □ 三角筋下包　　　　□ Subdeltoid bursa
⑤ □ 棘上筋の腱　　　　□ Tendon of supraspinatus
⑥ □ 肩峰　　　　　　　□ Acromion

棘上筋は主として肩関節における外転運動の開始(最初の10°)に関与する．したがって，棘上筋腱の断裂(肩回旋腱板の断裂のうち一般的なもの)により，棘上筋による外転開始機能が損なわれる．棘上筋腱は肩峰の下にできる狭い空間を通過するので，この腱に石灰化や退行性変性が生じ，腱の厚みが増すと，肩峰の直下で腱が損傷を受ける．

Anterior Muscles of the Shoulder & Arm I

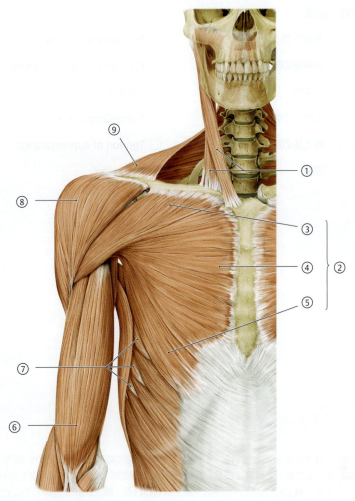

Q 大胸筋の作用は何か？

肩と上腕の筋（前面）1

右側，前面

① □ 胸鎖乳突筋　　□ Sternocleidomastoid
② □ 大胸筋　　　　□ Pectoralis major
③ □ 鎖骨部　　　　□ Clavicular part
④ □ 胸肋部　　　　□ Sternocostal part
⑤ □ 腹部　　　　　□ Abdominal part
⑥ □ 上腕二頭筋　　□ Biceps brachii
⑦ □ 前鋸筋　　　　□ Serratus anterior
⑧ □ 三角筋　　　　□ Deltoid
⑨ □ 僧帽筋　　　　□ Trapezius

A　大胸筋は上腕の内転と内旋に関与する強力な筋である．また，大胸筋の鎖骨部は肩関節を屈曲させ，胸肋部は屈曲位からの伸展に関与する．

Anterior Muscles of the Shoulder & Arm II

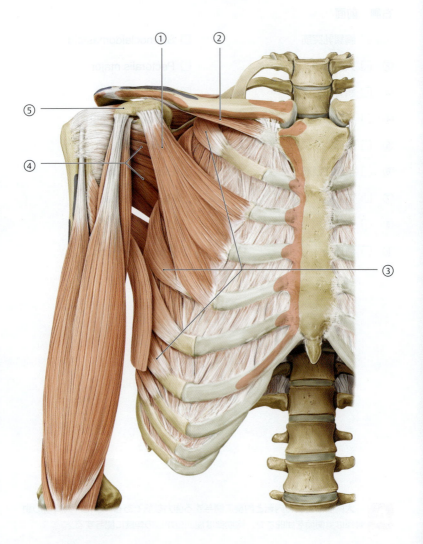

肩と上腕の筋（前面）2

胸鎖乳突筋，僧帽筋，大胸筋，三角筋，および腹斜筋を完全に取り除き，広背筋を部分的に取り除いてある

① □ 小胸筋　　　　　　　□ Pectoralis minor

② □ 鎖骨下筋　　　　　　□ Subclavius

③ □ 前鋸筋　　　　　　　□ Serratus anterior

④ □ 肩甲下筋　　　　　　□ Subscapularis

⑤ □ 烏口突起　　　　　　□ Coracoid process

Anterior Muscles of the Shoulder & Arm III

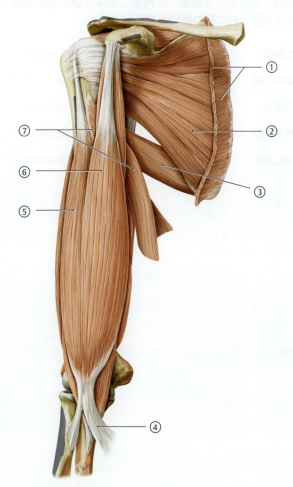

Q 上腕二頭筋の長頭の起始はどこか？

肩と上腕の筋(前面) 3

胸郭の骨格を取り除いてある．また，広背筋と前鋸筋を停止部を残して取り除いてある

① □ 前鋸筋　　　　　　□ Serratus anterior
② □ 肩甲下筋　　　　　□ Subscapularis
③ □ 大円筋　　　　　　□ Teres major
④ □ 上腕二頭筋腱膜　　□ Bicipital aponeurosis
⑤ □ 上腕二頭筋の長頭　□ Long head of biceps brachii
⑥ □ 上腕二頭筋の短頭　□ Short head of biceps brachii
⑦ □ 広背筋　　　　　　□ Latissimus dorsi

 　上腕二頭筋の長頭は肩甲骨の関節上結節から起始する．長頭の腱は滑膜に包まれた状態で肩関節腔を通過し，上腕骨の転子間溝に現れる．一方，上腕二頭筋の短頭は，小胸筋や烏口腕筋とともに，肩甲骨の烏口突起から起始する．

Anterior Muscles of the Shoulder & Arm IV

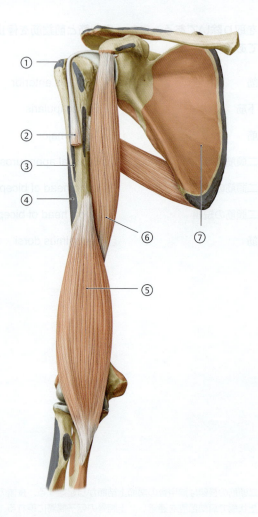

Q 上腕筋の作用は何か？

肩と上腕の筋(前面) 4

広背筋と前鋸筋をすべて取り除いたところ

① □ 棘上筋（筋の停止）　　　　□ Supraspinatus (insertion)
② □ 上腕二頭筋の長頭　　　　□ Long head of biceps brachii
③ □ 大胸筋（筋の停止）　　　　□ Pectoralis major (insertion)
④ □ 三角筋（筋の停止）　　　　□ Deltoid (insertion)
⑤ □ 上腕筋　　　　　　　　　　□ Brachialis
⑥ □ 烏口腕筋　　　　　　　　　□ Coracobrachialis
⑦ □ 肩甲下筋（筋の起始）　　　□ Subscapularis (origin)

A 　上腕筋は肘関節の屈曲に関与する．上腕二頭筋も肘関節を屈曲するが，上腕二頭筋は橈骨に停止するので，前腕の回外にも関与する．上腕筋は尺骨に停止するため，上腕二頭筋のような回外作用を持たない．

Posterior Muscles of the Shoulder & Arm I

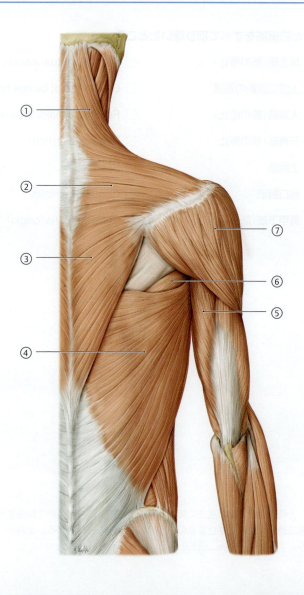

肩と上腕の筋(後面) 1

浅層

① □ 僧帽筋の下行部　　□ Descending part of trapezius
② □ 僧帽筋の横行部(水平部)　　□ Transverse part of trapezius
③ □ 僧帽筋の上行部　　□ Ascending part of trapezius
④ □ 広背筋　　□ Latissimus dorsi
⑤ □ 上腕三頭筋，長頭　　□ Long head of triceps brachii
⑥ □ 大円筋　　□ Teres major
⑦ □ 三角筋　　□ Deltoid

> **解説**
>
> 僧帽筋は胸鎖乳突筋と同様に頭に由来する上肢帯筋に属する(pp.376, 377参照).

Posterior Muscles of the Shoulder & Arm II

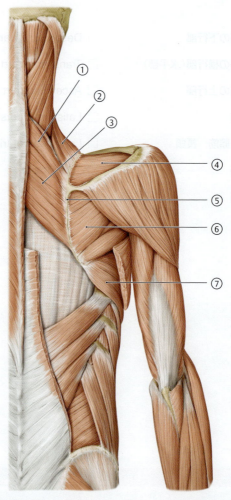

 翼状肩甲（肩甲骨の内側縁が後方に突出した状態）が見られる場合，どの筋の障害が示唆されるか？

肩と上腕の筋（後面）2

深層

① □ 小菱形筋　　　　□ Rhomboid minor
② □ 肩甲挙筋　　　　□ Levator scapulae
③ □ 大菱形筋　　　　□ Rhomboid major
④ □ 棘上筋　　　　　□ Supraspinatus
⑤ □ 肩甲骨の内側縁　□ Medial border of scapula
⑥ □ 棘下筋　　　　　□ Infraspinatus
⑦ □ 前鋸筋　　　　　□ Serratus anterior

　　前鋸筋や大・小菱形筋が麻痺すると，肩甲骨の内側縁が胸郭から遊離して，後方に突出し，翼のような外観（翼状肩甲）を呈する．

Posterior Muscles of the Shoulder & Arm III

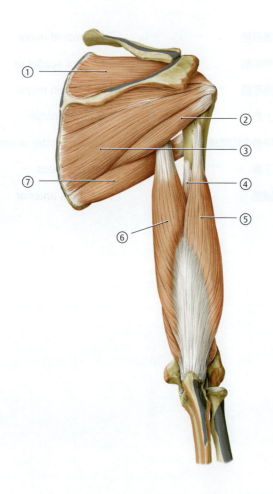

Q 回旋筋腱板を形成する筋はどれか？ また，これらの筋の支配神経は何か？

肩と上腕の筋（後面）3

僧帽筋を取り除いたところ．

① □ 棘上筋　　　　　　　　□ Supraspinatus

② □ 小円筋　　　　　　　　□ Teres minor

③ □ 棘下筋　　　　　　　　□ Infraspinatus

④ □ 上腕三頭筋の内側頭　　□ Medial head of triceps brachii

⑤ □ 上腕三頭筋の外側頭　　□ Lateral head of triceps brachii

⑥ □ 上腕三頭筋の長頭　　　□ Long head of triceps brachii

⑦ □ 大円筋　　　　　　　　□ Teres major

A 　回旋筋腱板を構成する筋（4種類）とその支配神経は以下のとおりである．これらの支配神経は，いずれも腕神経叢の後神経幹に由来する．
　棘上筋・棘下筋 ── 肩甲上神経
　小円筋 ──────── 腋窩神経
　肩甲下筋 ─────── 肩甲下神経

System of the Shoulder Girdle Muscles I

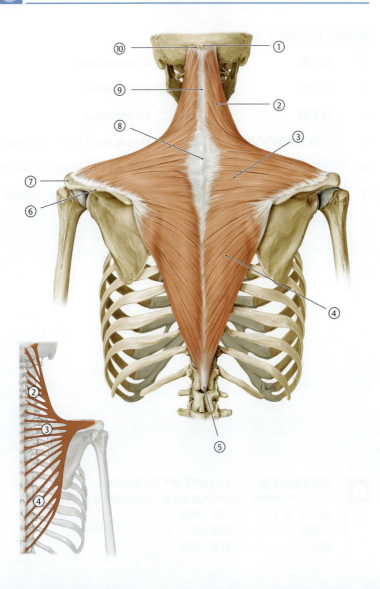

上肢帯の筋の区分 1

頭部から入り込んだ筋:僧帽筋

① ☐ 外後頭隆起 　　　　　　　　☐ External occipital protuberance

② ☐ 僧帽筋の下行部 　　　　　　☐ **Descending part of trapezius**

③ ☐ 僧帽筋の横行部 　　　　　　☐ **Transverse part of trapezius**

④ ☐ 僧帽筋の上行部 　　　　　　☐ **Ascending part of trapezius**

⑤ ☐ 第12胸椎の棘突起 　　　　　☐ T12 spinous process

⑥ ☐ 肩甲棘 　　　　　　　　　　☐ Spine of scapula

⑦ ☐ 肩峰 　　　　　　　　　　　☐ Acromion

⑧ ☐ 第7頸椎の棘突起 　　　　　☐ C7 spinous process

⑨ ☐ 項靱帯 　　　　　　　　　　☐ Nuchal ligament

⑩ ☐ 上項線 　　　　　　　　　　☐ Superior nuchal line

筋	起始	停止	各部位の作用	筋全体の作用	神経支配
僧帽筋の下行部	・後頭骨(上項線と外後頭隆起) ・項靱帯を介し頸椎の棘突起	鎖骨(外側1/3)	・肩甲骨を上内側に引き,外旋する(前鋸筋の下部と協同する) ・頭を同側に傾け,対側に回旋する(肩が固定されているとき)	胸部に肩甲骨を固定する	副神経(CN XI),頸神経(C2-C4)
僧帽筋の横行部	胸椎の棘突起の高さの腱膜	肩峰	肩甲骨を内側に引く		
僧帽筋の上行部	T5-T12の棘突起	肩甲棘	肩甲骨を下内側に引く(下行部の回旋作用の補助)		

System of the Shoulder Girdle Muscles II

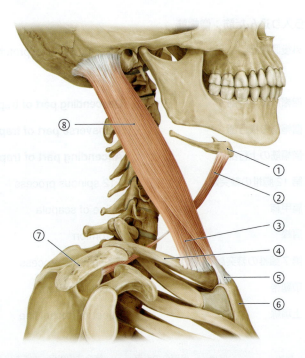

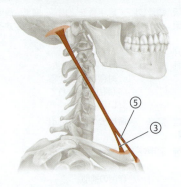

上肢帯の筋の区分 2

頭部から入り込んだ筋：胸鎖乳突筋

①	□ 舌骨	□ Hyoid bone
②	□ 肩甲舌骨筋*	□ Omohyoid
③	□ 胸鎖乳突筋の鎖骨頭	□ **Clavicular head of sternocleidomastoid**
④	□ 鎖骨	□ Clavicle
⑤	□ 胸鎖乳突筋の胸骨頭	□ **Sternal head of sternocleidomastoid**
⑥	□ 胸骨	□ Sternum
⑦	□ 肩峰	□ Acromion
⑧	□ 胸鎖乳突筋	□ **Sternocleidomastoid**

筋	起始	停止	作用	神経支配
胸鎖乳突筋の胸骨頭	胸骨柄	乳様突起, 上項線	・片側：同側に頭部を傾け, 対側に回転させる ・両側：頭部を上に向け, 頭部が固定されている場合には呼吸を助ける	副神経（CN Ⅺ）, 頸神経叢（C1-C2）
胸鎖乳突筋の鎖骨頭	鎖骨の内側 1/3			

*肩甲舌骨筋は, 胸鎖乳突筋と同様に, 頭部から入り込んだ上肢帯筋に属している.

System of the Shoulder Girdle Muscles III

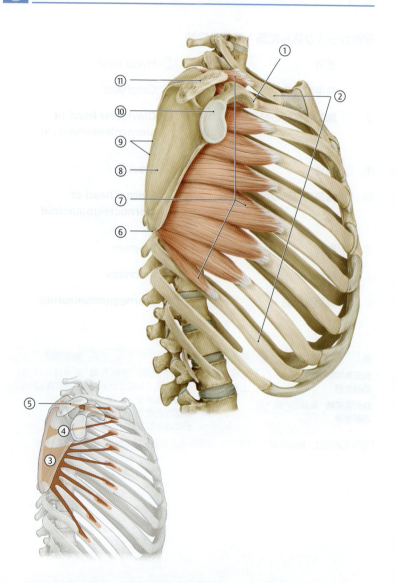

上肢帯の筋の区分 3

腹側の筋：前鋸筋

① □ 烏口突起　　　　　　□ Coracoid process

② □ 第 1-9 肋骨　　　　　□ 1st through 9th ribs

③ □ 前鋸筋の下部　　　　□ **Inferior part of serratus anterior**

④ □ 前鋸筋の中間部　　　□ **Intermediate part of serratus anterior**

⑤ □ 前鋸筋の上部　　　　□ **Superior part of serratus anterior**

⑥ □ 下角　　　　　　　　□ Inferior angle

⑦ □ 前鋸筋　　　　　　　□ Serratus anterior

⑧ □ 肩甲骨　　　　　　　□ Scapula

⑨ □ 内側縁　　　　　　　□ Medial border

⑩ □ 関節窩　　　　　　　□ Glenoid cavity

⑪ □ 肩峰　　　　　　　　□ Acromion

筋	起始	停止	各部位の作用	筋全体の作用	神経支配
前鋸筋の上部	第 1-9 肋骨	上角	挙上した上腕を下げる（前鋸筋の下部と拮抗する）	肩甲骨を前外側に引く、肩が固定されている場合には肋骨を挙上する（呼吸の補助）	長胸神経 (C5-C7)
前鋸筋の中間部		内側縁			
前鋸筋の下部		下角と内側縁	肩甲骨の下角を前外側に引く（腕の 90°以上の挙上を可能にする）		

System of the Shoulder Girdle Muscles IV

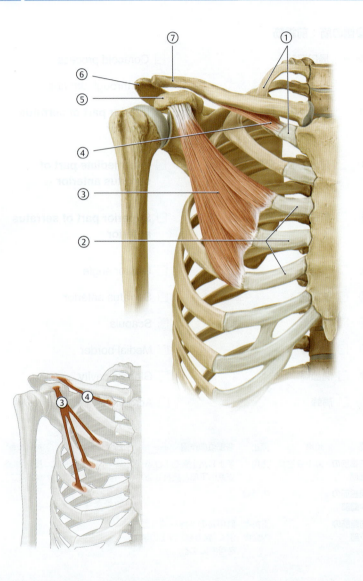

上肢帯の筋の区分 4

腹側の筋：鎖骨下筋と小胸筋

① ☐ 第 1 肋骨　　　　　　　　☐ 1st rib

② ☐ 第 3-5 肋骨　　　　　　　☐ 3rd through 5th ribs

③ ☐ 小胸筋　　　　　　　　　☐ **Pectoralis minor**

④ ☐ 鎖骨下筋　　　　　　　　☐ **Subclavius**

⑤ ☐ 烏口突起　　　　　　　　☐ Coracoid process

⑥ ☐ 肩峰　　　　　　　　　　☐ Acromion

⑦ ☐ 鎖骨　　　　　　　　　　☐ Clavicle

筋	起始	停止	作用	神経支配
鎖骨下筋	第 1 肋骨	鎖骨下面の外側	胸鎖関節において鎖骨を安定に保つ	鎖骨下筋神経（C5-C6）
小胸筋	第 3-5 肋骨	肩甲骨，烏口突起	・肩甲骨を引き下げ，下角を後内側に引く（挙上した上腕を下げる） ・呼吸の補助	内側・外側胸筋神経（C6-T1）

System of the Shoulder Girdle Muscles V

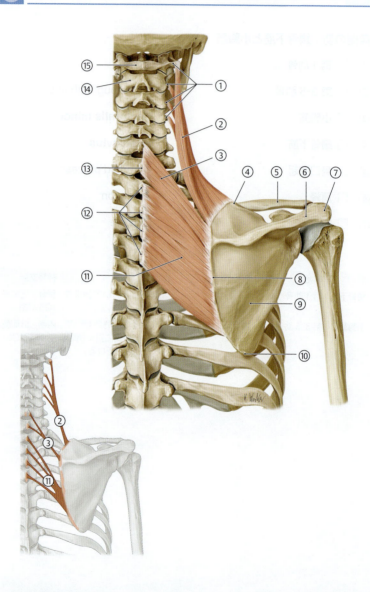

上肢帯の筋の区分 5

背側の筋：肩甲挙筋，大菱形筋，小菱形筋

① □ 第1-4頸椎の横突起
② □ 肩甲挙筋
③ □ 小菱形筋
④ □ 上角
⑤ □ 鎖骨
⑥ □ 肩甲棘
⑦ □ 肩峰
⑧ □ 内側縁
⑨ □ 肩甲骨の後面
⑩ □ 下角
⑪ □ 大菱形筋
⑫ □ 第1-4胸椎の棘突起
⑬ □ 第7頸椎の棘突起
⑭ □ 軸椎（第2頸椎）
⑮ □ 環椎（第1頸椎）

□ C1-C4 transverse processes
□ **Levator scapulae**
□ **Rhomboid minor**
□ Superior angle
□ Clavicle
□ Spine of scapula
□ Acromion
□ Medial border
□ Posterior surface of scapula
□ Inferior angle
□ **Rhomboid major**
□ T1-T4 spinous processes
□ C7 spinous process
□ Axis（C2）
□ Atlas（C1）

筋	起始	停止	作用	神経支配
肩甲挙筋	C1-C4の横突起	肩甲骨（上角）	・肩甲骨を上内側に引き，下角を内側に動かす ・首を同側に曲げる（肩甲骨が固定されている場合）	肩甲背神経（C4-C5）
小菱形筋	C6-C7の棘突起	肩甲骨の内側縁（肩甲棘より上の部分）	・肩甲骨を安定させる ・肩甲骨を上内側に引く	
大菱形筋	T1-T4の棘突起	肩甲骨の内側縁（肩甲棘より下の部分）		

System of the Shoulder Joint Muscles I

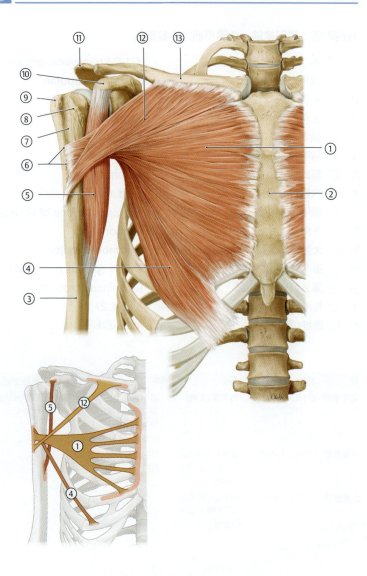

肩関節の筋の区分 1

腹側の筋：大胸筋と烏口腕筋

①	☐ **大胸筋の胸肋部**	☐	**Sternocostal head of pectoralis major**
②	☐ 胸骨	☐	Sternum
③	☐ 上腕骨	☐	Humerus
④	☐ **大胸筋の腹部**	☐	**Abdominal part of pectoralis major**
⑤	☐ **烏口腕筋**	☐	**Coracobrachialis**
⑥	☐ 大結節稜	☐	Crest of greater tubercle
⑦	☐ 結節間溝	☐	Intertubercular sulcus
⑧	☐ 小結節	☐	Lesser tubercle
⑨	☐ 大結節	☐	Greater tubercle
⑩	☐ 烏口突起	☐	Coracoid process
⑪	☐ 肩峰	☐	Acromion
⑫	☐ **大胸筋の鎖骨部**	☐	**Clavicular head of pectoralis major**
⑬	☐ 鎖骨	☐	Clavicle

筋	起始	停止	作用	神経支配
大胸筋の鎖骨部	鎖骨（内側半分）	上腕骨（大結節稜）	・内転・内旋 ・上肢帯を固定した際には呼吸の補助 ・鎖骨部と胸肋部のみ内旋	内側・外側胸筋神経（C5-T1）
大胸筋の胸肋部	胸骨と第2-6肋軟骨			
大胸筋の腹部	腹直筋鞘（前葉）			
烏口腕筋	肩甲骨（烏口突起）	上腕骨（小結節稜の下方に続く線）	・前方挙上 ・内転 ・内旋	筋皮神経（C6-C7）

System of the Shoulder Joint Muscles II

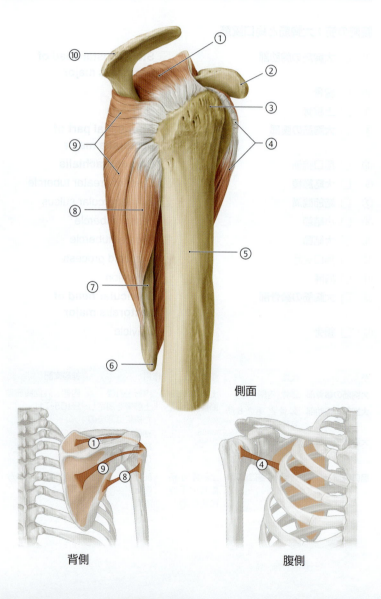

側面

背側

腹側

肩関節の筋の区分 2

背側の筋，回旋筋腱板：棘上筋，棘下筋，小円筋，肩甲下筋

① ☐ 棘上筋　　　　　☐ **Supraspinatus**
② ☐ 烏口突起　　　　☐ Coracoid process
③ ☐ 大結節　　　　　☐ Greater tubercle
④ ☐ 肩甲下筋　　　　☐ **Subscapularis**
⑤ ☐ 上腕骨体　　　　☐ Shaft of humerus
⑥ ☐ 下角　　　　　　☐ Inferior angle
⑦ ☐ 外側縁　　　　　☐ Lateral border
⑧ ☐ 小円筋　　　　　☐ **Teres minor**
⑨ ☐ 棘下筋　　　　　☐ **Infraspinatus**
⑩ ☐ 肩峰　　　　　　☐ Acromion

筋	起始	停止	作用	神経支配
棘上筋	肩甲骨の棘上窩	上腕骨の大結節	外転	肩甲上神経 (C4-C6)
棘下筋	肩甲骨の棘下窩		外旋	
小円筋	肩甲骨の外側縁		・外旋 ・弱い内転作用もある	腋窩神経 (C5-C6)
肩甲下筋	肩甲骨の肩甲下窩	上腕骨の小結節	内旋	肩甲下神経 (C5-C8)

System of the Shoulder Joint Muscles III

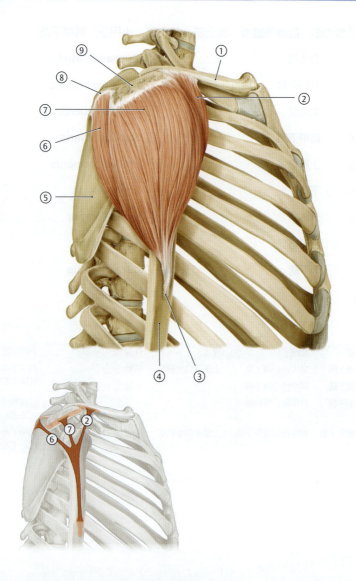

肩関節の筋の区分 3

背側の筋：三角筋

① ☐ 鎖骨　　　　　　　　　　☐ Clavicle
② ☐ 三角筋の鎖骨部　　　　　☐ **Clavicular part of deltoid**
③ ☐ 三角筋粗面　　　　　　　☐ Deltoid tuberosity
④ ☐ 上腕骨体　　　　　　　　☐ Shaft of humerus
⑤ ☐ 肩甲骨　　　　　　　　　☐ Scapula
⑥ ☐ 三角筋の肩甲棘部　　　　☐ **Spinal part of deltoid**
⑦ ☐ 三角筋の肩峰部　　　　　☐ **Acromial part of deltoid**
⑧ ☐ 肩甲棘　　　　　　　　　☐ Spine of scapula
⑨ ☐ 肩峰　　　　　　　　　　☐ Acromion

筋	起始	停止	作用	神経支配
三角筋の鎖骨部	鎖骨の外側 1/3	上腕骨の三角筋粗面	・前方挙上 ・内旋 ・外転(60-90°の外転位では肩峰部の外転作用を補助する)	腋窩神経(C5-C6)
三角筋の肩峰部	肩峰		外転	
三角筋の肩甲棘部	肩甲棘		・後方挙上 ・外旋 ・外転(60-90°の外転位では肩峰部の外転作用を補助する)	

System of the Shoulder Joint Muscles IV

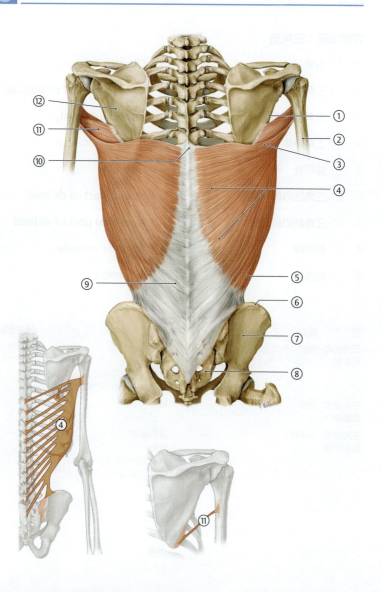

肩関節の筋の区分 4

背側の筋：広背筋と大円筋

① □ 外側縁 □ Lateral border
② □ 上腕骨 □ Humerus
③ □ 広背筋の肩甲骨部 □ **Scapular part of latissimus dorsi**
④ □ 広背筋の椎骨部 □ **Vertebral part of latissimus dorsi**
⑤ □ 広背筋の腸骨部 □ **Iliac part of latissimus dorsi**
⑥ □ 腸骨稜 □ Iliac crest
⑦ □ 腸骨 □ Ilium
⑧ □ 仙骨 □ Sacrum
⑨ □ 胸腰筋膜（広背筋の起始腱膜） □ Thoracolumbar fascia
⑩ □ 第 7 胸椎の棘突起 □ T7 spinous process
⑪ □ **大円筋** □ Teres major
⑫ □ 肩甲骨 □ Scapula

筋	起始	停止	作用	神経支配
広背筋の椎骨部	・T7-T12 の棘突起 ・全腰椎間板棘突起および仙骨（仙骨背側面）の胸腰筋膜上	上腕骨，小結節稜	・内旋 ・内転 ・後方挙上 ・第 9-12 肋骨の肋骨部を介して，呼息の補助をする	胸背神経（C5-C8）
広背筋の腸骨部	腸骨稜（後 1/3）			
広背筋の肩甲骨部	肩甲骨（下角）			
大円筋	肩甲骨（下角）		・内旋 ・内転 ・後方挙上	肩甲下神経（C5-C8）

System of the Muscles of the Upper Arm I

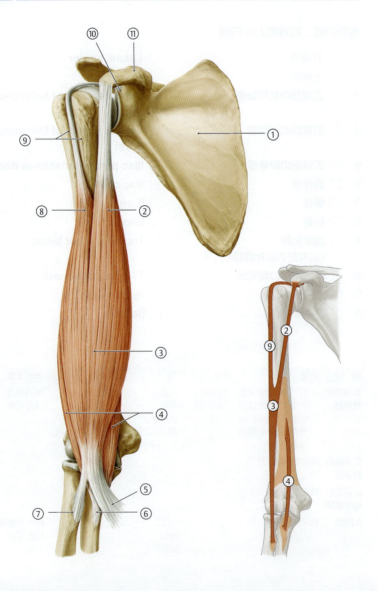

上腕の筋の区分 1

上腕前面の筋：上腕二頭筋と上腕筋

① □ 肩甲骨の肋骨面　　　　　　　□ Costal surface of scapula
② □ **上腕二頭筋の短頭**　　　　　□ **Short head of biceps brachii**
③ □ **上腕二頭筋**　　　　　　　　□ **Biceps brachii**
④ □ **上腕筋**　　　　　　　　　　□ **Brachialis**
⑤ □ 上腕二頭筋腱膜　　　　　　　□ Bicipital aponeurosis
⑥ □ 尺骨粗面（上腕筋の停止腱）　□ Tuberosity of ulna (brachialis tendon of insertion)
⑦ □ 橈骨粗面（上腕二頭筋の停止腱）　□ Radial tuberosity (biceps brachii tendon of insertion)
⑧ □ **上腕二頭筋の長頭**　　　　　□ **Long head of biceps brachii**
⑨ □ 結節間溝　　　　　　　　　　□ Intertubercular sulcus
⑩ □ 関節上結節　　　　　　　　　□ Supraglenoid tubercle
⑪ □ 烏口突起　　　　　　　　　　□ Coracoid process

筋	起始	停止	作用	神経支配
上腕二頭筋の長頭	肩甲骨の関節上結節	橈骨粗面	・肘関節：屈曲，回外（肘が屈曲している場合） ・肩関節：外転と内旋（長頭），前方挙上（長頭と短頭）	筋皮神経（C5-C7）
上腕二頭筋の短頭	肩甲骨の烏口突起	上腕二頭筋腱膜		
上腕筋	上腕骨の前面の遠位半分（内側・外側筋間中隔）	尺骨粗面	肘関節の屈曲	・筋皮神経（C5-C7） ・橈骨神経（C5-C6）

System of the Muscles of the Upper Arm II

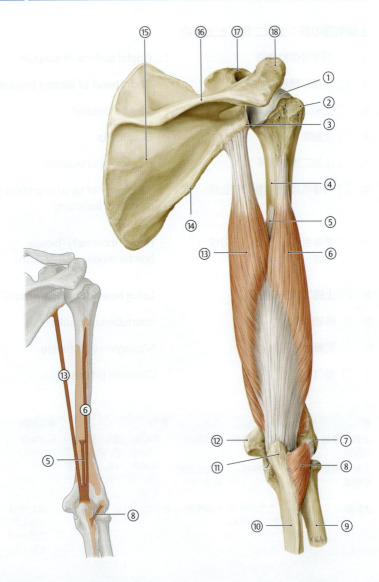

上腕の筋の区分 2

上腕後面の筋：上腕三頭筋と肘筋．後方から見たところ

①	□ 上腕骨頭	□ Head of humerus
②	□ 大結節	□ Greater tubercle
③	□ 関節下結節	□ Infraglenoid tubercle
④	□ 上腕骨体	□ Shaft of humerus
⑤	□ 上腕三頭筋の内側頭	□ **Medial head of triceps brachii**
⑥	□ 上腕三頭筋の外側頭	□ **Lateral head of triceps brachii**
⑦	□ 外側上顆	□ Lateral epicondyle
⑧	□ 肘筋	□ **Anconeus**
⑨	□ 橈骨	□ Radius
⑩	□ 尺骨	□ Ulna
⑪	□ 肘頭	□ Olecranon
⑫	□ 内側上顆	□ Medial epicondyle
⑬	□ 上腕三頭筋の長頭	□ **Long head of triceps brachii**
⑭	□ 外側縁	□ Lateral border
⑮	□ 肩甲骨の後面	□ Posterior surface of scapula
⑯	□ 肩甲棘	□ Spine of scapula
⑰	□ 烏口突起	□ Coracoid process
⑱	□ 肩峰	□ Acromion

筋	起始	停止	作用	神経支配
上腕三頭筋の長頭	肩甲骨（関節下結節）	尺骨の肘頭	・肘関節：伸展 ・肩関節（長頭の作用）：上腕の後方挙上と内転	橈骨神経 (C6-C8)
上腕三頭筋の内側頭	上腕骨の後面（橈骨神経溝の遠位），内側筋間中隔			
上腕三頭筋の外側頭	上腕骨の後面（橈骨神経溝の近位），外側筋間中隔			
肘筋	上腕骨の外側上顆（肘関節包の後部から起始することもある）	尺骨の肘頭（橈側面）	・伸展 ・関節包の伸展補助	

Radius & Ulna

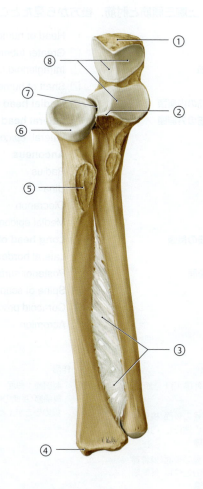

Q 上・下橈尺関節で行われる運動は何か？

橈骨と尺骨

右前腕，前上方面

① □ 肘頭　　　　　　　□ Olecranon
② □ 鉤状突起　　　　　□ Coronoid process
③ □ 前腕骨間膜　　　　□ Interosseous membrane of forearm
④ □ 橈骨の茎状突起　　□ Radial styloid process
⑤ □ 橈骨粗面　　　　　□ Radial tuberosity
⑥ □ 橈骨頭　　　　　　□ Head of radius
⑦ □ 上橈尺関節　　　　□ Proximal radio-ulnar joint
⑧ □ 滑車切痕　　　　　□ Trochlear notch

A 回内と回外が上・下橈尺関節で行われる．

Joint Capsule of the Elbow I

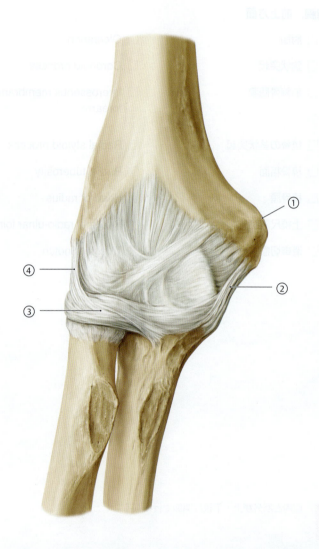

肘関節 1

右肘，伸展位，前面

① ☐ 内側上顆 ☐ Medial epicondyle
② ☐ 内側側副靱帯 ☐ Ulnar collateral ligament
③ ☐ 橈骨輪状靱帯 ☐ Annular ligament of radius
④ ☐ 外側側副靱帯 ☐ Radial collateral ligament

Joint Capsule of the Elbow II

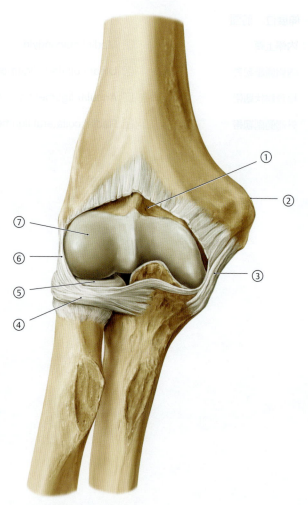

Q 肘内障(子守り肘)とは何か?

肘関節 2

右肘，伸展位，前面

① □ 鈎突窩　　　　　　　□ Coronoid fossa
② □ 内側上顆　　　　　　□ Medial epicondyle
③ □ 内側側副靱帯　　　　□ Ulnar collateral ligament
④ □ 橈骨輪状靱帯　　　　□ Annular ligament of radius
⑤ □ 橈骨頭　　　　　　　□ Head of radius
⑥ □ 外側側副靱帯　　　　□ Radial collateral ligament
⑦ □ 上腕骨小頭　　　　　□ Capitellum

　肘内障は小児によく見られ，手や手首を引っ張られた際に生じやすい．未成熟な橈骨頭が橈骨輪状靱帯よりも下方に偏位し，回外運動が強く制限される．上肢は一見麻痺したようになるが，簡単に整復できる．

Muscles of the Anterior Forearm I

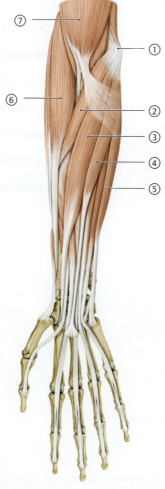

Q 腕橈骨筋の支配神経は何か？

前腕の筋（前面） 1

右腕，腹側から見た図．浅指屈筋と橈側筋群

①	□ 内側上顆（前腕屈筋の共通頭）	□ Medial epicondyle (common head of flexors)
②	□ 円回内筋	□ Pronator teres
③	□ 橈側手根屈筋	□ Flexor carpi radialis
④	□ 長掌筋	□ Palmaris longus
⑤	□ 尺側手根屈筋	□ Flexor carpi ulnaris
⑥	□ 腕橈骨筋	□ Brachioradialis
⑦	□ 上腕二頭筋	□ Biceps brachii

A 　腕橈骨筋は前腕の後区画の筋であり，橈骨神経に支配される．しかし，他の後区画の筋と異なり，前腕の前面に位置し，肘関節の屈筋として働く．

Muscles of the Anterior Forearm II

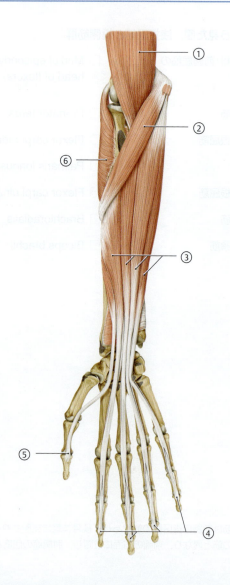

前腕の筋（前面） 2

右腕．腹側から見た図．橈側筋群を取り除いたところ

① □ 上腕筋 　　　　　　　　□ Brachialis

② □ 円回内筋 　　　　　　　□ Pronator teres

③ □ 浅指屈筋 　　　　　　　□ Flexor digitorum superficialis

④ □ 深指屈筋の腱 　　　　　□ Flexor digitorum profundus tendons

⑤ □ 長母指屈筋の腱 　　　　□ Flexor pollicis longus tendon

⑥ □ 回外筋 　　　　　　　　□ Supinator

Muscles of the Anterior Forearm III

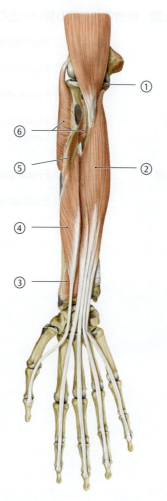

Q 回外に関与する筋は何か？（図示されていないものも含む）

前腕の筋（前面）3

右腕．腹側から見た図．円回内筋と浅指屈筋を取り除いたところ

① ☐ 浅指屈筋の上腕尺骨頭（筋の起始）　☐ Flexor digitorum superficialis, humero-ulnar head (origin)

② ☐ 深指屈筋　☐ Flexor digitorum profundus

③ ☐ 方形回内筋　☐ Pronator quadratus

④ ☐ 長母指屈筋　☐ Flexor pollicis longus

⑤ ☐ 浅指屈筋の橈骨頭（筋の起始）　☐ Flexor digitorum superficialis, radial head (origin)

⑥ ☐ 回外筋　☐ Supinator

A 回外筋と上腕二頭筋が回外に関与する．

Muscles of the Posterior Forearm I

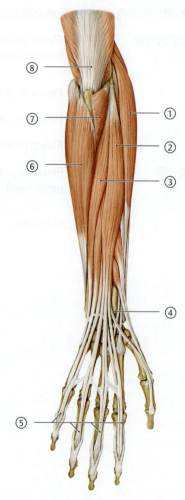

Q 複数の伸筋腱を有する指はどれか？

前腕の筋(後面) 1

右腕,背側から見た図.浅層の伸筋群と橈側筋群

① □ 長橈側手根伸筋 □ Extensor carpi radialis longus

② □ [総]指伸筋 □ Extensor digitorum
③ □ 尺側手根伸筋 □ Extensor carpi ulnaris
④ □ (橈骨の)背側結節 □ Dorsal tubercle
⑤ □ [総]指伸筋の腱,指背腱膜 □ Extensor digitorum tendons, dorsal digital expansion

⑥ □ 尺側手根屈筋 □ Flexor carpi ulnaris
⑦ □ 肘筋 □ Anconeus
⑧ □ 上腕三頭筋 □ Triceps brachii

A 第1指〔母指(親指)〕,第2指〔示指(人差し指)〕,第5指(小指)には2本の伸筋腱が停止する.

Muscles of the Posterior Forearm II

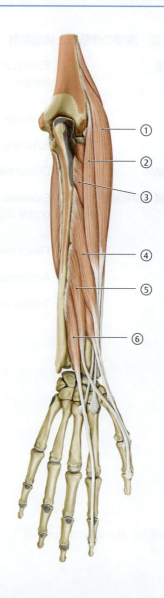

①
②
③
④
⑤
⑥

前腕の筋（後面）2

右腕．背側から見た図．上腕三頭筋，肘筋，尺側手根屈筋，尺側手根伸筋および指伸筋を取り除いたところ

① □ 長橈側手根伸筋 　　　　　　□ Extensor carpi radialis longus

② □ 短橈側手根伸筋 　　　　　　□ Extensor carpi radialis brevis

③ □ 回外筋 　　　　　　□ Supinator

④ □ 長母指外転筋 　　　　　　□ Abductor pollicis longus

⑤ □ 長母指伸筋 　　　　　　□ Extensor pollicis longus

⑥ □ 示指伸筋 　　　　　　□ Extensor indicis

System of the Muscles of the Forearm I

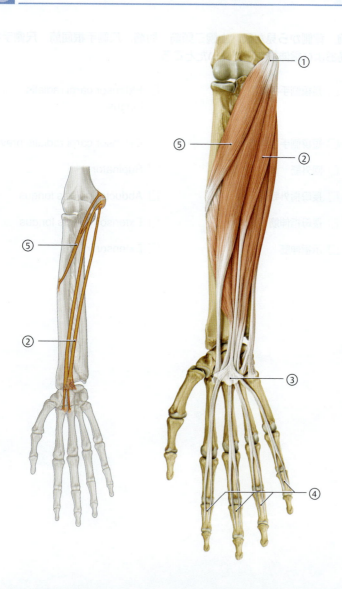

前腕の筋の区分 1

前腕前面の筋，浅層筋群：円回内筋と長掌筋

① □ 内側上顆（前腕屈筋の共通頭） □ Medial epicondyle (common head of flexors)

② □ **長掌筋** □ **Palmaris longus**

③ □ 手掌腱膜 □ Palmar aponeurosis

④ □ 第 2-5 中節骨 □ 2nd through 5th middle phalanges

⑤ □ **円回内筋** □ **Pronator teres**

筋	起始	停止	作用	神経支配
円回内筋の上腕頭	上腕骨の内側上顆	橈骨の外側面（回外筋の停止部よりも遠位）	・肘関節：弱い屈曲作用 ・前腕の関節：回内	正中神経(C6)
円回内筋の尺骨頭	尺骨の鉤状突起			
長掌筋	上腕骨の内側上顆	手掌腱膜	・肘関節：弱い屈曲作用 ・手首：屈曲・手掌腱膜を緊張させる	正中神経(C8-T1)

System of the Muscles of the Forearm II

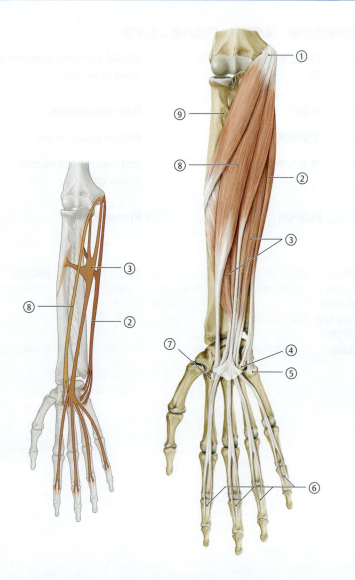

前腕の筋の区分 2

前腕前面の筋, 浅層筋群：浅指屈筋, 橈側手根屈筋, 尺側手根屈筋

① □ 内側上顆（前腕屈筋の共通頭）　□ Medial epicondyle (common head of flexors)
② □ 尺側手根屈筋　□ **Flexor carpi ulnaris**
③ □ 浅指屈筋　□ **Flexor digitorum superficialis**
④ □ 有鈎骨鈎　□ Hook of hamate
⑤ □ 第5中手骨の底　□ Base of 5th metacarpal
⑥ □ 第2-5中節骨　□ 2nd through 5th middle phalanges
⑦ □ 第2中手骨の底　□ Base of 2nd metacarpal
⑧ □ 橈側手根屈筋　□ **Flexor carpi radialis**
⑨ □ 橈骨粗面　□ Radial tuberosity

筋	起始	停止	作用	神経支配
浅指屈筋の上腕頭	上腕骨の内側上顆	第2-5指の中節骨（両縁）	・肘関節：弱い屈曲作用 ・手首, 第2-5指のMCP関節・PIP関節：屈曲	正中神経 (C7-T1)
浅指屈筋の尺骨頭	尺骨の鈎状突起 (pp.418, 419を参照)			
浅指屈筋の橈骨頭	橈骨の前面（橈骨粗面の下方）			
橈側手根屈筋	上腕骨の内側上顆	第2中手骨底（変異：第3中手底）	・手首：屈曲, 外転（橈側偏位） ・肘関節：弱い回内	正中神経 (C6-C8)
尺側手根屈筋の上腕頭	上腕骨の内側上顆	・第5中手骨底 ・有鈎骨鈎	手首：屈曲, 外転（尺側偏位）	尺骨神経 (C8-T1)
尺側手根屈筋の尺骨頭	尺骨の肘頭			

MCP関節：中手指節関節　PIP関節：近位指節間関節

System of the Muscles of the Forearm III

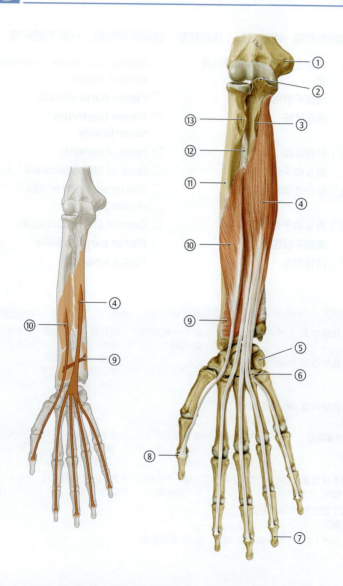

前腕の筋の区分 3

前腕前面の筋,深層筋群：深指屈筋,長母指屈筋,方形回内筋

① ☐ 上腕骨の内側上顆 ☐ Medial epicondyle of humerus
② ☐ 鈎状突起 ☐ Coronoid process
③ ☐ 尺骨粗面 ☐ Tuberosity of ulna
④ ☐ 深指屈筋 ☐ **Flexor digitorum profundus**
⑤ ☐ 豆状骨 ☐ Pisiform
⑥ ☐ 有鈎骨鈎 ☐ Hook of hamate
⑦ ☐ 第 4 末節骨 ☐ 4th distal phalanx
⑧ ☐ 第 1 末節骨の底 ☐ Base of 1st distal phalanx
⑨ ☐ 方形回内筋 ☐ **Pronator quadratus**
⑩ ☐ 長母指屈筋 ☐ **Flexor pollicis longus**
⑪ ☐ 橈骨 ☐ Radius
⑫ ☐ 前腕骨間膜 ☐ Interosseous membrane of forearm
⑬ ☐ 橈骨粗面 ☐ Radial tuberosity

筋	起始	停止	作用	神経支配
深指屈筋	・尺骨前面(中央) ・隣接する骨間膜	第 2-5 指の末節骨(掌側面)	手首,第 2-5 指の MCP 関節・PIP 関節・DIP 関節：屈曲	・第 2, 3 指の橈側部：正中神経(C8-T1) ・第 4, 5 指の尺側部：尺骨神経(C8-T1)
長母指屈筋	・橈骨前面(中央) ・隣接する骨間膜	母指の末節骨(掌側面)	・手首：屈曲・外転(橈側偏位) ・母指の手根中手関節：対立 ・母指の MCP 関節・IP 関節：屈曲	正中神経(C6-C8)
方形回内筋	尺骨前面(遠位 1/4)	橈骨前面(遠位 1/4)	・回内 ・下橈尺関節を安定させる	正中神経(C8-T1)

DIP 関節：遠位指節間関節　IP 関節：指節間関節　MCP 関節：中手指節関節　PIP 関節：近位指節間関節.

System of the Muscles of the Forearm IV

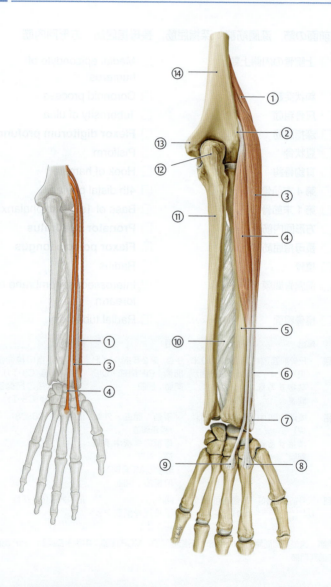

前腕の筋の区分 4

右前腕の橈側筋群：腕橈骨筋，長橈側手根伸筋，短橈側手根伸筋．後方から見たところ

①	□ 腕橈骨筋	□	**Brachioradialis**
②	□ 外側上顆	□	Lateral epicondyle
③	□ 長橈側手根伸筋	□	**Extensor carpi radialis longus**
④	□ 短橈側手根伸筋	□	**Extensor carpi radialis brevis**
⑤	□ 橈骨	□	Radius
⑥	□ 腕橈骨筋の停止腱	□	Brachioradialis tendon of insertion
⑦	□ 橈骨の茎状突起	□	Radial styloid process
⑧	□ 第2中手骨の底	□	Base of 2nd metacarpal
⑨	□ 第3中手骨の底	□	Base of 3rd metacarpal
⑩	□ 前腕骨間膜	□	Interosseous membrane of forearm
⑪	□ 尺骨	□	Ulna
⑫	□ 肘頭	□	Olecranon
⑬	□ 内側上顆	□	Medial epicondyle
⑭	□ 上腕骨	□	Humerus

筋	起始	停止	作用	神経支配
腕橈骨筋	上腕骨遠位部（外側面），外側筋間中隔	橈骨の茎状突起	・肘関節：屈曲 ・前腕の関節：半回内	橈骨神経 (C5-C7)
長橈側手根伸筋	上腕骨遠位部（外側上顆稜），外側筋間中隔	第2中手骨底背側	・肘関節：弱い屈曲作用 ・手首：背屈，外転（橈側偏位）	
短橈側手根伸筋	上腕骨の外側上顆	第3中手骨底背側		

System of the Muscles of the Forearm V

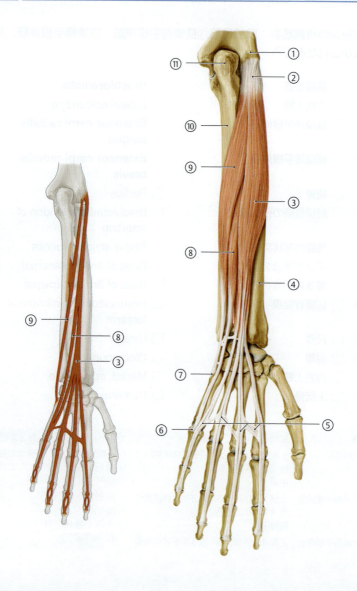

上肢 423

前腕の筋の区分 5

前腕後面の筋，浅層筋群：[総]指伸筋，小指伸筋，尺側手根伸筋．後方から見たところ．

① ☐ 外側上顆
② ☐ [総]指伸筋，小指伸筋，尺側手根伸筋の共通頭
③ ☐ [総]指伸筋
④ ☐ 橈骨
⑤ ☐ 指背腱膜 / 腱間結合
⑥ ☐ 第 5 基節骨の底
⑦ ☐ 第 5 中手骨の底
⑧ ☐ 小指伸筋
⑨ ☐ 尺側手根伸筋
⑩ ☐ 尺骨
⑪ ☐ 肘頭

☐ Lateral epicondyle
☐ Common head of extensor digitorum, extensor digiti minimi, and extensor carpi ulnaris
☐ **Extensor digitorum**
☐ Radius
☐ Dorsal digital expansion/ intertendinous connections
☐ Base of 5th proximal phalanx
☐ Base of 5th metacarpal
☐ **Extensor digiti minimi**
☐ **Extensor carpi ulnaris**
☐ Ulna
☐ Olecranon

筋	起始	停止	作用	神経支配
総指伸筋	上腕骨の外側上顆	第 2-5 指の指背腱膜	・手首：背屈 ・第 2-5 指の MCP 関節・PIP 関節・DIP 関節：伸展，指を広げる	橈骨神経 (C5-C8)
小指伸筋		第 5 指の指背腱膜	・手首：背屈，内転(尺側偏位) ・第 5 指の MCP 関節・PIP 関節・DIP 関節：伸展，指を広げる	
尺側手根伸筋		第 5 中手骨底	手首：背屈，内転(尺側偏位)	

DIP 関節：遠位指節間関節　MCP 関節：中手指節関節　PIP 関節：近位指節間関節

System of the Muscles of the Forearm VI

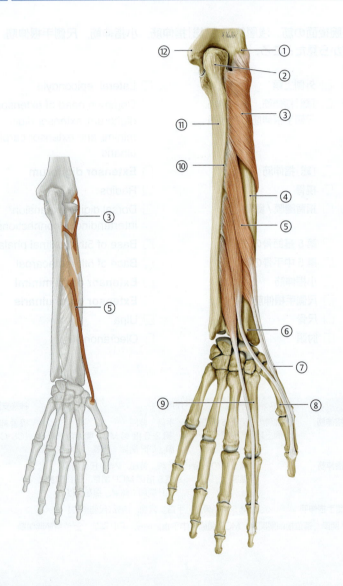

前腕の筋の区分 6

前腕後面の筋，深層筋群：回外筋と長母指外転筋

① □ 外側上顆　　　　　　　　　□ Lateral epicondyle
② □ 肘頭　　　　　　　　　　　□ Olecranon
③ □ **回外筋**　　　　　　　　　□ **Supinator**
④ □ 橈骨　　　　　　　　　　　□ Radius
⑤ □ **長母指外転筋**　　　　　　□ **Abductor pollicis longus**
⑥ □ 背側結節　　　　　　　　　□ Dorsal tubercle
⑦ □ 第1中手骨の底　　　　　　□ Base of 1st metacarpal
⑧ □ 第1中手骨　　　　　　　　□ 1st metacarpal
⑨ □ 第2中手骨　　　　　　　　□ 2nd metacarpal
⑩ □ 尺骨の後縁　　　　　　　　□ Posterior border of ulna
⑪ □ 尺骨　　　　　　　　　　　□ Ulna
⑫ □ 内側上顆　　　　　　　　　□ Medial epicondyle

筋	起始	停止	作用	神経支配
回外筋	・尺骨の回外筋稜 ・上腕骨の外側上顆	橈骨 (橈骨前面)	前腕の関節：回外	橈骨神経(C5-C6)
長母指外転筋	・橈骨と尺骨の背側面 ・骨間膜	第1中手骨底	・手関節近位部：外転(橈側偏位) ・母指の手根中手関節：外転 ・回外の補助	橈骨神経(C6-8)

System of the Muscles of the Forearm VII

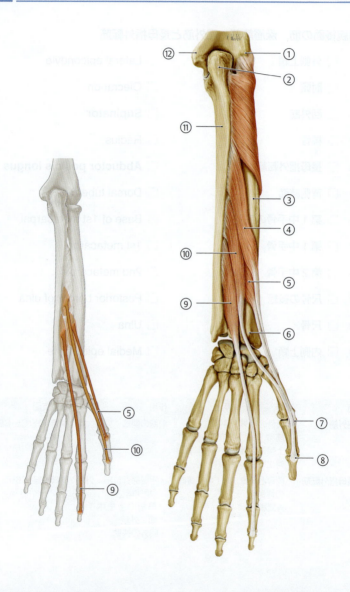

前腕の筋の区分 7

前腕後面の筋，深層筋群：短母指伸筋と長母指伸筋

① ☐ 外側上顆　　　　　☐ Lateral epicondyle
② ☐ 肘頭　　　　　　　☐ Olecranon
③ ☐ 橈骨　　　　　　　☐ Radius
④ ☐ 長母指外転筋　　　☐ Abductor pollicis longus
⑤ ☐ **短母指伸筋**　　☐ **Extensor pollicis brevis**
⑥ ☐ 背側結節　　　　　☐ Dorsal tubercle
⑦ ☐ 第1基節骨の底　　☐ Base of 1st proximal phalanx
⑧ ☐ 第1末節骨の底　　☐ Base of 1st distal phalanx
⑨ ☐ 示指伸筋　　　　　☐ **Extensor indicis**
⑩ ☐ **長母指伸筋**　　☐ **Extensor pollicis longus**
⑪ ☐ 尺骨　　　　　　　☐ Ulna
⑫ ☐ 内側上顆　　　　　☐ Medial epicondyle

筋	起始	停止	作用	神経支配
短母指伸筋*	・橈骨の背側面 ・骨間膜(長母指外転筋の遠位)	母指の基節骨底	・手関節近位部：外転(橈側偏位) ・母指の手根中手関節・MCP関節：伸展	橈骨神経 (C6-C8)
長母指伸筋*	・尺骨の背側面 ・骨間膜	母指の末節骨底	・手首：背屈と外転(橈側偏位) ・母指の手根中手関節：内転 ・母指のMCP関節・IP関節：伸展	
示指伸筋*		示指の指背腱膜	・手首：背屈 ・示指のMCP関節・PIP関節・DIP関節：背屈	

DIP関節：遠位指節間関節　IP関節：指節間関節　MCP関節：中手指節関節　PIP関節：近位指節間関節
*回外を補助する

Bones of the Wrist & Hand I

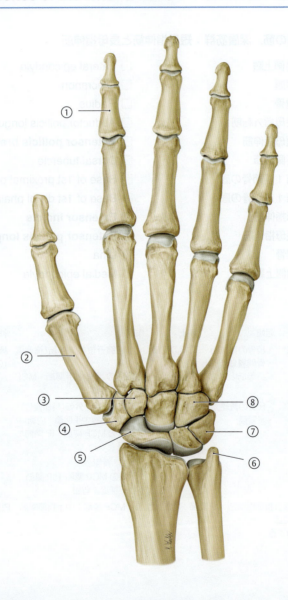

手首と手の骨格 1

右手，後面（背側面）

① □ 第2中節骨　　　　□ 2nd middle phalanx
② □ 第1中手骨　　　　□ 1st metacarpal
③ □ 小菱形骨　　　　　□ Trapezoid
④ □ 大菱形骨　　　　　□ Trapezium
⑤ □ 舟状骨　　　　　　□ Scaphoid
⑥ □ 尺骨の茎状突起　　□ Ulnar styloid process
⑦ □ 三角骨　　　　　　□ Triquetrum
⑧ □ 有鈎骨　　　　　　□ Hamate

臨床

　舟状骨骨折は，手根骨骨折の中で最もよく見られ，近位端と遠位端の間にあるくびれた部分で折れる場合が多い．舟状骨を栄養する動脈は遠位端から入るので，舟状骨骨折の際には近位端へ血流が途絶し，骨折が治癒せず，しばしば近位端の無血管性壊死をきたす．

Bones of the Wrist & Hand II

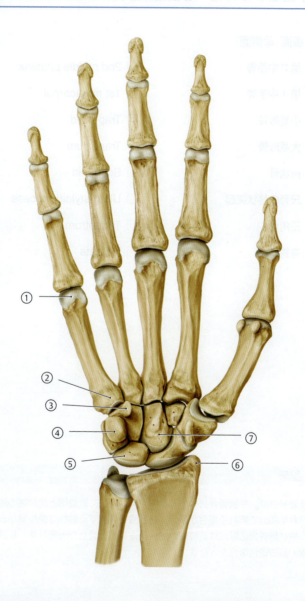

手首と手の骨格 2

右手, 前面(掌側面)

① □ 中手骨の頭　　　　　□ Head of metacarpal

② □ 中手骨の底　　　　　□ Base of metacarpal

③ □ 有鈎骨鈎　　　　　　□ Hook of hamate

④ □ 豆状骨　　　　　　　□ Pisiform

⑤ □ 月状骨　　　　　　　□ Lunate

⑥ □ 橈骨の茎状突起　　　□ Radial styloid process

⑦ □ 有頭骨　　　　　　　□ Capitate

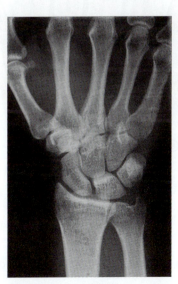

右手(後面)のX線像

Joints of the Wrist & Hand

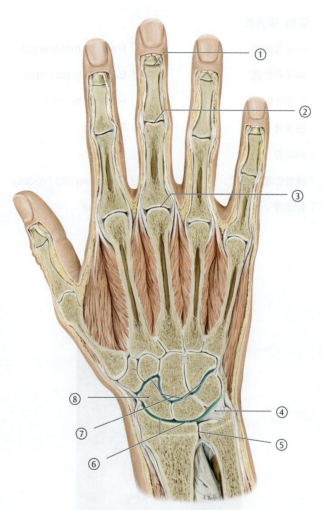

 手根骨のうち,第1指(母指)の中手骨と関節をなすのはどれか?

手首と手の関節

右手，後面（背側面）

① ☐ 遠位指節間（DIP）関節 ☐ Distal interphalangeal joint
② ☐ 近位指節間（PIP）関節 ☐ Proximal interphalangeal joint
③ ☐ 中手指節（MCP）関節 ☐ Metacarpophalangeal joint
④ ☐ 関節円板 ☐ Articular disc
⑤ ☐ 下橈尺関節 ☐ Distal radioulnar joint
⑥ ☐ 橈骨手根関節 ☐ Wrist joint
⑦ ☐ 手根中央関節 ☐ Midcarpal joint
⑧ ☐ 舟状骨 ☐ Scaphoid

A 大菱形骨が第1指（母指）の中手骨と関節をなす．

Muscles of the Hand I

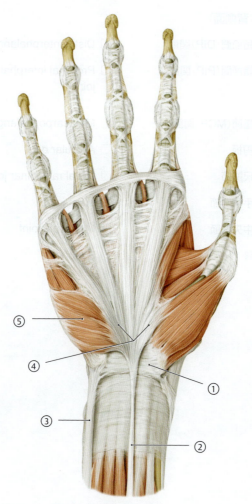

 デュプイトラン拘縮とは何か？

手の筋 1

右手,前面(掌側面)

① ☐ 屈筋支帯　　　　　☐ Flexor retinaculum

② ☐ 長掌筋の腱　　　　☐ Palmaris longus tendon

③ ☐ 尺側手根屈筋　　　☐ Flexor carpi ulnaris

④ ☐ 手掌腱膜　　　　　☐ Palmar aponeurosis

⑤ ☐ 短掌筋　　　　　　☐ Palmaris brevis

A 　デュプイトラン拘縮は手掌腱膜が徐々に萎縮することで生じる.萎縮により手掌腱膜は短縮し,主に第4・5指〔環指(薬指)・小指〕が屈曲位の状態で拘縮し,手の把握機能が著しく損なわれる.

Muscles of the Hand II

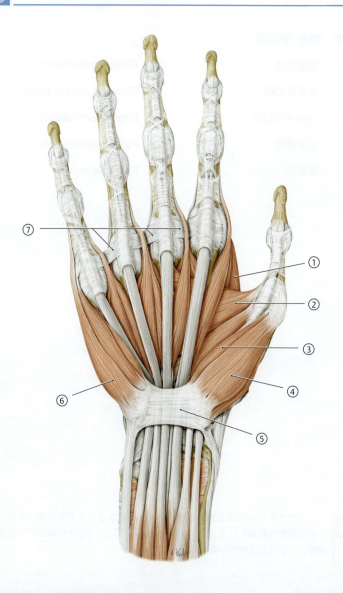

手の筋 2

右手，前面（掌側面）．手掌腱膜，前腕筋膜，掌側手根腱鞘，短掌筋および長掌筋を取り除いたところ

① □ 第1背側骨間筋 □ 1st dorsal interosseus
② □ 母指内転筋の横頭 □ Transverse head of adductor pollicis
③ □ 短母指屈筋の浅頭 □ Superficial head of flexor pollicis brevis
④ □ 短母指外転筋 □ Abductor pollicis brevis
⑤ □ 屈筋支帯 □ Flexor retinaculum
⑥ □ 小指外転筋 □ Abductor digiti minimi
⑦ □ 深横中手靱帯 □ Deep transverse metacarpal ligament

臨床

第1指（母指）の腱鞘は，長母指屈筋の腱鞘を介して，指屈筋の総腱鞘と連絡している．母指以外の指でも指の腱鞘と総腱鞘が連絡している場合がある．刺創によって指の腱鞘に感染が生じると，連絡部を介して感染が総腱鞘に広がることがある．

Muscles of the Hand III

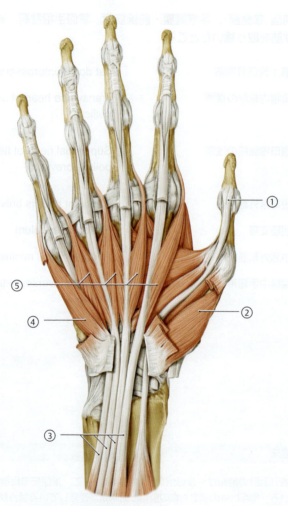

虫様筋の起始と停止はどこか？

手の筋 3

右手，前面（掌側面）．浅指屈筋を完全に取り除き，屈筋支帯，短母指外転筋，短母指屈筋，および小指外転筋を部分的に取り除いたところ．

① □ 長母指屈筋の腱　　　□ Flexor pollicis longus tendon

② □ 母指対立筋　　　　　□ Opponens pollicis

③ □ 深指屈筋　　　　　　□ Flexor digitorum profundus

④ □ 短小指屈筋　　　　　□ Flexor digiti minimi brevis

⑤ □ 虫様筋　　　　　　　□ Lumbricals

A 虫様筋は手掌において深指屈筋腱から起始し，指の背側面において指背腱膜に停止する．

Muscles of the Hand IV

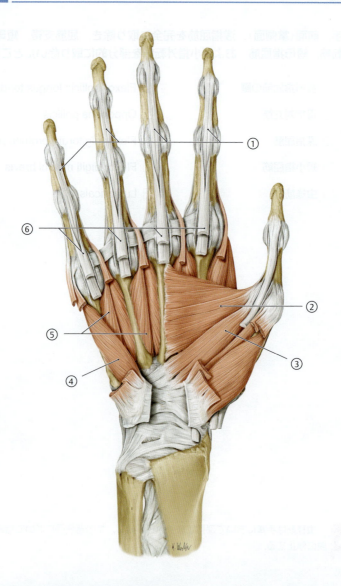

手の筋 4

右手，前面（掌側面）．母指外転筋，長指屈筋の起始腱および輪状靱帯を完全に取り除き，母指対立筋および小指対立筋を部分的に取り除いたところ

① □ 深指屈筋の腱 □ Flexor digitorum profundus tendons

② □ 母指内転筋の横頭 □ Transverse head of adductor pollicis

③ □ 母指内転筋の斜頭 □ Oblique head of adductor pollicis

④ □ 小指対立筋 □ Opponens digiti minimi

⑤ □ 第2・3掌側骨間筋 □ 2nd and 3rd palmar interossei

⑥ □ 浅指屈筋の腱 □ Flexor digitorum superficialis tendons

Dorsum of the Hand

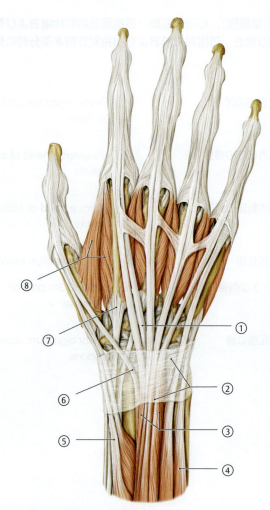

Q 背側骨間筋の支配神経は何か？

手背

右手の甲，後面（背側面）

① □ 示指伸筋の腱 □ Extensor indicis tendon
② □ 伸筋支帯 □ Extensor retinaculum
③ □ ［総］指伸筋 □ Extensor digitorum
④ □ 尺側手根伸筋 □ Extensor carpi ulnaris
⑤ □ 長母指外転筋 □ Abductor pollicis longus
⑥ □ 長母指伸筋の腱 □ Extensor pollicis longus tendon
⑦ □ 長橈側手根伸筋の腱 □ Extensor carpi radialis longus tendon
⑧ □ 第1背側骨間筋 □ 1st dorsal interosseous

A 背側骨間筋，掌側骨間筋はともに尺骨神経によって支配される．橈骨神経は上腕と前腕の後面にある筋を支配するが，手の筋（手内筋）には分布しない．

System of the Muscles of the Hand I

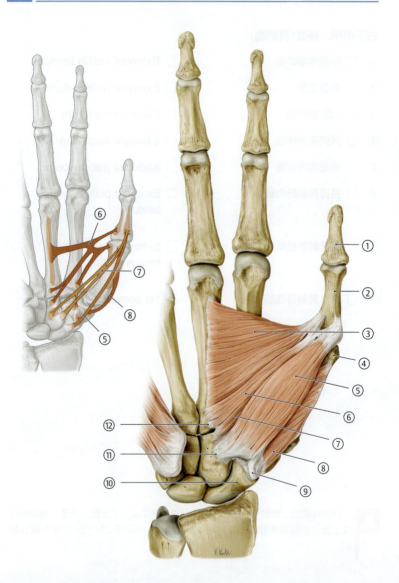

手の筋の区分 1

手内筋，母指球筋：短母指外転筋，母指内転筋，短母指屈筋，母指対立筋

① □ 第1末節骨 — □ 1st distal phalanx
② □ 第1基節骨 — □ 1st proximal phalanx
③ □ **母指内転筋の横頭** — □ **Transverse head of adductor pollicis**
④ □ 第1中手骨の頭 — □ Head of 1st metacarpal
⑤ □ **短母指外転筋** — □ **Abductor pollicis brevis**
⑥ □ **母指内転筋の斜頭** — □ **Oblique head of adductor pollicis**
⑦ □ **短母指屈筋の浅頭** — □ **Superficial head of flexor pollicis brevis**
⑧ □ **母指対立筋** — □ **Opponens pollicis**
⑨ □ 大菱形骨 — □ Trapezium
⑩ □ 舟状骨 — □ Scaphoid
⑪ □ 有頭骨 — □ Capitate
⑫ □ 第3中手骨の底 — □ Base of 3rd metacarpal

筋	起始	停止	作用	神経支配
短母指外転筋	舟状骨，屈筋支帯	母指の基節骨底（橈側の種子骨を介して）	・母指の手根中手関節：外転 ・母指のMCP関節：屈曲	正中神経（C6-C7）
母指内転筋の横頭	第3中手骨（掌側面）	母指の基節骨底（尺側の種子骨を介して）	・母指の手根中手関節：内転，対立 ・母指のMCP関節：屈曲	尺骨神経（C8-T1）
母指内転筋の斜頭	有頭骨，第2・3中手骨底			
短母指屈筋の浅頭	屈筋支帯	母指の基節骨底（橈側の種子骨を介して）	・母指の手根中手関節：屈曲，対立 ・母指のMCP関節：屈曲	正中神経（C6-T1）
短母指屈筋の深頭	有頭骨，大菱形骨			尺骨神経（C8-T1）
母指対立筋	大菱形骨	第1中手骨（橈側縁）	母指の手根中手関節：対立	正中神経（C6-C7）

MCP関節：中手指節関節

System of the Muscles of the Hand II

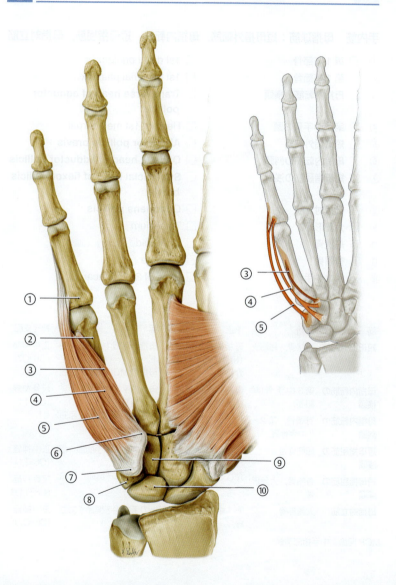

上肢 447

手の筋の区分 2

手内筋，小指球筋：小指外転筋，短小指屈筋，小指対立筋

① □ 第5基節骨の底　　　　　□ Base of 5th proximal phalanx
② □ 第5中手骨　　　　　　　□ 5th metacarpal
③ □ 小指対立筋　　　　　　　□ **Opponens digiti minimi**
④ □ 短小指屈筋　　　　　　　□ **Flexor digiti minimi brevis**
⑤ □ 小指外転筋　　　　　　　□ **Abductor digiti minimi**
⑥ □ 有鈎骨鈎　　　　　　　　□ Hook of hamate
⑦ □ 豆状骨　　　　　　　　　□ Pisiform
⑧ □ 三角骨　　　　　　　　　□ Triquetrum
⑨ □ 有鈎骨　　　　　　　　　□ Hamate
⑩ □ 月状骨　　　　　　　　　□ Lunate

筋	起始	停止	作用	神経支配
小指外転筋	豆状骨	第5基節骨底（尺側），小指の指背腱膜	・小指のMCP関節：屈曲，指を広げる（外転） ・小指のPIP・DIP関節：伸展	尺骨神経（C8-T1）
短小指屈筋	有鈎骨鈎，屈筋支帯	第5基節骨底	小指のMCP関節：屈曲	
小指対立筋	有鈎骨鈎	第5中手骨（尺側縁）	中手骨を手掌方向に引き寄せる（対立）	
*短掌筋 （pp.434, 435参照）	手掌腱膜（尺側縁）	小指球の皮膚	手掌腱膜を緊張させる（保護的機能）	

DIP関節：遠位指節間関節　MCP関節：中手指節関節　PIP関節：近位指節間関節
*図には描かれていない

System of the Muscles of the Hand III

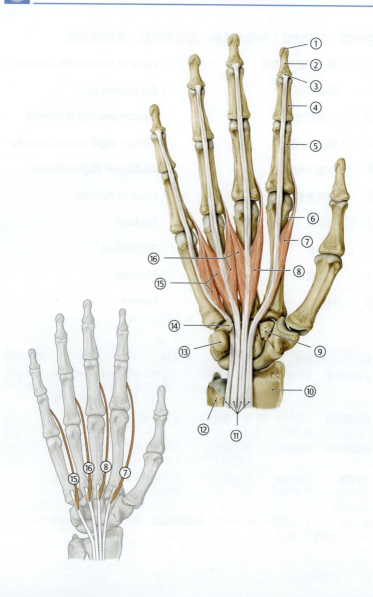

手の筋の区分 3

手内筋，中手筋：第 1-4 虫様筋

① □ 第 2 末節骨の頭
② □ 第 2 末節骨の体
③ □ 第 2 末節骨の底
④ □ 第 2 中節骨
⑤ □ 第 2 基節骨
⑥ □ 第 2 中手骨
⑦ □ **第 1 虫様筋**
⑧ □ **第 2 虫様筋**
⑨ □ 小菱形骨
⑩ □ 橈骨
⑪ □ 深指屈筋の腱
⑫ □ 尺骨
⑬ □ 豆状骨
⑭ □ 有鈎骨鈎
⑮ □ **第 4 虫様筋**（しばしば 2 頭で起始）
⑯ □ **第 3 虫様筋**（しばしば 2 頭で起始）

□ Head of 2nd distal phalanx
□ Shaft of 2nd distal phalanx
□ Base of 2nd distal phalanx
□ 2nd middle phalanx
□ 2nd proximal phalanx
□ 2nd metacarpal
□ **1st lumbrical**
□ **2nd lumbrical**
□ Trapezoid
□ Radius
□ Flexor digitorum profundus tendons
□ Ulna
□ Pisiform bone
□ Hook of hamate
□ **4th lumbrical** (often arises by two heads)
□ **3rd lumbrical** (often arises by two heads)

筋	起始	停止	作用	神経支配
第 1 虫様筋	深指屈筋腱の橈側縁	第 2 指の指背腱膜	・第 2-5 指の MCP 関節：屈曲 ・第 2-5 指の PIP・DIP 関節：伸展	正中神経 (C8-T1)
第 2 虫様筋		第 3 指の指背腱膜		
第 3 虫様筋		第 4 指の指背腱膜		尺骨神経 (C8-T1)
第 4 虫様筋		第 5 指の指背腱膜		

DIP 関節：遠位指節間関節　MCP 関節：中手指節関節　PIP 関節：近位指節間関節

System of the Muscles of the Hand IV

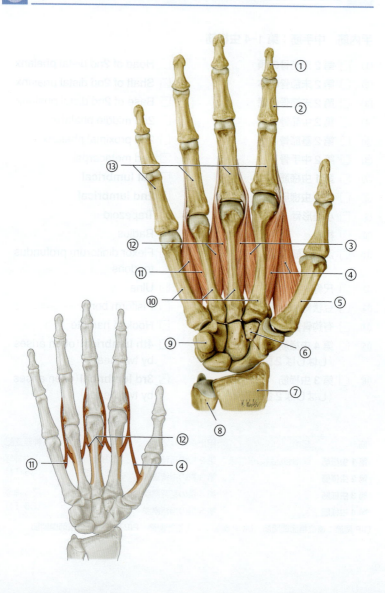

手の筋の区分 4

手内筋，中手筋：第 1-4 背側骨間筋

① □ 第 2 末節骨の体　　　　　　□ Shaft of 2nd distal phalanx
② □ 第 2 中節骨　　　　　　　　□ 2nd middle phalanx
③ □ **第 2 背側骨間筋**　　　　　**□ 2nd dorsal interosseous**
④ □ **第 1 背側骨間筋**　　　　　**□ 1st dorsal interosseous**
⑤ □ 第 1 中手骨　　　　　　　　□ 1st metacarpal
⑥ □ 小菱形骨　　　　　　　　　□ Trapezoid
⑦ □ 橈骨　　　　　　　　　　　□ Radius
⑧ □ 尺骨　　　　　　　　　　　□ Ulna
⑨ □ 豆状骨　　　　　　　　　　□ Pisiform bone
⑩ □ 第 2-5 中手骨　　　　　　　□ 2nd through 5th metacarpals
⑪ □ **第 4 背側骨間筋**　　　　　**□ 4th dorsal interosseous**
⑫ □ **第 3 背側骨間筋**　　　　　**□ 3rd dorsal interosseous**
⑬ □ 第 2-5 基節骨　　　　　　　□ 2nd through 5th proximal phalanges

筋	起始	停止(すべての筋)	停止(個々の筋)	作用	神経支配
第 1 背側骨間筋	第 1-5 中手骨の相対する面，2 頭	第 2-4 指の基節骨底，指背腱膜	第 2 指の基節骨底(橈側)	・第 2-4 指の MCP 関節：屈曲 ・第 2-4 指の PIP・DIP 関節：伸展，指の又を広げる(第 3 指を中心とした第 2，4 指の外転)	尺骨神経(C8-T1)
第 2 背側骨間筋			第 3 指の基節骨底(橈側)		
第 3 背側骨間筋			第 3 指の基節骨底(尺側)		
第 4 背側骨間筋			第 4 指の基節骨底(尺側)		

DIP 関節：遠位指節間関節　MCP 関節：中手指節関節　PIP 関節：近位指節間関節

System of the Muscles of the Hand V

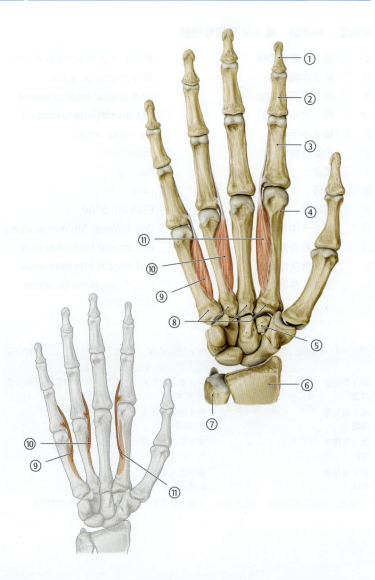

手の筋の区分 5

手内筋，中手筋：第 1-3 掌側骨間筋

① □ 第 2 末節骨の体 □ Shaft of 2nd distal phalanx
② □ 第 2 中節骨 □ 2nd middle phalanx
③ □ 第 2 基節骨 □ 2nd proximal phalanx
④ □ 第 2 中手骨 □ 2nd metacarpal
⑤ □ 小菱形骨 □ Trapezoid
⑥ □ 橈骨 □ Radius
⑦ □ 尺骨 □ Ulna
⑧ □ 第 2-5 中手骨 □ 2nd through 5th metacarpals
⑨ □ **第 3 掌側骨間筋** □ **3rd palmar interosseous**
⑩ □ **第 2 掌側骨間筋** □ **2nd palmar interosseous**
⑪ □ **第 1 掌側骨間筋** □ **1st palmar interosseous**

筋	起始	停止	作用	神経支配
第 1 掌側骨間筋	第 2 中手骨（尺側面）	第 2, 4, 5 各指の基節骨底と指背腱膜	・第 2, 4, 5 指の MCP 関節：屈曲 ・第 2, 4, 5 指の PIP・DIP 関節：伸展，広げた指の又を閉じる（第 2, 4, 5 指の第 3 指への内転）	尺骨神経（C8-T1）
第 2 掌側骨間筋	第 4 中手骨（橈側面）			
第 3 掌側骨間筋	第 5 中手骨（橈側面）			

DIP 関節：遠位指節間関節　MCP 関節：中手指節関節　PIP 関節：近位指節間関節

Arteries of the Upper Limb

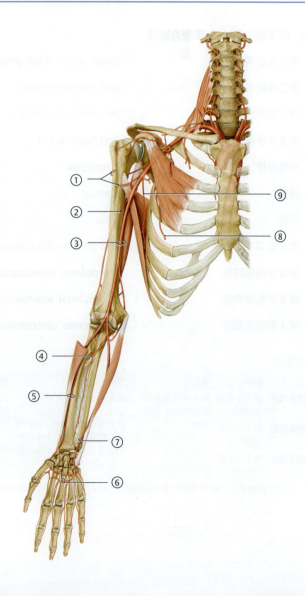

上肢の動脈

右上肢，前面

① □ 前・後上腕回旋動脈　　□ Anterior and posterior circumflex humeral arteries
② □ 上腕深動脈　　□ Profunda brachii artery
③ □ 上腕動脈　　□ Brachial artery
④ □ 後骨間動脈　　□ Posterior interosseous artery
⑤ □ 橈骨動脈　　□ Radial artery
⑥ □ 浅掌動脈弓　　□ Superficial palmar arch
⑦ □ 尺骨動脈　　□ Ulnar artery
⑧ □ 外側胸動脈　　□ Lateral thoracic artery
⑨ □ 胸背動脈　　□ Thoracodorsal artery

解説

　上肢に分布する動脈は鎖骨下動脈およびその枝である．鎖骨下動脈は第1肋骨の外側縁を越えたところで，腋窩動脈となる．また，腋窩動脈は大円筋の下縁を過ぎると上腕動脈となる．上腕動脈は肘窩で橈骨動脈と尺骨動脈に分かれる．この2つの動脈は手掌において，2つの動脈弓（浅・深掌動脈弓）を形成する．

Superficial Veins of the Upper Limb

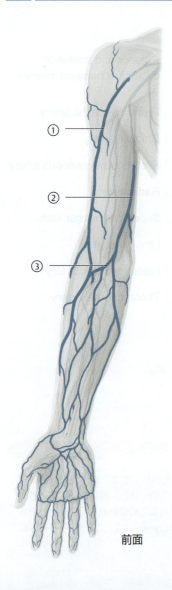

前面

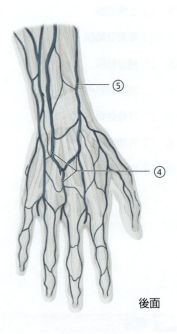

後面

上肢の皮静脈

右上肢，左：前面，右：後面

① □ 橈側皮静脈　　　　　　□ Cephalic vein
② □ 尺側皮静脈　　　　　　□ Basilic vein
③ □ 肘正中皮静脈　　　　　□ Median cubital vein
④ □ 手背静脈網　　　　　　□ Dorsal venous network
⑤ □ 橈側皮静脈　　　　　　□ Cephalic vein

臨床

　肘窩の静脈は採血の際に頻繁に利用される．採血の準備として上腕に駆血帯を巻く．この操作では皮静脈は容易に圧迫されるが，深部にある動脈は比較的圧迫を受けない．したがって，皮静脈はうっ滞した血液により怒張し，静脈の視認や触知が容易になる．

Structure of the Brachial Plexus

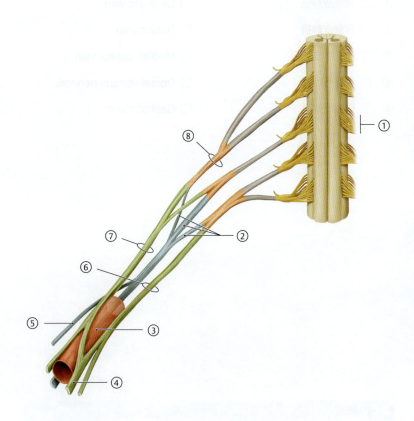

Q 後神経束に含まれる神経はどの根に由来するか？

腕神経叢の構造

右側,前面

①	□ 第7頸神経	□ C7 spinal nerve
②	□ 腕神経叢の後部	□ Posterior divisions of brachial plexus
③	□ 腋窩動脈	□ Axillary artery
④	□ 正中神経	□ Median nerve
⑤	□ 腋窩神経	□ Axillary nerve
⑥	□ 内側神経束	□ Medial cord
⑦	□ 外側神経束	□ Lateral cord
⑧	□ 上神経幹(第5・6頸神経)	□ Upper trunk(C5-C6 spinal nerve)

A 腕神経叢を構成する根(C5-T1)のすべてが後神経側の形成に関与する.

Course of the Brachial Plexus

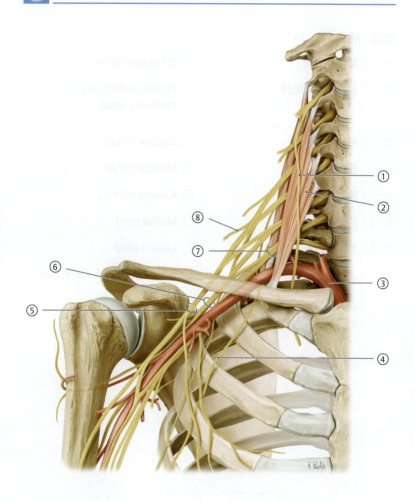

Q 腕神経叢のうち，鎖骨のすぐ後ろに存在するのは何か？

腕神経叢の走行

右側,前面

① □ 横隔神経　　　　　　□ Phrenic nerve
② □ 前斜角筋　　　　　　□ Scalenus anterior (anterior scalene)
③ □ 鎖骨下動脈　　　　　□ Subclavian artery
④ □ 長胸神経　　　　　　□ Long thoracic nerve
⑤ □ 外側神経束　　　　　□ Lateral cord
⑥ □ 後神経束　　　　　　□ Posterior cord
⑦ □ 下神経幹　　　　　　□ Lower trunk
⑧ □ 肩甲上神経　　　　　□ Suprascapular nerve

鎖骨の後ろには,腕神経叢の3本の神経束が存在する.

Nerves of the Brachial Plexus I

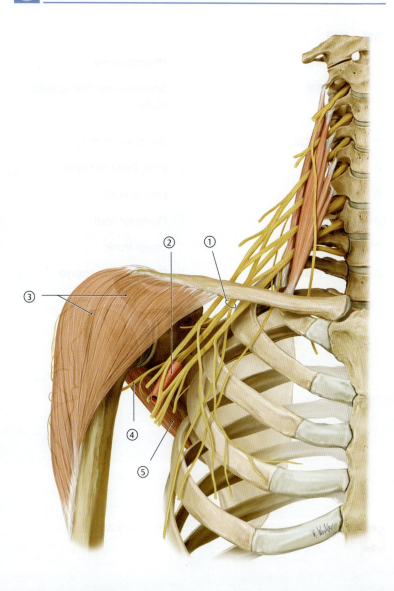

腕神経叢からの神経 1（腋窩神経）

右側，前面

① □ 後神経束　　　　　□ Posterior cord

② □ 腋窩動脈　　　　　□ Axillary artery

③ □ 三角筋　　　　　　□ Deltoid

④ □ 腋窩神経　　　　　□ Axillary nerve

⑤ □ 小円筋　　　　　　□ Teres minor

臨床

腋窩神経は上腕骨近位部の骨折に伴って損傷される場合がある．腋窩神経の損傷では，上肢の外転が制限され，三角筋による肩の盛り上がりが失われる．

Nerves of the Brachial Plexus II

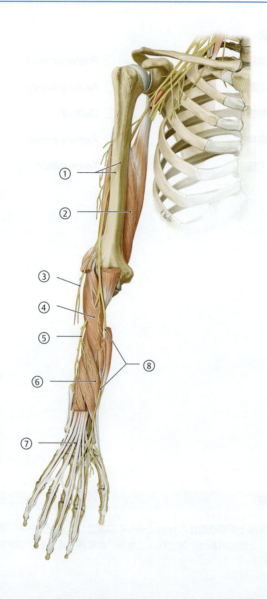

腕神経叢からの神経 2（橈骨神経）

右上肢，回内位，前面

① ☐ 橈骨神経（橈骨神経溝を通る） ☐ Radial nerve (in radial groove)

② ☐ 上腕三頭筋 ☐ Triceps brachii

③ ☐ 後前腕皮神経 ☐ Posterior antebrachial cutaneous nerve

④ ☐ 回外筋 ☐ Supinator

⑤ ☐ 後［前腕］骨間神経 ☐ Posterior interosseous nerve

⑥ ☐ 長母指外転筋 ☐ Abductor pollicis longus

⑦ ☐ ［総］指伸筋の腱 ☐ Extensor digitorum tendon

⑧ ☐ 橈骨神経の浅枝 ☐ Superficial branch of radial nerve

臨床

腋窩において橈骨神経が慢性的な圧迫を受けると（例えば，松葉杖の不適切な使用），上腕，前腕，手の感覚および運動機能が広範囲にわたって損なわれる場合がある．橈骨神経がより遠位で障害された場合，影響を受ける筋の数は少なくなり，上腕三頭筋の機能は正常だが，下垂手が見られるといった状態となる．

Nerves of the Brachial Plexus III

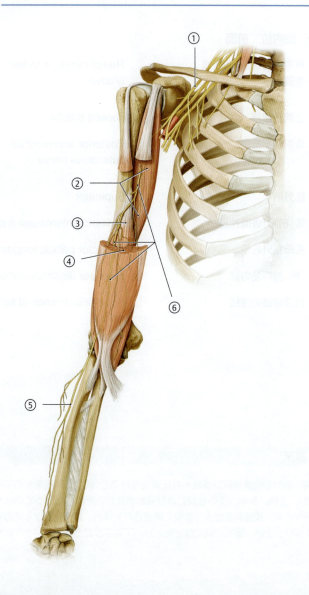

腕神経叢からの神経 3（筋皮神経）

右上肢，前面

① □ 外側神経束　　　　□ Lateral cord
② □ 烏口腕筋　　　　　□ Coracobrachialis
③ □ 上腕筋　　　　　　□ Brachialis
④ □ 上腕二頭筋　　　　□ Biceps brachii
⑤ □ 外側前腕皮神経　　□ Lateral antebrachial cutaneous nerve
⑥ □ 筋皮神経　　　　　□ Musculocutaneous nerve

Nerves of the Brachial Plexus IV

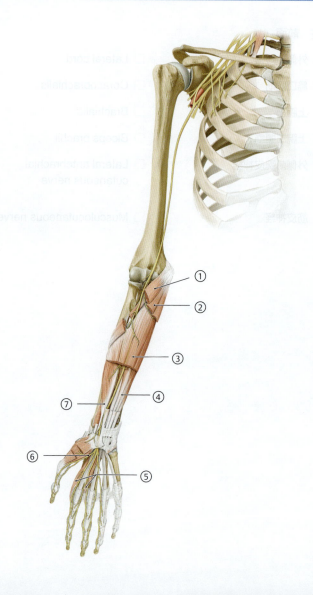

腕神経叢からの神経 4（正中神経）

右上肢，前面

① ☐ 円回内筋の上腕頭　　　　　☐ Humeral head of pronator teres

② ☐ 橈側手根屈筋　　　　　　　☐ Flexor carpi radialis

③ ☐ 浅指屈筋　　　　　　　　　☐ Flexor digitorum superficialis

④ ☐ 深指屈筋　　　　　　　　　☐ Flexor digitorum profundus

⑤ ☐ 第1・2虫様筋　　　　　　　☐ 1st and 2nd lumbricals

⑥ ☐ 母指球筋への筋枝　　　　　☐ Thenar muscular branch

⑦ ☐ 長母指屈筋　　　　　　　　☐ Flexor pollicis longus

臨床

　正中神経は腕神経叢から出る主要な神経であり，内側神経束と外側神経束の両方の成分からなる．肘関節の骨折や脱臼によって正中神経が損傷されると，手の把握機能と指先の感覚が損なわれる．

Nerves of the Brachial Plexus V

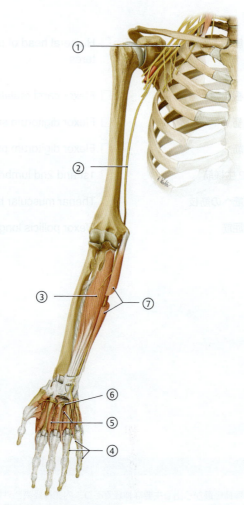

①
②
③
④
⑤
⑥
⑦

尺骨神経損傷の主要な特徴は何か？

腕神経叢からの神経 5（尺骨神経）

右上肢，前面

① □ 内側神経束　　　　□ Medial cord
② □ 尺骨神経　　　　　□ Ulnar nerve
③ □ 深指屈筋　　　　　□ Flexor digitorum profundus
④ □ 固有掌側指神経　　□ Proper palmar digital nerves
⑤ □ 骨間筋　　　　　　□ Interossei
⑥ □ 深枝　　　　　　　□ Deep branch
⑦ □ 尺側手根屈筋　　　□ Flexor carpi ulnaris

A 尺骨神経の損傷では，いわゆる「鷲手」が見られる．鷲手は，骨間筋（尺骨神経支配）の萎縮により，指が中手指節関節で過伸展位，近位および遠位指節間関節で軽い屈曲位をとるようになった状態を指す．

Neurovasculature of the Posterior Shoulder I

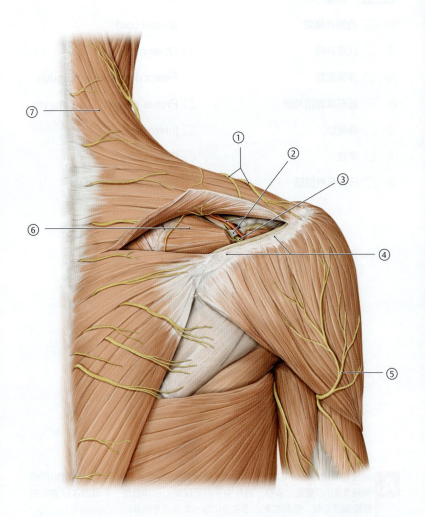

肩の後部における神経・血管 1

右肩，後面

①	□ 鎖骨上神経	□ Supraclavicular nerves
②	□ 肩甲上動脈（上肩甲横靭帯の上を通る）	□ Suprascapular artery (with superior transverse scapular ligament)
③	□ 肩甲上神経（肩甲切痕を通る）	□ Suprascapular nerve (in scapular notch)
④	□ 肩甲棘	□ Spine of scapular
⑤	□ 上外側上腕皮神経（腋窩神経の枝）	□ Superior lateral brachial cutaneous nerve (axillary nerve)
⑥	□ 棘上筋	□ Supraspinatus
⑦	□ 僧帽筋の下行部	□ Descending part of trapezius

Neurovasculature of the Posterior Shoulder II

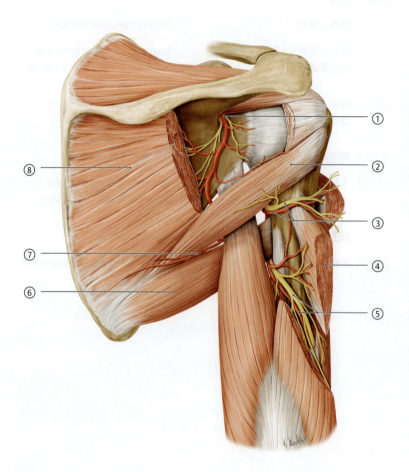

Q 肩甲骨動脈網に加わる主要な動脈は何か？

肩の後部における神経・血管 2

右肩，後面

① □ 肩甲上動脈・神経 □ Suprascapular artery and nerve

② □ 小円筋 □ Teres minor

③ □ 腋窩神経と後上腕回旋動脈 □ Axillary nerve and posterior circumflex humeral artery

④ □ 上腕三頭筋の外側頭 □ Lateral head of triceps brachii

⑤ □ 上腕深動脈と橈骨神経（橈骨神経溝を通る） □ Profunda brachii artery and radial nerve (in radial groove)

⑥ □ 大円筋 □ Teres major

⑦ □ 肩甲回旋動脈 □ Circumflex scapular artery

⑧ □ 棘下筋 □ Infraspinatus

肩甲骨動脈網を形成する主要な動脈は，甲状頸動脈から出る肩甲上動脈と頸横動脈（枝である肩甲背動脈を介して），腋窩動脈から出る肩甲下動脈の3種である．

Neurovasculature of the Axilla I

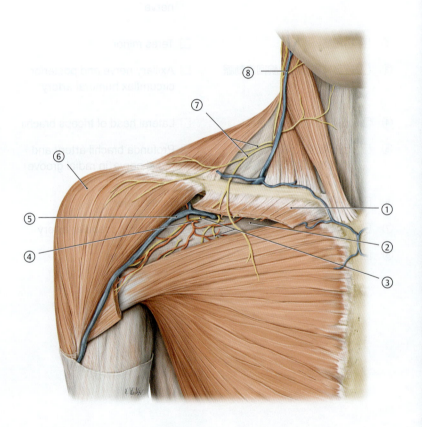

腋窩の神経・血管 1

右肩，前面

① ☐ 大胸筋の鎖骨部 　　　　☐ Clavicular part of pectoralis major

② ☐ 鎖骨胸筋筋膜 　　　　☐ Clavipectoral fascia

③ ☐ 内側・外側胸筋神経 　　　　☐ Medial and lateral pectoral nerves

④ ☐ 胸肩峰動脈 　　　　☐ Thoraco-acromial artery

⑤ ☐ 橈側皮静脈（三角筋胸筋溝を通る） 　　　　☐ Cephalic vein (in deltopectoral groove)

⑥ ☐ 三角筋 　　　　☐ Deltoid

⑦ ☐ 鎖骨上神経 　　　　☐ Supraclavicular nerves

⑧ ☐ 外頸静脈 　　　　☐ External jugular vein

Neurovasculature of the Axilla II

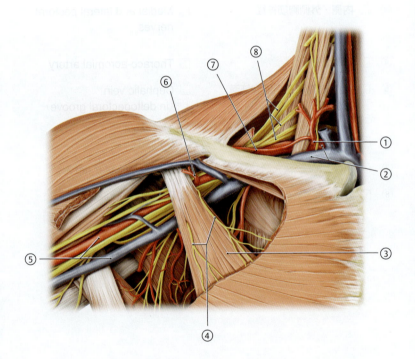

腋窩の神経・血管 2

右肩，前面

①	□ 甲状頸動脈	□ Thyrocervical trunk
②	□ 鎖骨下動脈・静脈	□ Subclavian artery and vein
③	□ 小胸筋	□ Pectoralis minor
④	□ 内側・外側胸筋神経	□ Medial and lateral pectoral nerves
⑤	□ 腋窩動脈・静脈	□ Axillary artery and vein
⑥	□ 胸肩峰動脈	□ Thoraco-acromial artery
⑦	□ 肩甲上動脈	□ Suprascapular artery
⑧	□ 腕神経叢（斜角筋隙から出る）	□ Brachial plexus（emerging from interscalene space）

Neurovasculature of the Axilla III

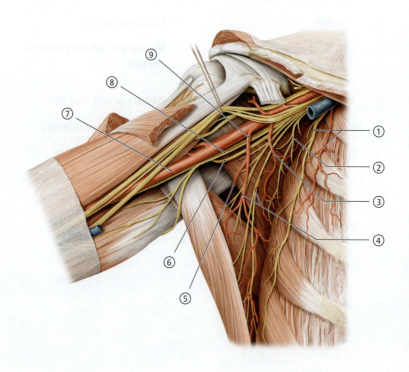

Q 長胸神経の起始はどこか？

腋窩の神経・血管 3

右肩，前面

① ☐ 長胸神経，最上胸動脈　　☐ Long thoracic nerve, superior thoracic artery

② ☐ 上肩甲下神経　　☐ Upper subscapular nerve
③ ☐ 外側胸動脈　　☐ Lateral thoracic artery
④ ☐ 胸背動脈・神経　　☐ Thoracodorsal artery and nerve

⑤ ☐ 肩甲回旋動脈　　☐ Circumflex scapular artery
⑥ ☐ 腋窩神経　　☐ Axillary nerve
⑦ ☐ 上腕動脈　　☐ Brachial artery
⑧ ☐ 橈骨神経　　☐ Radial nerve
⑨ ☐ 肩甲下動脈　　☐ Subscapular artery

A 長胸神経は腕神経叢の根（C5-C7）から起始する．

Neurovasculature of the Brachial Region

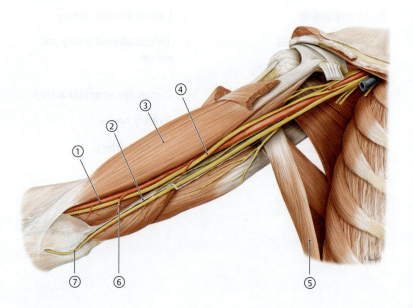

上腕の神経・血管

右上腕,前面

① □ 上腕動脈   □ Brachial artery
② □ 内側上腕筋間中隔   □ Medial intermuscular septum
③ □ 上腕二頭筋   □ Biceps brachii
④ □ 正中神経   □ Median nerve
⑤ □ 広背筋   □ Latissimus dorsi
⑥ □ 下尺側側副動脈   □ Inferior ulnar collateral artery
⑦ □ 尺骨神経(尺骨神経溝を通る)   □ Ulnar nerve (in ulnar groove)

Neurovasculature of the Forearm

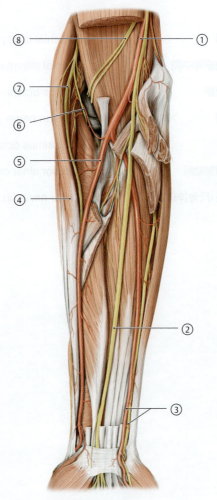

 前腕の筋のうち，尺骨神経に支配されるのはどれか？

前腕の神経・血管

右前腕，前面

① □ 上腕動脈 □ Brachial artery
② □ 正中神経 □ Median nerve
③ □ 尺骨動脈・神経 □ Ulnar artery and nerve
④ □ 腕橈骨筋 □ Brachioradialis
⑤ □ 橈骨動脈 □ Radial artery
⑥ □ 橈骨神経の深枝 □ Deep branch of radial nerve
⑦ □ 橈骨神経の浅枝 □ Superficial branch of radial nerve
⑧ □ 筋皮神経（外側前腕皮神経） □ Musculocutaneous nerve (lateral antebrachial cutaneous nerve)

 尺骨神経は，前腕では尺側手根屈筋と深指屈筋の尺側半分（第4・5指に腱を送る）を支配する．前腕の前区画に位置する残りの筋は正中神経によって支配される．

The Carpal Tunnel

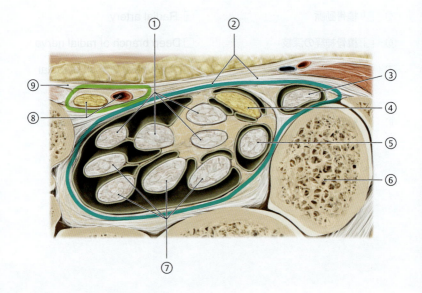

手根管

右手首の横断面，近位面（上面）

① □ 浅指屈筋の腱　　　□ Flexor digitorum superficialis tendons
② □ 屈筋支帯　　　　　□ Flexor retinaculum
③ □ 橈側手根屈筋の腱　□ Flexor carpi radialis tendon
④ □ 正中神経　　　　　□ Median nerve
⑤ □ 長母指屈筋の腱　　□ Flexor pollicis longus tendon
⑥ □ 舟状骨　　　　　　□ Scaphoid
⑦ □ 深指屈筋の腱　　　□ Flexor digitorum profundus tendons
⑧ □ 尺骨動脈・神経　　□ Ulnar artery and nerve
⑨ □ 掌側手根靱帯　　　□ Palmar carpal ligament

解説

　手根管は屈筋支帯と手根骨によって囲まれた空間である．正中神経や屈筋腱は手根管を通って手掌に達する．尺骨管は屈筋支帯と掌側手根靱帯によって囲まれた空間であり，ここを尺骨神経と尺骨動脈が通る．

Superficial Palmar Arch

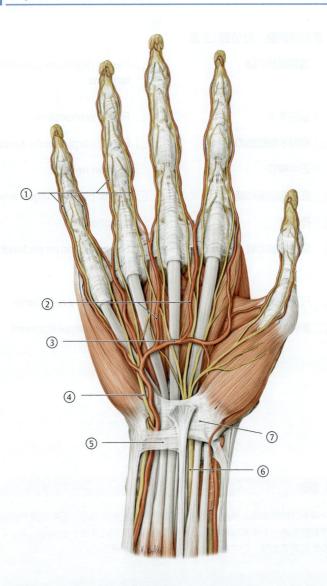

浅掌動脈弓

右手,前面(掌側面)

① □ 固有掌側指動脈・神経 □ Proper palmar digital arteries and nerves

② □ 総掌側指動脈 □ Common palmar digital arteries

③ □ 浅掌動脈弓 □ Superficial palmar arch

④ □ 尺骨神経の浅枝 □ Superficial branch of ulnar nerve

⑤ □ 掌側手根靱帯 □ Palmar carpal ligament

⑥ □ 正中神経 □ Median nerve

⑦ □ 屈筋支帯 □ Flexor retinaculum

臨床

手根管症候群では,感覚障害は指に現れるが,手掌の感覚は保たれる.これは,指に分布する正中神経の枝(総掌側指神経)が手根管よりも遠位で分かれるためである.正中神経の掌枝は手根管よりも近位で分かれ,手根管を通らずに手に達する.

Deep Palmar Arch

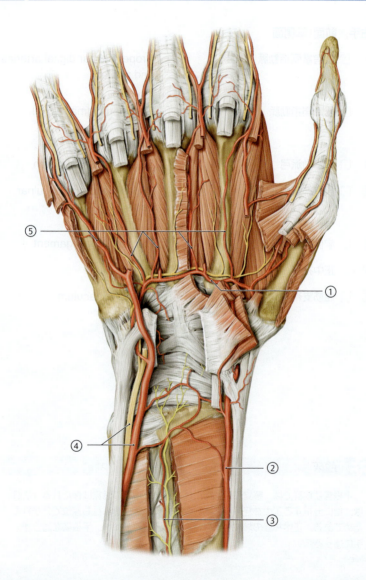

深掌動脈弓

右手，前面（掌側面）

① □ 深掌動脈弓　　　　　　□ Deep palmar arch
② □ 橈骨動脈　　　　　　　□ Radial artery
③ □ 前骨間動脈　　　　　　□ Anterior interosseous artery
④ □ 尺骨動脈・神経　　　　□ Ulnar artery and nerve
⑤ □ 掌側中手動脈　　　　　□ Palmar metacarpal arteries

Anatomic Snuffbox

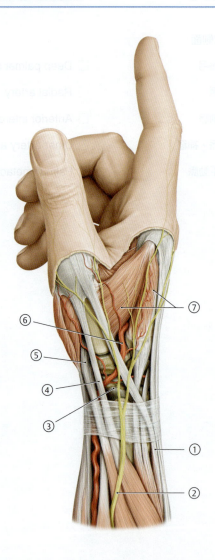

解剖学的嗅ぎタバコ入れ

右手，橈側面（内側面）

① ☐ 長母指伸筋の腱 ☐ Extensor pollicis longus tendon

② ☐ 橈骨神経の浅枝 ☐ Superficial branch of radial nerve

③ ☐ 舟状骨 ☐ Scaphoid

④ ☐ 短母指伸筋の腱 ☐ Extensor pollicis brevis tendon

⑤ ☐ 長母指外転筋の腱 ☐ Abductor pollicis longus tendon

⑥ ☐ 橈骨動脈 ☐ Radial artery

⑦ ☐ 第1背側骨間筋 ☐ 1st dorsal interosseous

臨床

　解剖学的嗅ぎタバコ入れは，手首の橈側面（外側面）に位置した小区画であり，境界は長母指伸筋腱，短母指伸筋腱，長母指外転筋腱によって形成される．嗅ぎタバコ入れの床の大部分は舟状骨からなるので，舟状骨骨折では嗅ぎタバコ入れに自発痛や圧痛が見られる．

Sensory Innervation of the Hand I

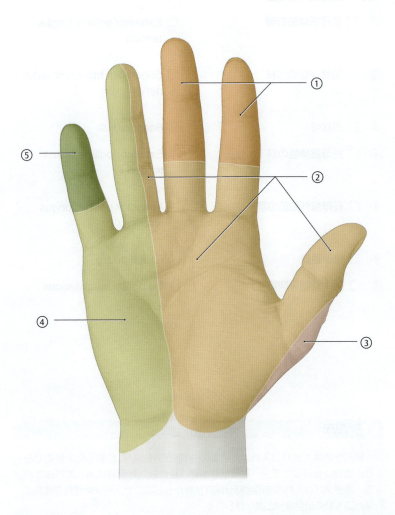

手における感覚神経の分布 1

右手，前面（掌側面）

① ☐ 掌側指神経（正中神経の固有領域） ☐ Palmar digital nerves (exclusive area of median nerve)

② ☐ 正中神経の掌枝 ☐ Palmar branch of median nerve

③ ☐ 橈骨神経，背側指神経 ☐ Radial nerve, dorsal digital nerve

④ ☐ 尺骨神経の掌枝 ☐ Palmar branch of ulnar nerve

⑤ ☐ 掌側指神経（尺骨神経の固有領域） ☐ Palmar digital nerve (exclusive area of ulnar nerve)

Sensory Innervation of the Hand II

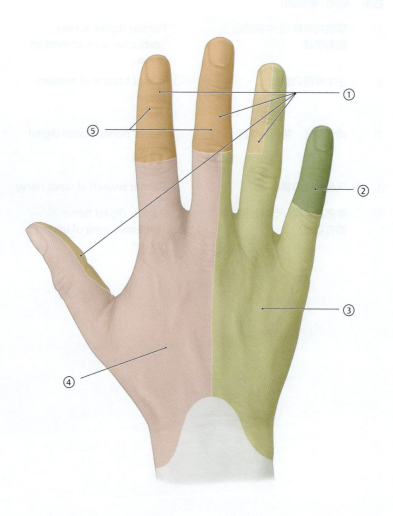

手における感覚神経の分布 2

右手，後面（背側面）

① □ 正中神経と掌側指神経の背側枝 　　　□ Median nerve and dorsal branches of palmar digital nerves

② □ 背側指神経（尺骨神経の固有領域） 　　　□ Dorsal digital nerve (exclusive area of ulnar nerve)

③ □ 尺骨神経の背側枝 　　　□ Dorsal branch of ulnar nerve

④ □ 橈骨神経の浅枝と背側指神経 　　　□ Superficial branch of radial nerve and dorsal digital nerves

⑤ □ 正中神経の固有領域 　　　□ Exclusive area of median nerve

Transverse Section of the Arm

背側

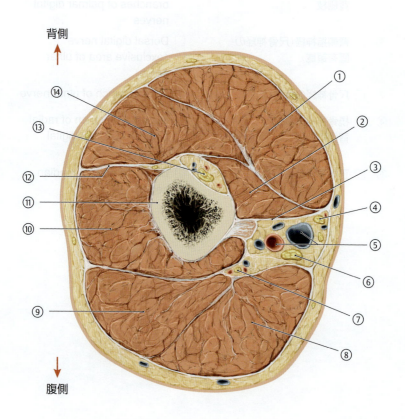

腹側

上腕の横断面

右上腕，近位方向（上方）から見たところ

① □ 上腕三頭筋の長頭　　□ Long head of triceps brachii
② □ 上腕三頭筋の内側頭　□ Medial head of triceps brachii
③ □ 内側上腕筋間中隔　　□ Medial intermuscular septum
④ □ 尺骨神経　　　　　　□ Ulnar nerve
⑤ □ 上腕動脈・静脈　　　□ Brachial artery and vein
⑥ □ 正中神経　　　　　　□ Median nerve
⑦ □ 筋皮神経　　　　　　□ Musculocutaneus nerve
⑧ □ 上腕二頭筋の短頭　　□ Short head of biceps brachii
⑨ □ 上腕二頭筋の長頭　　□ Long head of biceps brachii
⑩ □ 上腕筋　　　　　　　□ Brachialis
⑪ □ 上腕骨　　　　　　　□ Humerus
⑫ □ 外側上腕筋間中隔　　□ Lateral intermuscular septum
⑬ □ 橈骨神経　　　　　　□ Radial nerve
⑭ □ 上腕三頭筋の外側頭　□ Lateral head of triceps brachii

解説

　上・下肢の筋は筋間中隔によって，区画化されている．各区画に入る筋どうしは同様の機能を有し，多くの場合，同じ神経と血管が分布する．

Transverse Section of the Forearm

背側

腹側

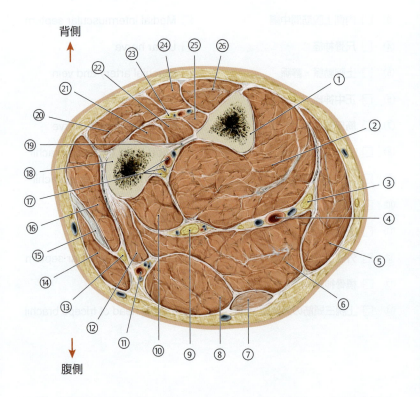

前腕の横断面

右前腕，近位方向（上方）から見たところ

① ☐ 尺骨 — ☐ Ulna
② ☐ 深指屈筋 — ☐ Flexor digitorum profundus
③ ☐ 尺骨神経 — ☐ Ulnar nerve
④ ☐ 尺骨動脈 — ☐ Ulnar artery
⑤ ☐ 尺側手根屈筋 — ☐ Flexor carpi ulnaris
⑥ ☐ 浅指屈筋 — ☐ Flexor digitorum superficialis
⑦ ☐ 長掌筋 — ☐ Palmaris longus
⑧ ☐ 橈側手根屈筋 — ☐ Flexor carpi radialis
⑨ ☐ 正中神経 — ☐ Median nerve
⑩ ☐ 長母指屈筋 — ☐ Flexor pollicis longus
⑪ ☐ 橈骨動脈 — ☐ Radial artery
⑫ ☐ 円回内筋 — ☐ Pronetor teres
⑬ ☐ 橈骨神経の浅枝 — ☐ Superficial branch of radial nerve
⑭ ☐ 腕橈骨筋 — ☐ Brachioradialis
⑮ ☐ 長橈側手根伸筋 — ☐ Extensor carpi radialis longus
⑯ ☐ 短橈側手根伸筋 — ☐ Extensor carpi radialis brevis
⑰ ☐ 前骨間動脈・静脈・神経 — ☐ Anterior interosseous artery, vein, and nerve
⑱ ☐ 橈骨 — ☐ Radius
⑲ ☐ 前腕骨間膜 — ☐ Interosseous membrane
⑳ ☐ ［総］指伸筋 — ☐ Extensor digitorum
㉑ ☐ 長母指外転筋 — ☐ Abductor pollicis longus
㉒ ☐ 短母指伸筋 — ☐ Extensor pollicis brevis
㉓ ☐ 後骨間神経 — ☐ Posterior interosseous nerve
㉔ ☐ 小指伸筋 — ☐ Extensor digiti minimi
㉕ ☐ 長母指伸筋 — ☐ Extensor pollicis longus
㉖ ☐ 尺側手根伸筋 — ☐ Extensor carpi ulnaris

Surface Anatomy

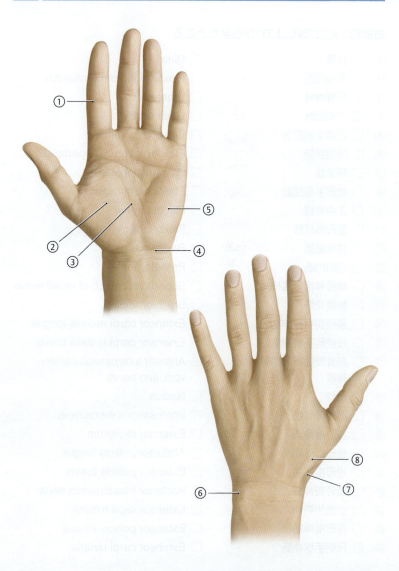

手の体表解剖

左手，上：前面（掌側面），下：後面（背側面）

① □ 近位指節間（PIP）関節線 □ Proximal interphalangeal joint crease

② □ 母指球 □ Thenar eminence

③ □ 母指線（"生命線"） □ Thenar crease（"life line"）

④ □ 遠位手根線 □ Distal wrist crease

⑤ □ 小指球 □ Hypothenar eminence

⑥ □ 尺骨の茎状突起 □ Ulnar styloid process

⑦ □ 解剖学的嗅ぎタバコ入れ □ Anatomic snuffbox

⑧ □ 長母指伸筋の腱 □ Extensor pollicis longus tendon

手の体表解剖

下肢 Lower Limb

下肢の骨格 ………………………… *506*
寛骨の構成 ………………………… *508*
大腿骨 ……………………………… *510*
股関節 1, 2 ………………………… *512*
股関節の靱帯 1, 2 ………………… *516*
骨盤と大腿の筋 1-8 ……………… *520*
骨盤と殿部の筋の区分 1-7 ……… *536*
大腿の筋の区分 1-4 ……………… *550*
脛骨と腓骨 ………………………… *558*
膝関節 1, 2 ………………………… *560*
膝関節の靱帯 1-3 ………………… *564*
下腿の筋 1-5 ……………………… *570*
下腿の筋の区分 1-4 ……………… *580*
足の骨格 1, 2 ……………………… *588*
足首と足の関節 1-3 ……………… *592*
足首と足の靱帯 1-3 ……………… *598*
足底の筋 1-4 ……………………… *604*
足首と足 …………………………… *612*
足の筋の区分 1-7 ………………… *614*

下肢の動脈 1, 2 …………………… *628*
腰仙骨神経叢 1, 2 ………………… *632*
腰神経叢からの神経 1, 2 ………… *636*
仙骨神経叢からの神経 1, 2 ……… *640*
皮静脈と皮神経 …………………… *644*
鼡径部 ……………………………… *646*
坐骨孔 ……………………………… *648*
大腿前面の神経・血管 …………… *650*
大腿後面の神経・血管 …………… *652*
下腿後面の神経・血管 …………… *654*
足根管 ……………………………… *656*
下腿外側の神経・血管 …………… *658*
下腿前面の神経・血管 …………… *660*
足背の神経・血管 ………………… *662*
足底の神経・血管 ………………… *664*
大腿の横断面 ……………………… *666*
下腿の横断面 ……………………… *668*
下肢の体表解剖 …………………… *670*

Bones of the Lower Limb

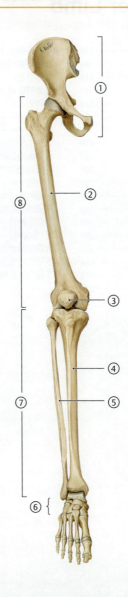

下肢の骨格

右下肢，前面

① □ 下肢帯　　　　　□ Pelvic girdle

② □ 大腿骨　　　　　□ Femur

③ □ 膝蓋骨　　　　　□ Patella

④ □ 脛骨　　　　　　□ Tibia

⑤ □ 腓骨　　　　　　□ Fibula

⑥ □ 足根骨　　　　　□ Tarsal bones

⑦ □ 下腿　　　　　　□ Lower leg

⑧ □ 大腿　　　　　　□ Thigh

Components of the Hip Bone

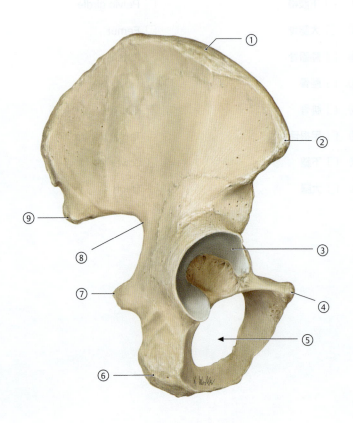

Q 寛骨は3つの骨が寛骨臼で融合してできる．この3つの骨とは何か？

寛骨の構成

右寛骨，外側面

① □ 腸骨稜　　　　　□ Iliac crest
② □ 上前腸骨棘　　　□ Anterior superior iliac spine
③ □ 寛骨臼　　　　　□ Acetabulum
④ □ 恥骨結節　　　　□ Pubic tubercle
⑤ □ 閉鎖孔　　　　　□ Obturator foramen
⑥ □ 坐骨結節　　　　□ Ischial tuberosity
⑦ □ 坐骨棘　　　　　□ Ischial spine
⑧ □ 大坐骨切痕　　　□ Greater sciatic notch
⑨ □ 下後腸骨棘　　　□ Posterior inferior iliac spine

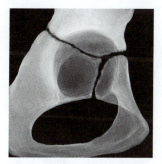

小児における右寛骨臼のX線像

寛骨は腸骨，坐骨，恥骨が融合してできる．融合は14〜16歳の間に起こる．

Femur

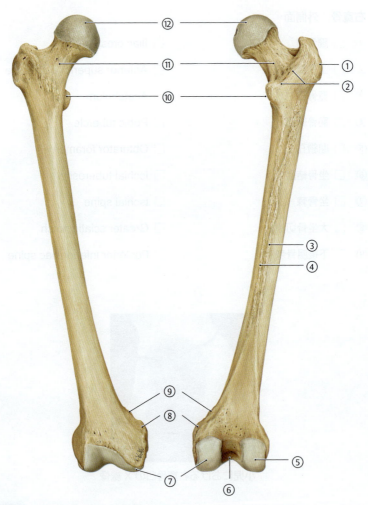

骨粗鬆症患者の大腿骨骨折はどの部位に起こりやすいか？

大腿骨

右大腿骨，左：前面，右：後面

① ☐ 大転子　　　　　　　　☐ Greater trochanter
② ☐ 転子間稜　　　　　　　☐ Intertrochanteric crest
③ ☐ 粗線の外側唇　　　　　☐ Lateral lip of linea aspera
④ ☐ 粗線の内側唇　　　　　☐ Medial lip of linea aspera
⑤ ☐ 外側顆　　　　　　　　☐ Lateral condyle
⑥ ☐ 顆間窩　　　　　　　　☐ Intercondylar notch
⑦ ☐ 内側顆　　　　　　　　☐ Medial condyle
⑧ ☐ 内側上顆　　　　　　　☐ Medial epicondyle
⑨ ☐ 内転筋結節　　　　　　☐ Adductor tubercle
⑩ ☐ 小転子　　　　　　　　☐ Lesser trochanter
⑪ ☐ 大腿骨頸　　　　　　　☐ Neck of femur
⑫ ☐ 大腿骨頭　　　　　　　☐ Head of femur

A 骨粗鬆症患者の大腿骨骨折は大腿骨頸に起こりやすい．

Hip Joint I

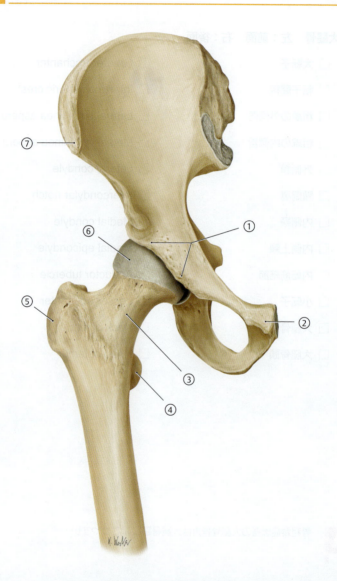

股関節 1

右股関節,前面

① □ 寛骨臼縁　　　　　　□ Bony acetabular rim

② □ 恥骨結節　　　　　　□ Pubic tubercle

③ □ 大腿骨頚　　　　　　□ Neck of femur

④ □ 小転子　　　　　　　□ Lesser trochanter

⑤ □ 大転子　　　　　　　□ Greater trochanter

⑥ □ 大腿骨頭　　　　　　□ Head of femur

⑦ □ 上前腸骨棘　　　　　□ Anterior superior iliac spine

 解説

　大腿骨頭は寛骨の寛骨臼との間で,球関節の一種である股関節を形成する（球関節とは,ボールとソケットを組み合わせたような様式の関節を指す）.大腿骨頭はほぼ球状であり（平均曲率半径は約2.5 cm）,その大部分が寛骨臼内にはまり込む.

Hip Joint II

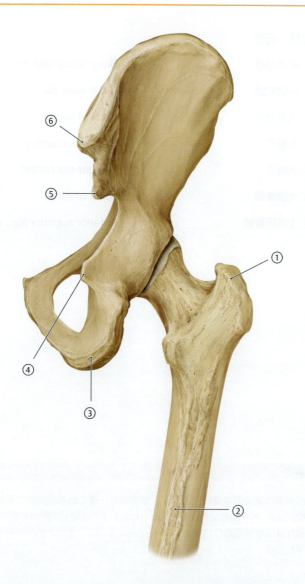

股関節 2

右股関節，後面

① □ 大転子 □ Greater trochanter
② □ 粗線 □ Linea aspera
③ □ 坐骨結節 □ Ischial tuberosity
④ □ 坐骨棘 □ Ischial spine
⑤ □ 下後腸骨棘 □ Posterior inferior iliac spine
⑥ □ 上後腸骨棘 □ Posterior superior iliac spine

臨床

乳幼児における股関節のスクリーニング検査において，超音波検査は最も重要なものである．この検査では，股関節の低形成や脱臼といった形態的な異常を見つけ出すことができる．股関節脱臼の患者では，股関節の不安定性や外転制限，殿溝の非対称を伴った下肢の短縮が見られる．

Ligaments of the Hip Joint I

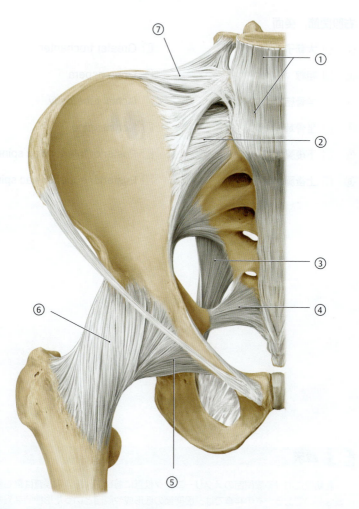

 股関節はどの肢位において最も不安定となるか(最も脱臼しやすいか)？

股関節の靱帯 1

右股関節,前面

① □ 前縦靱帯　　　　　　　□ Anterior longitudinal ligament
② □ 前仙腸靱帯　　　　　　□ Anterior sacro-iliac ligaments
③ □ 仙結節靱帯　　　　　　□ Sacrotuberous ligament
④ □ 仙棘靱帯　　　　　　　□ Sacrospinous ligament
⑤ □ 恥骨大腿靱帯　　　　　□ Pubofemoral ligament
⑥ □ 腸骨大腿靱帯　　　　　□ Iliofemoral ligament
⑦ □ 腸腰靱帯　　　　　　　□ Iliolumbar ligament

A 　股関節の関節包は,大腿骨頸をラセン状に取り巻く3つの靱帯(腸骨大腿靱帯,恥骨大腿靱帯,坐骨大腿靱帯)で補強されている.これらの靱帯は外転屈曲位において弛緩し,このとき股関節が最も不安定となる.

Ligaments of the Hip Joint II

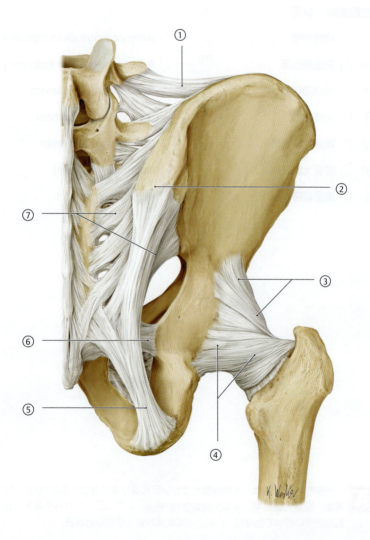

股関節の靱帯 2

右股関節, 後面

① ☐ 腸腰靱帯 ☐ Iliolumbar ligament
② ☐ 上後腸骨棘 ☐ Posterior superior iliac spine
③ ☐ 腸骨大腿靱帯 ☐ Iliofemoral ligament
④ ☐ 坐骨大腿靱帯 ☐ Ischiofemoral ligament
⑤ ☐ 仙結節靱帯 ☐ Sacrotuberous ligament
⑥ ☐ 仙棘靱帯 ☐ Sacrospinous ligament
⑦ ☐ 後仙腸靱帯 ☐ Posterior sacro-iliac ligaments

Muscles of the Hip & Thigh I

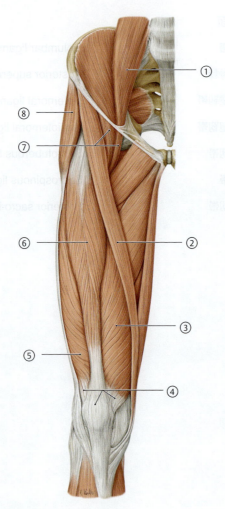

Q 大腿三角とはどこか？

骨盤と大腿の筋 1

右下肢，前面

① □ 大腰筋　　　　　　□ Psoas major

② □ 縫工筋　　　　　　□ Sartorius

③ □ 内側広筋　　　　　□ Vastus medialis

④ □ 大腿四頭筋の腱　　□ Quadriceps femoris tendon

⑤ □ 外側広筋　　　　　□ Vastus lateralis

⑥ □ 大腿直筋　　　　　□ Rectus femoris

⑦ □ 腸腰筋　　　　　　□ Iliopsoas

⑧ □ 大腿筋膜張筋　　　□ Tensor fasciae latae

　大腿三角は鼡径靱帯，縫工筋，長内転筋によって囲まれた大腿前面の領域であり，大腿動脈，大腿静脈，大腿神経がここを通過する．腸腰筋と恥骨筋は大腿三角の後壁（床）を形成する．

Muscles of the Hip & Thigh II

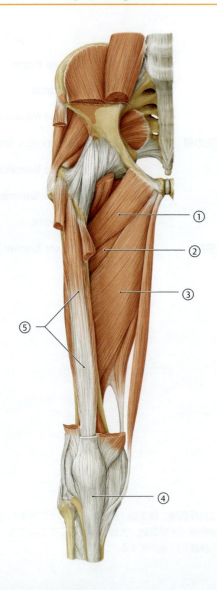

骨盤と大腿の筋 2

右下肢，前面．縫工筋，大腿直筋，外側広筋，内側広筋，腸腰筋と大腿筋膜張筋を取り除いたところ

① □ 恥骨筋　　　　　□ Pectineus
② □ 短内転筋　　　　□ Adductor brevis
③ □ 長内転筋　　　　□ Adductor longus
④ □ 膝蓋靱帯　　　　□ Patellar ligament
⑤ □ 中間広筋　　　　□ Vastus intermedius

Muscles of the Hip & Thigh III

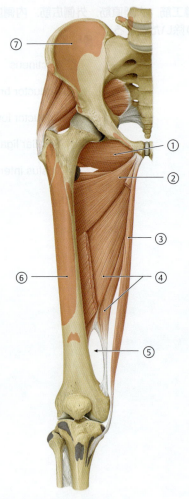

[内転筋]腱裂孔を通過する血管は何か？

骨盤と大腿の筋 3

右下肢，前面．大腿四頭筋，腸腰筋，大腿筋膜張筋を完全に取り除き，長内転筋の中央部分を取り除いたところ

① □ 外閉鎖筋　　　　　　　　□ Obturator externus
② □ 短内転筋　　　　　　　　□ Adductor brevis
③ □ 薄筋　　　　　　　　　　□ Gracilis
④ □ 大内転筋　　　　　　　　□ Adductor magnus
⑤ □ ［内転筋］腱裂孔　　　　□ Adductor hiatus
⑥ □ 中間広筋（筋の起始）　　□ Vastus intermedius（origin）
⑦ □ 腸骨筋（筋の起始）　　　□ Iliacus（origin）

A 　大腿動脈と大腿静脈が［内転筋］腱裂孔を通過し，大腿前面から膝窩に達する．

Muscles of the Hip & Thigh IV

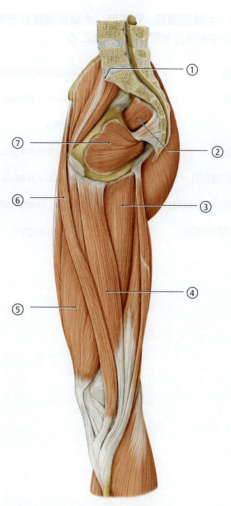

Q 縫工筋，薄筋，半腱様筋の共通停止腱は何と呼ばれるか？

骨盤と大腿の筋 4

右下肢,内側面

① □ 岬角 □ Promontory
② □ 梨状筋 □ Piriformis
③ □ 大内転筋 □ Adductor magnus
④ □ 薄筋 □ Gracilis
⑤ □ 内側広筋 □ Vastus medialis
⑥ □ 縫工筋 □ Sartorius
⑦ □ 内閉鎖筋 □ Obturator internus

A 　縫工筋,薄筋,半腱様筋は,鵞足と呼ばれる共通停止腱を形成する.鵞足の直下には鵞足包(滑液包の一種)が存在する.

Muscles of the Hip & Thigh V

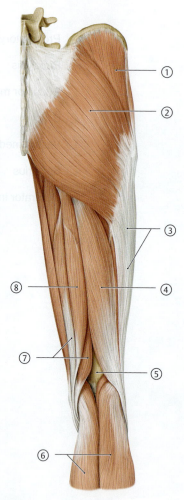

Q 大殿筋の機能は何か？

骨盤と大腿の筋 5

右下肢，後面

① ☐ 中殿筋　　☐ Gluteus medius
② ☐ 大殿筋　　☐ Gluteus maximus
③ ☐ 腸脛靱帯　　☐ Iliotibial tract
④ ☐ 大腿二頭筋の長頭　　☐ Long head of biceps femoris
⑤ ☐ 膝窩　　☐ Posterior part of knee
⑥ ☐ 腓腹筋の内側頭と外側頭　　☐ Medial and lateral heads of gastrocnemius
⑦ ☐ 半膜様筋　　☐ Semimembranosus
⑧ ☐ 半腱様筋　　☐ Semitendinosus

A 大殿筋は股関節を伸展・外旋する強力な筋である．また，大殿筋の上部は股関節の外転作用，下部は股関節の内転作用を有する．

Muscles of the Hip & Thigh VI

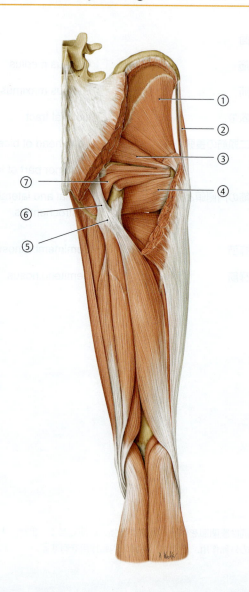

骨盤と大腿の筋 6

右下肢，後面．大殿筋と中殿筋を部分的に取り除いたところ

① □ 小殿筋　　　　　　　　□ Gluteus minimus

② □ 大腿筋膜張筋　　　　　□ Tensor fasciae latae

③ □ 梨状筋　　　　　　　　□ Piriformis

④ □ 大腿方形筋　　　　　　□ Quadratus femoris

⑤ □ 坐骨結節　　　　　　　□ Ischial tuberosity

⑥ □ 仙結節靱帯　　　　　　□ Sacrotuberous ligament

⑦ □ 内閉鎖筋　　　　　　　□ Obturator internus

解説

　ハムストリングス（半腱様筋，半膜様筋，大腿二頭筋の長頭）はすべてが坐骨結節から起始し，坐骨神経の脛骨神経部によって支配される．これらの筋は，股関節の伸筋ならびに膝関節の屈筋として働く．

Muscles of the Hip & Thigh VII

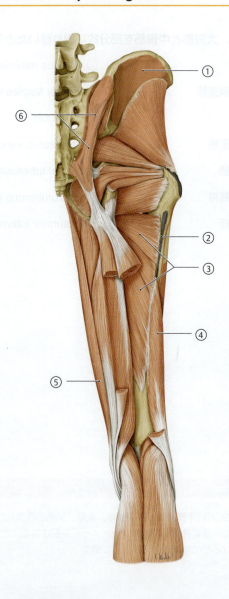

骨盤と大腿の筋 7

右下肢，後面．大殿筋と小殿筋を完全に取り除き，半腱様筋と大腿二頭筋を部分的に取り除いたところ

① □ 中殿筋（筋の起始）　　　□ Gluteus medius（origin）

② □ 大殿筋（筋の停止）　　　□ Gluteus maximus（insertion）

③ □ 大内転筋　　　　　　　　□ Adductor magnus

④ □ 大腿二頭筋の短頭　　　　□ Short head of biceps femoris

⑤ □ 薄筋　　　　　　　　　　□ Gracilis

⑥ □ 大殿筋（筋の起始）　　　□ Gluteus maximus（origin）

Muscles of the Hip & Thigh VIII

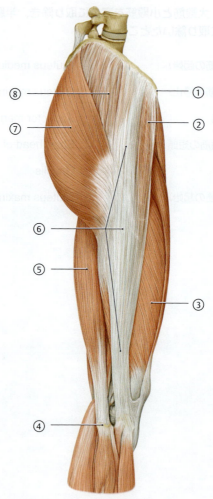

Q 腸脛靱帯とは何か？

骨盤と大腿の筋 8

右下肢,外側面

① ☐ 上前腸骨棘　　　　☐ Anterior superior iliac spine
② ☐ 大腿筋膜張筋　　　☐ Tensor fasciae latae
③ ☐ 外側広筋　　　　　☐ Vastus lateralis
④ ☐ 腓骨頭　　　　　　☐ Head of fibula
⑤ ☐ 大腿二頭筋の長頭　☐ Long head of biceps femoris
⑥ ☐ 腸脛靱帯　　　　　☐ Iliotibial tract
⑦ ☐ 大殿筋　　　　　　☐ Gluteus maximus
⑧ ☐ 中殿筋　　　　　　☐ Gluteus medius

　腸脛靱帯は大腿筋膜の外側部が肥厚したものであり,長軸方向に発達した線維によって補強されている.腸脛靱帯は幅の広い帯のようであり,腸骨稜と脛骨の前外側面の間に張っている.腸脛靱帯の上部は,大腿筋膜張筋を包み込むとともに,大殿筋腱膜の停止にもなっている.

System of the Muscles of the Hip & Gluteal Region I

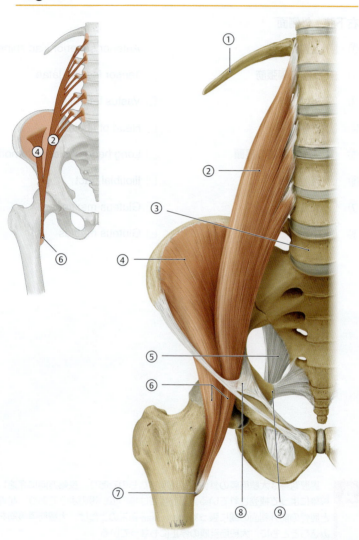

骨盤と殿部の筋の区分 1

骨盤内部の筋：大腰筋と腸骨筋

① ☐ 第 12 肋骨　　☐ 12th rib
② ☐ **大腰筋**　　☐ **Psoas major**
③ ☐ 第 5 腰椎　　☐ L5 vertebra
④ ☐ **腸骨筋**　　☐ **Iliacus**
⑤ ☐ 仙結節靱帯　　☐ Sacrotuberous ligament
⑥ ☐ 腸腰筋　　☐ Iliopsoas
⑦ ☐ 小転子　　☐ Lesser trochanter
⑧ ☐ 腸恥筋膜弓　　☐ Iliopectineal arch
⑨ ☐ 坐骨棘　　☐ Ischiadic spine

筋	起始	停止	作用	神経支配
大腰筋の浅層	T12-L4 の椎体と椎間円板（側面）	大腿骨の小転子（腸腰筋として）	・股関節：屈曲・外旋 ・腰部脊柱：大腿を固定した状態で片側が収縮すると体幹を同側に曲げる，仰臥位で両側が収縮すると体幹を引き起こす	・大腿神経（L2-L4） ・腰神経叢からの直接の枝
大腰筋の深層	L1-L5 の椎骨（肋骨突起）			
腸骨筋	腸骨窩			

System of the Muscles of the Hip & Gluteal Region II

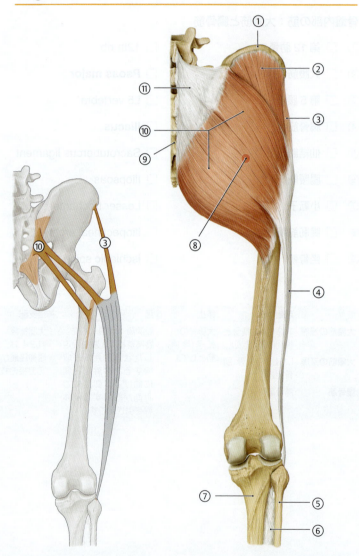

骨盤と殿部の筋の区分 2

縦方向に走る殿筋群：大殿筋と大腿筋膜張筋

① □ 腸骨稜　　　　　　　　□ Iliac crest

② □ 中殿筋　　　　　　　　□ Gluteus medius

③ □ **大腿筋膜張筋**　　　　□ **Tensor fasciae latae**

④ □ 腸脛靱帯　　　　　　　□ Iliotibial tract

⑤ □ 腓骨　　　　　　　　　□ Fibula

⑥ □ 下腿骨間膜　　　　　　□ Interosseous membrane

⑦ □ 脛骨　　　　　　　　　□ Tibia

⑧ □ 外転軸/内転軸　　　　　□ Axis of abduction/adduction

⑨ □ 仙骨　　　　　　　　　□ Sacrum

⑩ □ **大殿筋**　　　　　　　□ **Gluteus maximus**

⑪ □ 胸腰筋膜　　　　　　　□ Thoracolumbar fascia

筋	起始	停止	作用	神経支配
大殿筋	・仙骨（後面の外側部） ・腸骨の殿筋面の後部（後殿筋線の後部） ・胸腰筋膜 ・仙結節靱帯	・上部の筋束：腸脛靱帯 ・下部の筋束：殿筋粗面	・筋全体：股関節の伸展・外旋・矢状面および冠状面における股関節の安定化 ・上部の筋束：外転 ・下部の筋束：内転	下殿神経 (L4-S2)
大腿筋膜張筋	上前腸骨棘	腸脛靱帯	・大腿筋膜の緊張 ・股関節：外転・屈曲・内旋	上殿神経 (L4-S1)

System of the Muscles of the Hip & Gluteal Region III

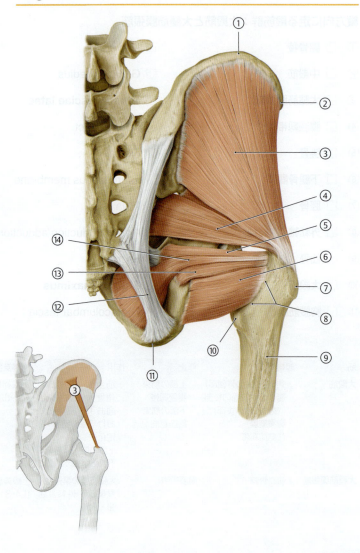

骨盤と殿部の筋の区分 3

縦方向に走る殿筋群：中殿筋

① ☐ 腸骨稜　　　　　☐ Iliac crest
② ☐ 上前腸骨棘　　　☐ Anterior superior iliac spine
③ ☐ **中殿筋**　　　　☐ **Gluteus medius**
④ ☐ 梨状筋　　　　　☐ Piriformis
⑤ ☐ 上双子筋　　　　☐ Gemellus superior
⑥ ☐ 大腿方形筋　　　☐ Quadratus femoris
⑦ ☐ 大転子　　　　　☐ Greater trochanter
⑧ ☐ 転子間稜　　　　☐ Intertrochanteric crest
⑨ ☐ 殿筋粗面　　　　☐ Gluteal tuberosity
⑩ ☐ 小転子　　　　　☐ Lesser trochanter
⑪ ☐ 坐骨結節　　　　☐ Ischial tuberosity
⑫ ☐ 仙結節靱帯　　　☐ Sacrotuberous ligament
⑬ ☐ 下双子筋　　　　☐ Gemellus inferior
⑭ ☐ 内閉鎖筋　　　　☐ Obturator internus

筋	起始	停止	作用	神経支配
中殿筋	腸骨の殿筋面（腸骨稜と前・後殿筋線に挟まれた部分）	大腿骨の大転子（外側面）	・筋全体：外転・冠状面における骨盤の安定化 ・前部：屈曲・内旋 ・後部：伸展・外旋	上殿神経（L4-S1）

System of the Muscles of the Hip & Gluteal Region IV

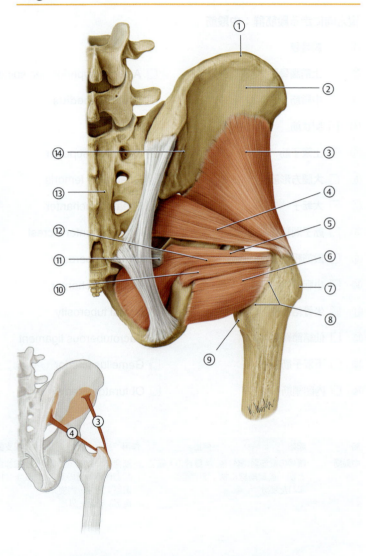

骨盤と殿部の筋の区分 4

縦方向に走る殿筋群：小殿筋と梨状筋

① ☐ 腸骨稜　　　　　　　　　☐ Iliac crest
② ☐ 腸骨の殿筋面　　　　　　☐ Gluteal surface of ilium
③ ☐ 小殿筋　　　　　　　　　☐ **Gluteus minimus**
④ ☐ 梨状筋　　　　　　　　　☐ **Piriformis**
⑤ ☐ 上双子筋　　　　　　　　☐ Gemellus superior
⑥ ☐ 大腿方形筋　　　　　　　☐ Quadratus femoris
⑦ ☐ 大転子　　　　　　　　　☐ Greater trochanter
⑧ ☐ 転子間稜　　　　　　　　☐ Intertrochanteric crest
⑨ ☐ 小転子　　　　　　　　　☐ Lesser trochanter
⑩ ☐ 下双子筋　　　　　　　　☐ Gemellus inferior
⑪ ☐ 坐骨棘　　　　　　　　　☐ Ischiadic spine
⑫ ☐ 内閉鎖筋　　　　　　　　☐ Obturator internus
⑬ ☐ 仙骨　　　　　　　　　　☐ Sacrum
⑭ ☐ 後殿筋線　　　　　　　　☐ Posterior gluteal line

筋	起始	停止	作用	神経支配
小殿筋	腸骨の殿筋面（中殿筋の起始部よりも下方の部分）	大腿骨の大転子（内側面）	・筋全体：外転・冠状面における骨盤の安定化 ・前部：屈曲・内旋 ・後部：伸展・外旋	上殿神経（L4-S1）
梨状筋	仙骨の前面	大腿骨の大転子（尖端）	・股関節の外旋・外転・伸展 ・股関節の安定化	仙骨神経叢からの直接の枝（L5-S2）

System of the Muscles of the Hip & Gluteal Region V

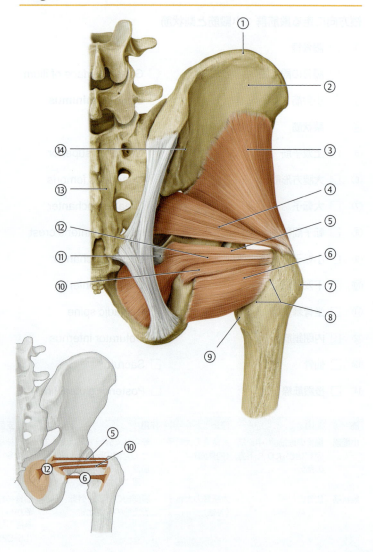

骨盤と殿部の筋の区分 5

水平方向に走る殿筋群：内閉鎖筋，上・下双子筋，大腿方形筋

① □ 腸骨稜 □ Iliac crest
② □ 腸骨の殿筋面 □ Gluteal surface of ilium
③ □ 小殿筋 □ Gluteus minimus
④ □ 梨状筋 □ Piriformis
⑤ □ 上双子筋 □ **Gemellus superior**
⑥ □ 大腿方形筋 □ **Quadratus femoris**
⑦ □ 大転子 □ Greater trochanter
⑧ □ 転子間稜 □ Intertrochanteric crest
⑨ □ 小転子 □ Lesser trochanter
⑩ □ 下双子筋 □ **Gemellus inferior**
⑪ □ 坐骨棘 □ Ischial spine
⑫ □ 内閉鎖筋 □ **Obturator internus**
⑬ □ 仙骨 □ Sacrum
⑭ □ 後殿筋線 □ Posterior gluteal line

筋	起始	停止	作用	神経支配
内閉鎖筋	閉鎖膜（内面）および閉鎖孔周辺の骨	大腿骨の転子窩	・股関節の外旋・内転・伸展 ・肢位によっては股関節の外転作用も持つ	仙骨神経叢からの直接の枝(L5-S2)
上双子筋	坐骨棘	大腿骨の転子窩（内閉鎖筋の腱とともに停止する）	・股関節の外旋・内転	
下双子筋	坐骨結節			
大腿方形筋	坐骨結節の外側縁	大腿骨の転子間稜		

System of the Muscles of the Hip & Gluteal Region VI

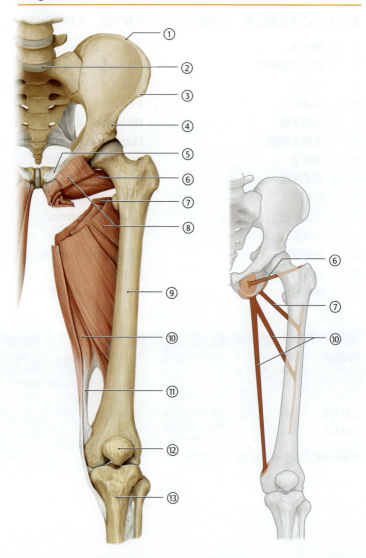

骨盤と殿部の筋の区分 6

内転筋：外閉鎖筋，大内転筋，小内転筋

①	☐ 腸骨稜	☐ Iliac crest	
②	☐ 岬角	☐ Promontory	
③	☐ 上前腸骨棘	☐ Anterior superior iliac spine	
④	☐ 下前腸骨棘	☐ Anterior inferior iliac spine	
⑤	☐ 恥骨上肢	☐ Superior pubic ramus	
⑥	☐ **外閉鎖筋**	☐ **Obturator externus**	
⑦	☐ **小内転筋**	☐ **Adductor minimus**	
⑧	☐ 恥骨筋	☐ Pectineus	
⑨	☐ 大腿骨	☐ Femur	
⑩	☐ **大内転筋**	☐ **Adductor magnus**	
⑪	☐ **大内転筋（腱性の停止部）**	☐ **Adductor magnus, tendon of insertion**	
⑫	☐ 膝蓋骨	☐ Patella	
⑬	☐ 脛骨粗面	☐ Tibial tuberosity	

筋	起始	停止	作用	神経支配
外閉鎖筋	閉鎖膜（外面）および閉鎖孔周辺の骨	大腿骨の転子窩	・股関節：内転・外旋 ・骨盤：矢状面における安定化	閉鎖神経（L2-L4）
大内転筋（筋性の停止部）	・恥骨下肢 ・坐骨枝 ・坐骨結節	大腿骨（粗線の内側唇）	・股関節：内転・外旋・伸展（腱性の停止部を介して内旋） ・骨盤：冠状面と矢状面における安定化	
大内転筋（腱性の停止部）		大腿骨の内側上顆		脛骨神経（L4-L5）
小内転筋（大内転筋の最上部）	恥骨下肢	大腿骨（粗線の内側唇）	股関節：内転・外旋・わずかな屈曲	閉鎖神経（L2-L4）

System of the Muscles of the Hip & Gluteal Region VII

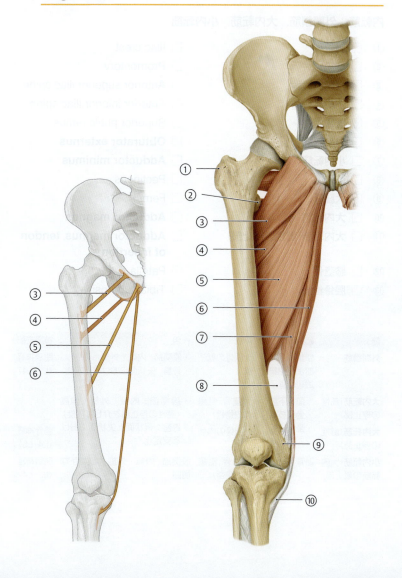

骨盤と殿部の筋の区分 7

内転筋：恥骨筋，長内転筋，短内転筋，薄筋

① □ 大転子　　　　　　　　　□ Greater trochanter
② □ 小転子　　　　　　　　　□ Lesser trochanter
③ □ 恥骨筋　　　　　　　　　□ **Pectineus**
④ □ 短内転筋　　　　　　　　□ **Adductor brevis**
⑤ □ 長内転筋　　　　　　　　□ **Adductor longus**
⑥ □ 薄筋　　　　　　　　　　□ **Gracilis**
⑦ □ 大内転筋　　　　　　　　□ Adductor magnus
⑧ □ ［内転筋］腱裂孔　　　　　□ Adductor hiatus
⑨ □ 内側上顆　　　　　　　　□ Medial epicondyle
⑩ □ 薄筋の停止腱　　　　　　□ Gracilis, tendon of insertion

筋	起始	停止	作用	神経支配
恥骨筋	恥骨櫛	大腿骨（恥骨筋線，粗線の近位部）	・股関節：内転・外旋・わずかな屈曲 ・骨盤：冠状面と矢状面における安定化	・大腿神経 ・閉鎖神経 （L2-L4）
長内転筋	恥骨上肢，恥骨結合の前面	大腿骨（粗線中央1/3の内側唇）	・股関節：内転・屈曲（70°までの屈曲位）・伸展（80°以上の屈曲位） ・骨盤：冠状面と矢状面における安定化	閉鎖神経 （L2-L4）
短内転筋	恥骨下肢	大腿骨（粗線上部1/3の内側唇）		
薄筋	恥骨下肢	鵞足（＝脛骨粗面よりも内側の部分）（縫工筋や半腱様筋の腱とともに停止する）	・股関節：内転・屈曲 ・膝関節：屈曲・内旋	

System of the Muscles of Thigh I

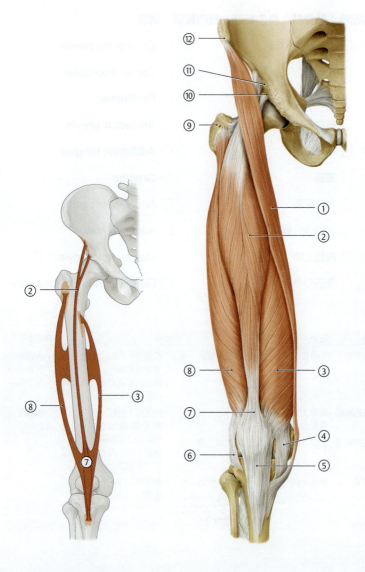

大腿の筋の区分 1

伸筋：大腿四頭筋（大腿直筋，内側広筋，外側広筋，中間広筋）

（中間広筋は pp.552, 553 参照）

① □ 縫工筋 □ Sartorius
② □ 大腿直筋 □ **Rectus femoris**
③ □ 内側広筋 □ **Vastus medialis**
④ □ 内側膝蓋支帯 □ Medial patellar retinaculum
⑤ □ 膝蓋靱帯 □ Patellar ligament
⑥ □ 外側膝蓋支帯 □ Lateral patellar retinaculum
⑦ □ 大腿四頭筋の停止腱 □ Quadriceps femoris, tendon of insertion
⑧ □ 外側広筋 □ **Vastus lateralis**
⑨ □ 大転子 □ Greater trochanter
⑩ □ 寛骨臼蓋 □ Acetabular roof
⑪ □ 下前腸骨棘 □ Anterior inferior iliac spine
⑫ □ 上前腸骨棘 □ Anterior superior iliac spine

筋	起始	停止	作用	神経支配
大腿直筋	・下前腸骨棘（直頭） ・寛骨臼蓋（反転頭）	脛骨粗面（膝蓋靱帯を介して停止する．大腿四頭筋の他の部分も同様）	・股関節：屈曲 ・膝関節：伸展	大腿神経 (L2-L4)
内側広筋	粗線（内側唇），転子間線（遠位部）	脛骨粗面，内側顆（内側膝蓋支帯を介して停止する）	膝関節：伸展	
外側広筋	粗線（外側唇），大転子（外側面）	脛骨粗面，外側顆（外側膝蓋支帯を介して停止する）		

 解説

　大腿四頭筋はその名が示すように，4 個の頭より構成される筋肉である（大腿直筋，内側広筋，外側広筋，中間広筋）．膝関節筋（pp.552, 553 参照）を，中間広筋の遠位筋束に所属させると，大腿四頭筋は五頭筋とみなすこともできる．

System of the Muscles of Thigh II

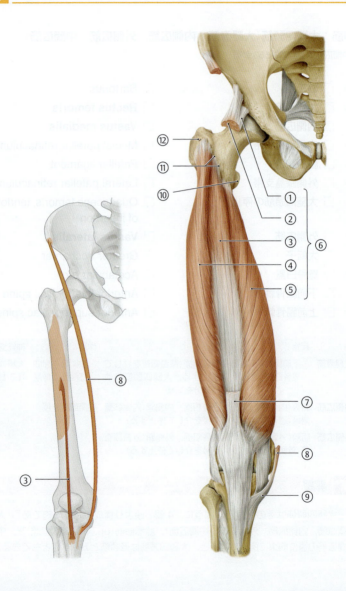

大腿の筋の区分 2

伸筋：大腿四頭筋，深層（中間広筋と膝関節筋），縫工筋

① ☐ 大腿直筋の反転頭　　☐ Reflected head of rectus femoris
② ☐ 大腿直筋の直頭　　　☐ Straight head of rectus femoris
③ ☐ 中間広筋　　　　　　☐ **Vastus intermedius**
④ ☐ 外側広筋　　　　　　☐ Vastus lateralis
⑤ ☐ 内側広筋　　　　　　☐ Vastus medialis
⑥ ☐ 大腿四頭筋　　　　　☐ Quadriceps femoris
⑦ ☐ 大腿直筋　　　　　　☐ Rectus femoris
⑧ ☐ **縫工筋**　　　　　　☐ **Sartorius**
⑨ ☐ 鵞足　　　　　　　　☐ Pes anserinus
⑩ ☐ 小転子　　　　　　　☐ Lesser trochanter
⑪ ☐ 転子間線　　　　　　☐ Intertrochanteric line
⑫ ☐ 大転子　　　　　　　☐ Greater trochanter

筋	起始	停止	作用	神経支配
中間広筋	大腿骨体（前面）	脛骨粗面（膝蓋靱帯を介して停止する）	・膝関節：伸展	大腿神経（L2-L4）
膝関節筋（中間広筋の遠位筋束）	大腿骨体（前面，膝蓋上陥凹の高さ）	膝関節包，膝蓋上陥凹	・股関節：屈曲 ・膝関節：伸展．関節包が巻き込まれるのを防ぐ	
縫工筋	上前腸骨棘	鵞足（＝脛骨粗面よりも内側の部分）（薄筋や半腱様筋の腱とともに停止する）	・股関節：屈曲・外転・外旋 ・膝関節：屈曲・内旋	

解説

　大腿四頭筋のその他の構成要素については pp.550, 551 で解説する．起始と付着が認められるだけの縫工筋についても同様に pp.550, 551 参照．

System of the Muscles of Thigh III

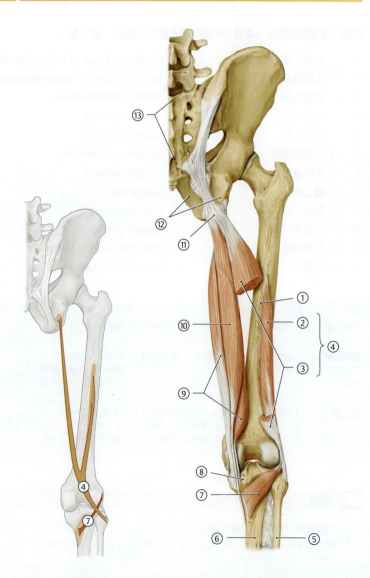

大腿の筋の区分 3

屈筋：大腿二頭筋と膝窩筋，右側．後方から見たところ

① ☐ 粗線 ☐ Linia aspera
② ☐ **大腿二頭筋の短頭** ☐ **Short head of biceps femoris**
③ ☐ **大腿二頭筋の長頭** ☐ **Long head of biceps femoris**
④ ☐ **大腿二頭筋** ☐ **Biceps femoris**
⑤ ☐ 腓骨 ☐ Fibula
⑥ ☐ 脛骨 ☐ Tibia
⑦ ☐ **膝窩筋** ☐ **Popliteus**
⑧ ☐ 脛骨の内側顆 ☐ Medial condyle of tibia
⑨ ☐ 半膜様筋 ☐ Semimembranosus
⑩ ☐ 半腱様筋 ☐ Semitendinosus
⑪ ☐ 仙結節靱帯（ハムストリングスの共通頭） ☐ Sacrotuberous ligament (common head of hamstrings)
⑫ ☐ 坐骨 ☐ Ischium
⑬ ☐ 仙骨 ☐ Sacrum

筋	起始	停止	作用	神経支配
大腿二頭筋の長頭	坐骨結節，仙結節靱帯(半腱様筋と共通頭を形成する．pp. 556, 557参照)	腓骨頭	・股関節：内転・伸展・矢状面で骨盤を安定化する ・膝関節：屈曲・外旋	脛骨神経 (L5-S2)
大腿二頭筋の短頭	粗線外側唇の中央1/3		膝関節：屈曲・外旋	総腓骨神経 (L5-S2)
膝窩筋	大腿骨の外側顆，外側半月の後角	脛骨後面(ヒラメ筋の起始部よりも上方．pp. 584, 585参照)	膝関節：屈曲・内旋	脛骨神経 (L5-S2)

System of the Muscles of Thigh IV

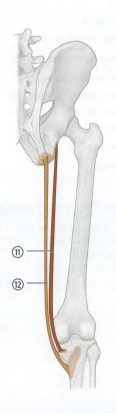
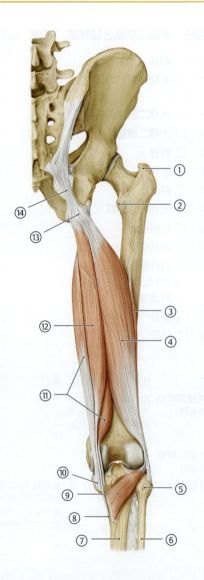

大腿の筋の区分 4

屈筋：半膜様筋と半腱様筋，右側．後方から見たところ

① □ 大転子　　　　　　　□ Greater trochanter
② □ 小転子　　　　　　　□ Lesser trochanter
③ □ 大腿二頭筋の短頭　　□ Short head of biceps femoris
④ □ 大腿二頭筋の長頭　　□ Long head of biceps femoris
⑤ □ 腓骨頭　　　　　　　□ Head of fibula
⑥ □ 腓骨　　　　　　　　□ Fibula
⑦ □ 脛骨　　　　　　　　□ Tibia
⑧ □ 浅鵞足　　　　　　　□ Pes anserinus superficialis
⑨ □ 膝窩筋　　　　　　　□ Popliteus
⑩ □ 半膜様筋の腱　　　　□ Semimembranosus tendon
⑪ □ 半膜様筋　　　　　　□ **Semimembranosus**
⑫ □ 半腱様筋　　　　　　□ **Semitendinosus**
⑬ □ 坐骨結節　　　　　　□ Ischial tuberosity
⑭ □ 仙結節靱帯　　　　　□ Sacrotuberous ligament

筋	起始	停止	作用	神経支配
半膜様筋	坐骨結節	脛骨の内側顆：斜膝窩靱帯，膝窩筋膜	・股関節：内転・伸展 ・骨盤：矢状面における安定化 ・膝関節：屈曲・内旋	脛骨神経 (L5-S2)
半腱様筋	坐骨結節，仙結節靱帯（大腿二頭筋の長頭と共通頭を形成する）	鵞足（薄筋や縫工筋の腱とともに停止する．pp.524, 525, pp.552, 553 参照）		

Tibia & Fibula

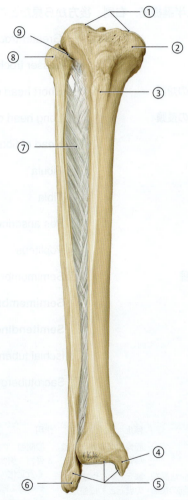

腓骨の役割は何か？

脛骨と腓骨

右下腿，前面

① □ 上関節面　　　　□ Tibial plateau
② □ 内側顆　　　　　□ Medial condyle
③ □ 脛骨粗面　　　　□ Tibial tuberosity
④ □ 内果　　　　　　□ Medial malleolus
⑤ □ 足関節窩　　　　□ Ankle mortise
⑥ □ 外果　　　　　　□ Lateral malleolus
⑦ □ 下腿骨間膜　　　□ Interosseous membrane of leg
⑧ □ 腓骨頭　　　　　□ Head of fibula
⑨ □ 脛腓関節　　　　□ Tibiofibular joint

 腓骨には体重を支える役割はないが，距腿関節の関節面の一部を形成し，関節の安定性を保つうえで重要な役割をはたす．また，腓骨には下肢のいくつかの筋が起始もしくは停止する．

Knee Joint I

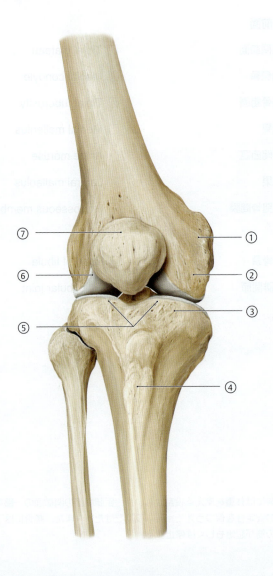

膝関節 1

右膝,前面

① □ 内側上顆　　　　　□ Medial epicondyle
② □ 大腿骨の内側顆　　□ Medial condyle of femur
③ □ 脛骨の内側顆　　　□ Medial condyle of tibia
④ □ 脛骨粗面　　　　　□ Tibial tuberosity
⑤ □ 上関節面　　　　　□ Tibial plateau
⑥ □ 大腿骨の外側顆　　□ Lateral condyle of femur
⑦ □ 膝蓋骨　　　　　　□ Patella

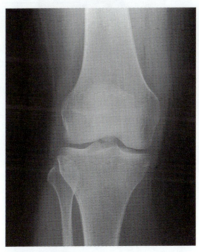

右膝の X 線像

Knee Joint II

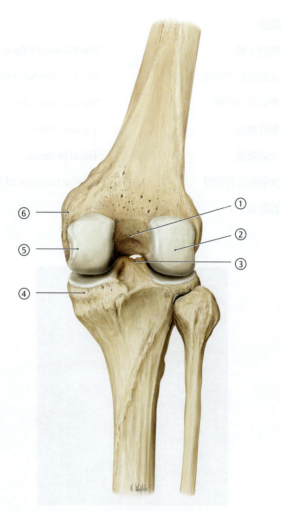

Q 膝関節を構成する骨は何か?

膝関節 2

右膝，後面

① □ 顆間窩　　　　　　　□ Intercondylar notch
② □ 大腿骨の外側顆　　　□ Lateral condyle of femur
③ □ 顆間隆起　　　　　　□ Intercondylar eminence
④ □ 脛骨の内側顆　　　　□ Medial condyle of tibia
⑤ □ 大腿骨の内側顆　　　□ Medial condyle of femur
⑥ □ 内側上顆　　　　　　□ Medial epicondyle

A　膝関節は3つの骨（大腿骨，脛骨，膝蓋骨）からなる．腓骨は膝関節には関与しないが，脛骨との間に脛腓関節と脛腓靱帯結合を形成する．

Ligaments of the Knee Joint I

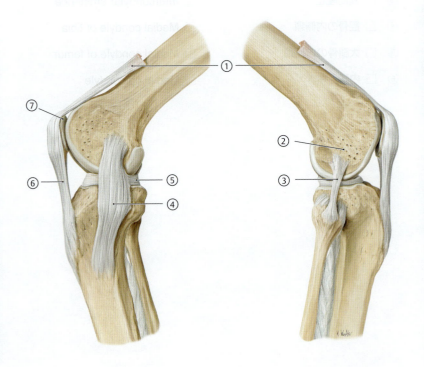

膝関節の靱帯 1

右膝，左：内側面，右：外側面

① □ 大腿四頭筋の腱　　□ Quadriceps femoris tendon
② □ 外側上顆　　　　　□ Lateral epicondyle
③ □ 外側側副靱帯　　　□ Lateral collateral ligament
④ □ 内側側副靱帯　　　□ Medial collateral ligament
⑤ □ 内側半月　　　　　□ Medial meniscus
⑥ □ 膝蓋靱帯　　　　　□ Patellar ligament
⑦ □ 膝蓋大腿関節　　　□ Femoropatellar joint

解説

　膝関節は内側および外側側副靱帯によって補強される．内側側副靱帯は関節包と内側半月に付着するが，外側側副靱帯は関節包と外側半月のどちらとも接触しない．膝関節の伸展位において，側副靱帯は緊張し，冠状断面内で膝関節を安定化する．

Ligaments of the Knee Joint II

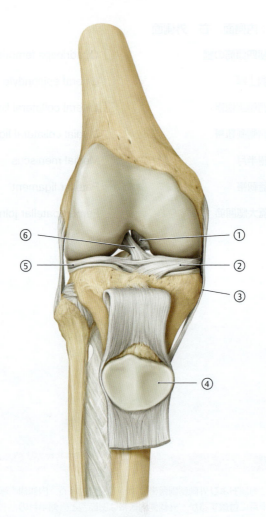

十字靱帯はどのようにして膝関節を安定化するか？

膝関節の靱帯 2

右膝，前面

① □ 後十字靱帯　　　　　□ Posterior cruciate ligament
② □ 内側半月　　　　　　□ Medial meniscus
③ □ 内側側副靱帯　　　　□ Medial collateral ligament
④ □ 膝蓋骨　　　　　　　□ Patella
⑤ □ 外側半月　　　　　　□ Lateral meniscus
⑥ □ 前十字靱帯　　　　　□ Anterior cruciate ligament

A 　十字靱帯は，大腿骨が脛骨に対して前方あるいは後方に偏位することを防ぎ，膝関節の安定化をはかっている．すべての肢位において，十字靱帯のどこかが緊張している．

Ligaments of the Knee Joint III

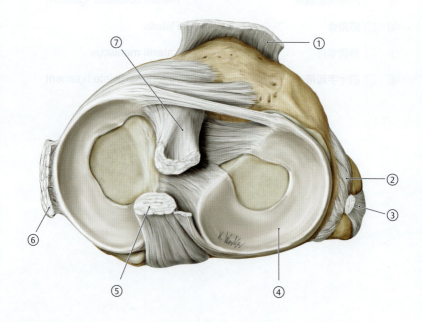

内側半月の外傷性断裂に伴いやすい膝構造の損傷は何か？

膝関節の靱帯 3

右脛骨の上関節面

① □ 膝蓋靱帯　　　□ Patellar ligament
② □ 脛腓関節　　　□ Tibiofibular joint
③ □ 外側側副靱帯　□ Lateral collateral ligament
④ □ 外側半月　　　□ Lateral meniscus
⑤ □ 後十字靱帯　　□ Posterior cruciate ligament
⑥ □ 内側側副靱帯　□ Medial collateral ligament
⑦ □ 前十字靱帯　　□ Anterior cruciate ligament

A 膝関節の外傷時(特に外側からの衝撃を受けた場合)には、内側半月の断裂、内側側副靱帯の断裂、前十字靱帯の断裂の3つがしばしば合併する。

Muscles of the Leg I

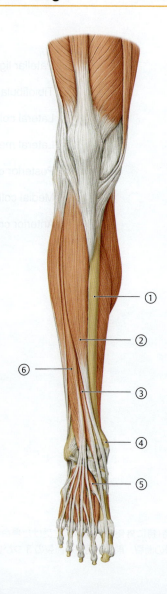

下腿の筋 1

右下腿，前面

① □ 脛骨　　　　　□ Tibia
② □ 前脛骨筋　　　□ Tibialis anterior
③ □ 長母趾伸筋　　□ Extensor hallucis longus
④ □ 内果　　　　　□ Medial malleolus
⑤ □ 短母趾伸筋　　□ Extensor hallucis brevis
⑥ □ 長趾伸筋　　　□ Extensor digitorum longus

Muscles of the Leg II

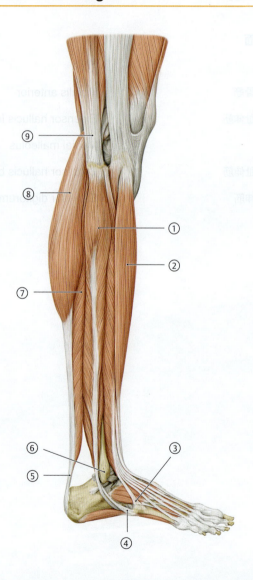

下腿の筋 2

右下腿，外側面

① □ 長腓骨筋 □ Fibularis longus
② □ 前脛骨筋 □ Tibialis anterior
③ □ 第3腓骨筋（欠く場合もある） □ Fibularis tertius (variable)
④ □ 短腓骨筋 □ Fibularis brevis
⑤ □ 踵骨腱（アキレス腱） □ Calcaneal (Achilles') tendon
⑥ □ 外果，腓骨 □ Lateral malleolus, fibula
⑦ □ ヒラメ筋 □ Soleus
⑧ □ 腓腹筋の外側頭 □ Lateral head of gastrocnemius
⑨ □ 大腿二頭筋の腱 □ Biceps femoris tendon

Muscles of the Leg III

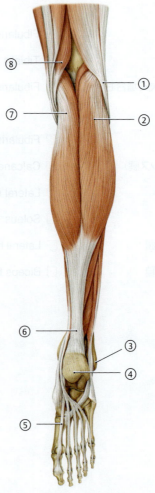

Q 下腿の後区画に存在する筋のうち，膝関節の運動に関与するものはどれか？

下腿の筋 3

右下腿，後面

① □ 大腿二頭筋の腱　　□ Biceps femoris tendon
② □ 腓腹筋の外側頭　　□ Lateral head of gastrocnemius
③ □ 外果　　□ Lateral malleolus
④ □ 踵骨　　□ Calcaneus
⑤ □ 長母趾屈筋の腱　　□ Flexor hallucis longus tendon
⑥ □ 踵骨腱（アキレス腱）　　□ Calcaneal (Achilles') tendon
⑦ □ 腓腹筋の内側頭　　□ Medial head of gastrocnemius
⑧ □ 半膜様筋　　□ Semimembranosus

 腓腹筋は，膝関節を乗り越える筋のうち，膝関節の屈曲作用を有する主要な筋である．足底筋も膝関節を乗り越えるが，小さな筋であるため，関節への影響はほとんど無視できる．

Muscles of the Leg IV

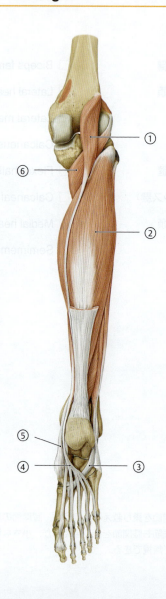

下腿の筋 4

右下腿，後面

① □ 足底筋 　　　　　□ Plantaris
② □ ヒラメ筋 　　　　□ Soleus
③ □ 長腓骨筋の腱 　　□ Fibularis longus tendon
④ □ 長趾屈筋の腱 　　□ Flexor digitorum longus tendon
⑤ □ 後脛骨筋の腱 　　□ Tibialis posterior tendon
⑥ □ 膝窩筋 　　　　　□ Popliteus

Muscles of the Leg V

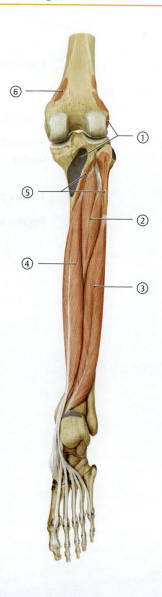

下腿の筋 5

右下腿，後面．下腿三頭筋，足底筋，膝窩筋を取り除いたところ

① □ 膝窩筋〔筋の起始（赤）・停止（青）〕　□ Popliteus (origin and insertion)

② □ 後脛骨筋　□ Tibialis posterior

③ □ 長母趾屈筋　□ Flexor hallucis longus

④ □ 長趾屈筋　□ Flexor digitorum longus

⑤ □ ヒラメ筋（筋の起始）　□ Soleus (origin)

⑥ □ 腓腹筋の内側頭（筋の起始）　□ Medial head of gastrocnemius (origin)

System of the Muscles of the Leg I

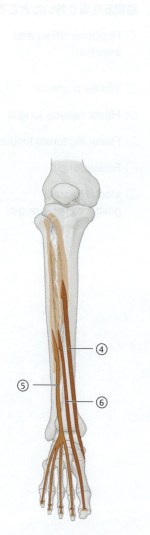
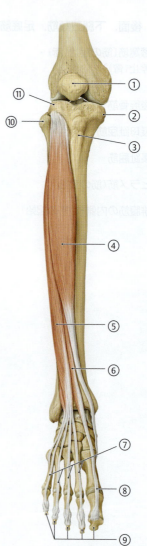

下腿の筋の区分 1

伸筋：前脛骨筋，長趾伸筋，長母趾伸筋

① □ 膝蓋骨 — □ Patella
② □ 脛骨の内側顆 — □ Medial tibial condyle
③ □ 脛骨粗面 — □ Tibial tuberosity
④ □ **前脛骨筋** — □ **Tibialis anterior**
⑤ □ **長趾伸筋** — □ **Extensor digitorum longus**
⑥ □ **長母趾伸筋** — □ **Extensor hallucis longus**
⑦ □ 長趾伸筋の腱 — □ Extensor digitorum longus tendons
⑧ □ 長母趾伸筋の腱 — □ Extensor hallucis longus tendon
⑨ □ 第1-5末節骨 — □ 1st through 5th distal phalanges
⑩ □ 腓骨頭 — □ Head of fibula
⑪ □ 脛骨の外側顆 — □ Lateral condyle of tibia

筋	起始	停止	作用	神経支配
前脛骨筋	・脛骨(外側面の上部2/3) ・骨間膜 ・下腿筋膜(最上部)	・内側楔状骨(内側面，足底面) ・第1中足骨底(内側面)	・距腿関節：背屈 ・距骨下関節：内反(回外)	深腓骨神経 (L4-L5)
長趾伸筋	・脛骨(外側顆) ・腓骨(頭と前縁) ・骨間膜	・第2-5趾の趾背腱膜(4本に分かれた細い腱の上) ・第2-5趾の末節骨底	・距腿関節：背屈 ・距骨下関節：外反(回内) ・第2-5趾のMTP関節とIP関節：伸展	
長母趾伸筋	・腓骨(内側面の中間1/3) ・骨間膜	・第1趾の趾背腱膜 ・第1趾の末節骨底	・距腿関節：背屈 ・距骨下関節：足の位置に応じ，内反と外反の両方に働く(回内/回外) ・第1趾のMTP関節とIP関節：伸展	深腓骨神経 (L5-S1)

IP関節：趾節間関節　MTP関節：中足趾節関節

System of the Muscles of the Leg II

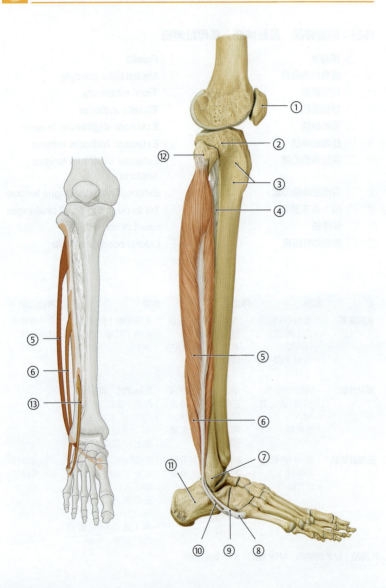

下腿の筋の区分 2

腓骨筋群：長腓骨筋，短腓骨筋，第 3 腓骨筋

① ☐ 膝蓋骨 ☐ Patella
② ☐ 脛骨の外側顆 ☐ Lateral condyle of tibia
③ ☐ 脛骨の外側面 ☐ Lateral surface of tibia
④ ☐ 下腿骨間膜 ☐ Interosseous membrane of leg
⑤ ☐ **長腓骨筋** ☐ **Fibularis longus**
⑥ ☐ **短腓骨筋** ☐ **Fibularis brevis**
⑦ ☐ 外果 ☐ Lateral malleolus
⑧ ☐ 第 5 中足骨粗面 ☐ Tuberosity of 5th metatarsal
⑨ ☐ 短腓骨筋の腱 ☐ Fibularis brevis tendon
⑩ ☐ 長腓骨筋の腱 ☐ Fibularis longus tendon
⑪ ☐ 踵骨 ☐ Calcaneus
⑫ ☐ 腓骨頭 ☐ Head of fibula
⑬ ☐ **第 3 腓骨筋** ☐ **Fibularis tertius**

筋	起始	停止	作用	神経支配
長腓骨筋	・腓骨(頭，外側面の近位 2/3) ・一部は筋間中隔からも起始する	・内側楔状骨(足底面) ・第 1 中足骨底	・距腿関節：底屈 ・距骨下関節：外反(回内) ・横足弓の保持	浅腓骨神経 (L5-S1)
短腓骨筋	・腓骨(外側面の遠位 1/2) ・一部は筋間中隔からも起始する	第 5 中足骨粗面(場合によっては第 5 趾の趾背腱膜へ分岐腱を伸ばす)	・距腿関節：底屈 ・距骨下関節：外反(回内)	
第 3 腓骨筋(長趾伸筋から分離．pp.612, 613 参照)	腓骨(前縁)の遠位部	第 5 中足骨底	・距腿関節：背屈 ・距骨下関節：外反(回内)	深腓骨神経 (L4-S1)

System of the Muscles of the Leg III

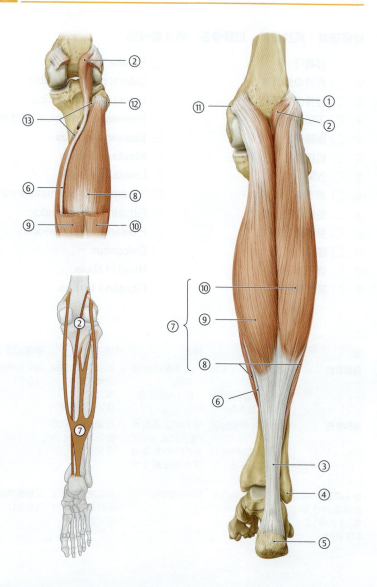

下腿の筋の区分 3

浅層の屈筋：下腿三頭筋（＝ヒラメ筋，腓腹筋），足底筋

① □ 大腿骨の外側上顆　　　□ Lateral epicondyle of femur
② □ 足底筋　　　　　　　　□ **Plantaris**
③ □ 踵骨腱（アキレス腱）　　□ Calcaneal (Achilles') tendon
④ □ 外果　　　　　　　　　□ Lateral malleolus
⑤ □ 踵骨隆起　　　　　　　□ Calcaneal tuberosity
⑥ □ 足底筋の腱　　　　　　□ Plantaris tendon
⑦ □ 下腿三頭筋　　　　　　□ Triceps surae
⑧ □ ヒラメ筋　　　　　　　□ **Soleus**
⑨ □ 腓腹筋の内側頭　　　　□ **Medial head of gastrocnemius**
⑩ □ 腓腹筋の外側頭　　　　□ **Lateral head of gastrocnemius**
⑪ □ 大腿骨の内側上顆　　　□ Medial epicondyle of femur
⑫ □ 腓骨頭　　　　　　　　□ Head of fibula
⑬ □ ヒラメ筋腱弓　　　　　□ Tendinous arch of soleus

筋	起始	停止	作用	神経支配
ヒラメ筋	腓骨頭，腓骨頸，ヒラメ筋腱弓，ヒラメ筋線（pp.586, 587参照）	踵骨腱（アキレス腱）を介して踵骨隆起に停止する	・距腿関節：底屈 ・距骨下関節：内反（回外） ・膝関節：屈曲（腓腹筋）	脛骨神経（S1-S2）
腓腹筋の内側頭	大腿骨の内側上顆			
腓腹筋の外側頭	大腿骨の外側上顆			
足底筋	腓腹筋外側頭の近位部		生理的横断面積が小さいことから無視することができる（膝屈曲の際に後頸骨脈管の圧迫が阻止される）	

System of the Muscles of the Leg IV

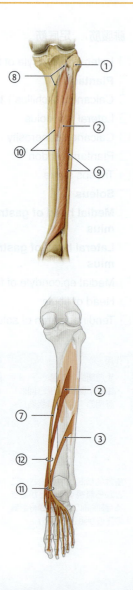
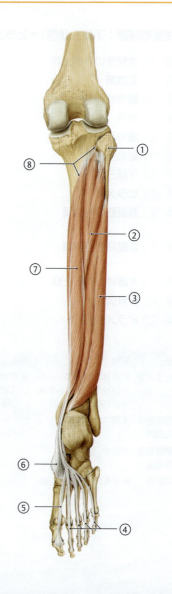

下腿の筋の区分 4

深層の屈筋：後脛骨筋，長趾屈筋，長母指屈筋

① ☐ 腓骨頭　　　　　　　☐ Head of fibula
② ☐ **後脛骨筋**　　　　　☐ **Tibialis posterior**
③ ☐ **長母趾屈筋**　　　　☐ **Flexor hallucis longus**
④ ☐ 長趾屈筋の腱　　　　☐ Flexor digitorum longus tendons
⑤ ☐ 長母趾屈筋の腱　　　☐ Flexor hallucis longus tendon
⑥ ☐ 後脛骨筋の腱　　　　☐ Tibialis posterior tendon
⑦ ☐ **長趾屈筋**　　　　　☐ **Flexor digitorum longus**
⑧ ☐ ヒラメ筋線　　　　　☐ Soleal line
⑨ ☐ 腓骨の後面　　　　　☐ Posterior surface of fibula
⑩ ☐ 脛骨の後面　　　　　☐ Posterior surface of tibia
⑪ ☐ 足底交叉　　　　　　☐ Plantar chiasm
⑫ ☐ 下腿交叉　　　　　　☐ Crural chiasm

筋	起始	停止	作用	神経支配
後脛骨筋	・骨間膜 ・脛骨と腓骨の隣接する部分	・舟状骨粗面 ・内側・中間・外側楔状骨 ・第2-4中足骨底	・距腿関節：底屈 ・距骨下関節：内反(回外) ・縦足弓と横足弓の保持	脛骨神経 (L5-S2)
長趾屈筋	脛骨(後面の中間1/3)	第2-5末節骨底	・距腿関節：底屈 ・距骨下関節：内反(回外) ・第2-5趾のMTP関節とIP関節：底屈	
長母趾屈筋	・腓骨(後面の遠位2/3) ・隣接する骨間膜	第1末節骨底	・距腿関節：底屈 ・距骨下関節：内反(回外) ・第1趾のMTP関節とIP関節：底屈 ・内側縦足弓の保持	

IP関節：趾節間関節　MTP関節：中足趾節関節

Bones of the Foot I

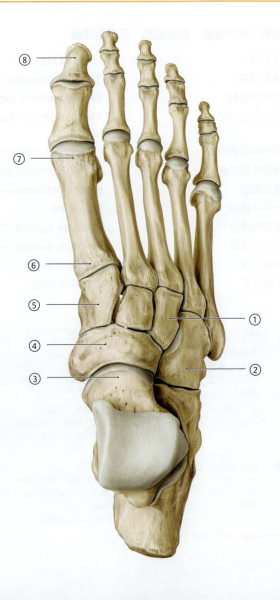

足の骨格 1

右足，背側面（上面）

① ☐ 外側楔状骨　　☐ Lateral cuneiform
② ☐ 立方骨　　　　☐ Cuboid
③ ☐ 距骨頭　　　　☐ Head of talus
④ ☐ 舟状骨　　　　☐ Navicular
⑤ ☐ 内側楔状骨　　☐ Medial cuneiform
⑥ ☐ 第1中足骨底　☐ Base of 1st metatarsal
⑦ ☐ 第1中足骨頭　☐ Head of 1st metatarsal
⑧ ☐ 第1末節骨　　☐ 1st distal phalanx

Bones of the Foot II

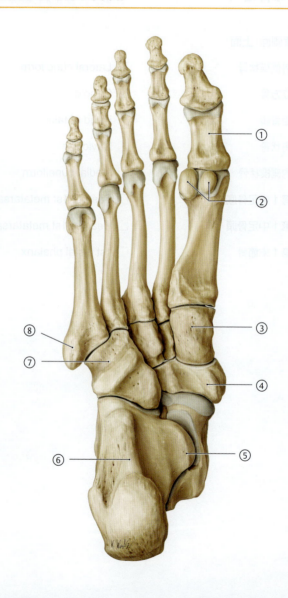

足の骨格 2

右足，足底面（下面）

① □ 第 1 基節骨 □ 1st proximal phalanx
② □ 種子骨 □ Sesamoid bones
③ □ 内側楔状骨 □ Medial cuneiform
④ □ 舟状骨 □ Navicular
⑤ □ 載距突起 □ Sustentaculum tali
⑥ □ 踵骨 □ Calcaneus
⑦ □ 長腓骨筋腱溝 □ Groove for fibularis longus tendon
⑧ □ 第 5 中足骨粗面 □ Tuberosity of 5th metatarsal

Joints of the Ankle & Foot I

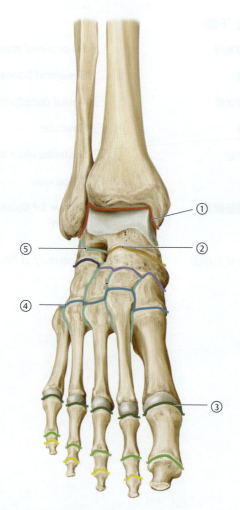

Q 足首が底屈位において損傷を受けやすい理由は何か？

足首と足の関節 1

右足，距腿関節の底屈位，前面

① □ 距腿関節　　　　　　□ Ankle joint
② □ 距舟関節　　　　　　□ Talonavicular joint
③ □ 中足趾節関節　　　　□ Metatarsophalangeal joints
④ □ 足根中足関節　　　　□ Tarsometatarsal joints
⑤ □ 距骨下関節　　　　　□ Subtalar (talocalcaneal) joint

 距骨滑車の後部は幅が狭く，底屈位では脛骨と腓骨からなる関節窩の中で距骨滑車の安定性（つまり，距腿関節の安定性）が低下する．このため，距腿関節は，背屈位よりも底屈位において損傷を受けやすい．

Joints of the Ankle & Foot II

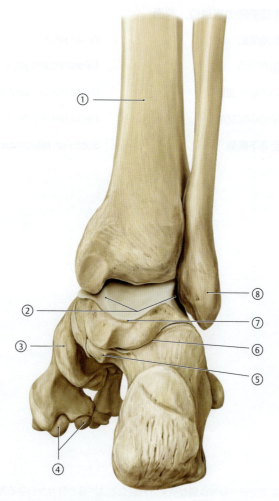

Q 距骨下関節で行われる運動は何か？

足首と足の関節 2

右足,後面

① □ 脛骨　　　　　　□ Tibia
② □ 距腿関節　　　　□ Ankle joint
③ □ 舟状骨　　　　　□ Navicular
④ □ 種子骨　　　　　□ Sesamoid bones
⑤ □ 載距突起　　　　□ Sustentaculum tali
⑥ □ 距骨下関節　　　□ Subtaler (talocalcaneal) joint
⑦ □ 距骨　　　　　　□ Talus
⑧ □ 外果　　　　　　□ Lateral malleolus

距骨下関節では,主として足の外反と内反が行われる.

Joints of the Ankle & Foot III

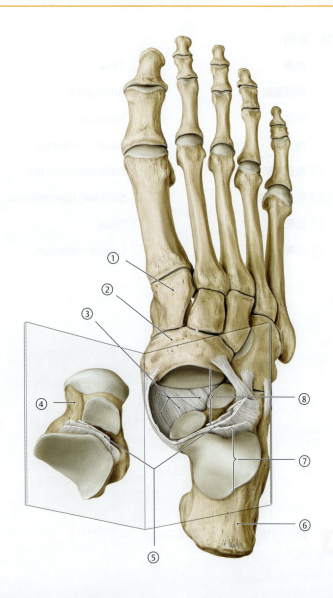

足首と足の関節 3

右足, 背側面（上面）

① ☐ 内側楔状骨　　　　☐ Medial cuneiform

② ☐ 舟状骨　　　　　　☐ Navicular

③ ☐ 底側踵舟靱帯　　　☐ Plantar calcaneonavicular ligament

④ ☐ 距骨　　　　　　　☐ Talus

⑤ ☐ 骨間距踵靱帯　　　☐ Interosseous talocalcanean ligament

⑥ ☐ 踵骨　　　　　　　☐ Calcaneus

⑦ ☐ 距骨下関節の後区　☐ Posterior compartment of subtalar joint
　　　（距踵関節）

⑧ ☐ 距骨下関節の前区　☐ Anterior compartment of subtalar joint
　　　（距踵舟関節）

解説

距骨下関節は，骨間距踵靱帯によって分けられた2つの関節（後区の距踵関節と前区の距踵舟関節）からなる．

Ligaments of the Ankle & Foot I

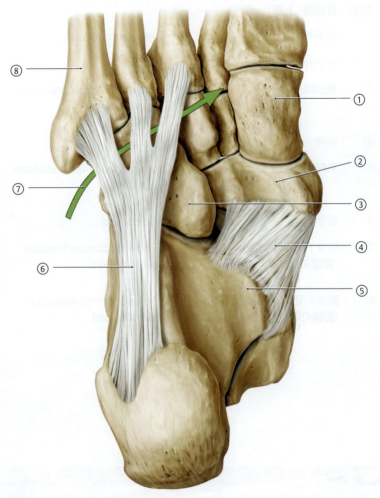

底側踵舟靭帯の機能は何か？

足首と足の靱帯 1

右足，足底面（下面）

① □ 内側楔状骨　　　　　　□ Medial cuneiform

② □ 舟状骨　　　　　　　　□ Navicular

③ □ 立方骨　　　　　　　　□ Cuboid

④ □ 底側踵舟靱帯　　　　　□ Plantar calcaneonavicular ligament

⑤ □ 載距突起　　　　　　　□ Sustentaculum tali

⑥ □ 長足底靱帯　　　　　　□ Long plantar ligament

⑦ □ 長腓骨筋の腱のトンネル　□ Tunnel for fibularis longus tendon

⑧ □ 第5中足骨　　　　　　　□ 5th metatarsal

底側踵舟靱帯（跳躍靱帯とも呼ばれる）は，距骨頭を下から支えるハンモックのような構造であり，内側縦足弓の最も高い部分を支えている．長足底靱帯は長腓骨筋腱を通すトンネルを形成し，外側縦足弓を支える．

Ligaments of the Ankle & Foot II

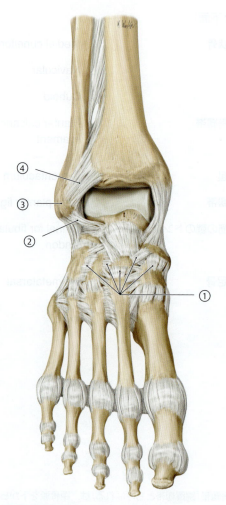

Q 足首の強制的な内反によって引き伸ばされる靱帯はどれか？

足首と足の靱帯 2

右足，前面

① □ 背側足根靱帯　　　　□ Dorsal tarsal ligaments

② □ 前距腓靱帯　　　　　□ Anterior talofibular ligament

③ □ 外果　　　　　　　　□ Lateral malleolus

④ □ 前脛腓靱帯　　　　　□ Anterior tibiofibular ligament

　足首の捻挫の大部分は足の強制的な内反によって生じ，外側側副靱帯（特に前距腓靱帯）が損傷を受ける．

Ligaments of the Ankle & Foot III

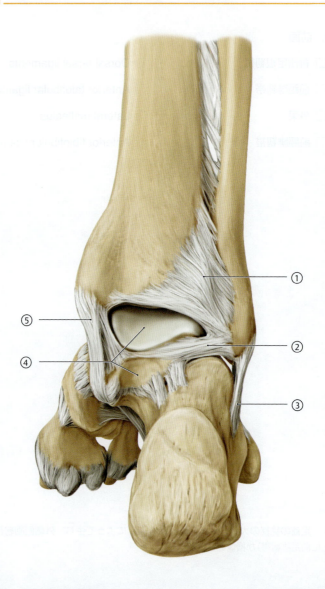

足首と足の靱帯 3

右足，足底を床につけた足位，後面

① □ 後脛腓靱帯　　　　　　　□ Posterior tibiofibular ligament

② □ 後距腓靱帯　　　　　　　□ Posterior talofibular ligament

③ □ 踵腓靱帯　　　　　　　　□ Calcaneofibular ligament

④ □ 距骨　　　　　　　　　　□ Talus

⑤ □ 三角靱帯　　　　　　　　□ Deltoid ligament

Muscles of the Sole of the Foot I

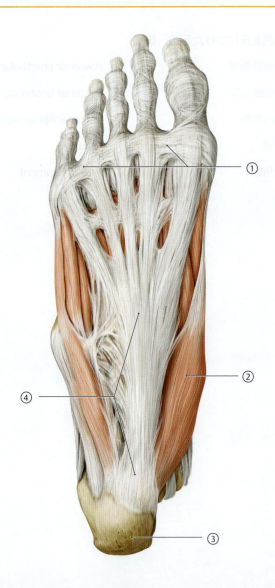

足底の筋 1

右足，足底面（下面）

① □ 浅横中足靱帯 □ Superficial transverse metacarpal ligament

② □ 母趾外転筋 □ Abductor hallucis

③ □ 踵骨隆起 □ Calcaneal tuberosity

④ □ 足底腱膜 □ Plantar aponeurosis

解説

足底腱膜は頑丈な腱膜であり，中央部が肥厚している．足の縁で足底腱膜は足背筋膜に移行する．

Muscles of the Sole of the Foot II

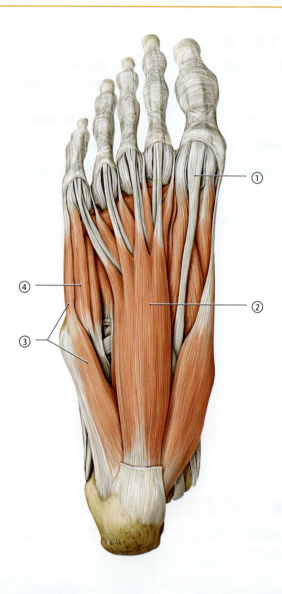

足底の筋 2

右足，足底面（下面），浅横中足靱帯を含む足底腱膜全体を取り除いたところ

① □ 長母趾屈筋の腱　　　□ Flexor hallucis longus tendon
② □ 短趾屈筋　　　　　　□ Flexor digitorum brevis
③ □ 小趾外転筋　　　　　□ Abductor digiti minimi
④ □ 短小趾屈筋　　　　　□ Flexor digiti minimi brevis

Muscles of the Sole of the Foot III

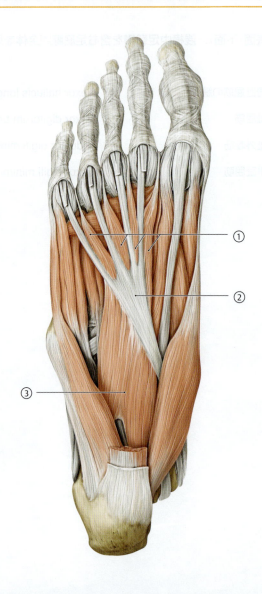

足底の筋 3

右足．足底面（下面）．足底腱膜と短趾屈筋を取り除いたところ

① ☐ 虫様筋 　　　　　　　　☐ Lumbricals

② ☐ 長趾屈筋の腱 　　　　　☐ Flexor digitorum longus tendon

③ ☐ 足底方形筋 　　　　　　☐ Quadratus plantae

Muscles of the Sole of the Foot IV

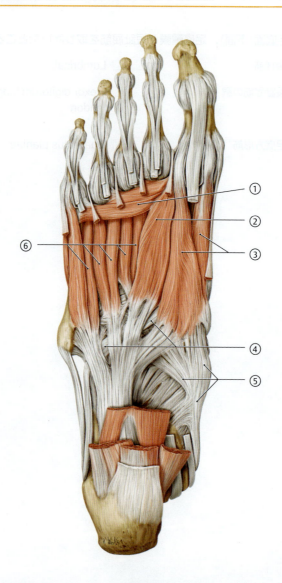

足底の筋 4

右足,足底面(下面).足底腱膜,短趾屈筋,小趾外転筋,母趾外転筋,足底方形筋,虫様筋,長趾屈筋腱,および長母趾屈筋腱を取り除いたところ

① ☐ 母趾内転筋の横頭 ☐ Transverse head of adductor hallucis

② ☐ 母趾内転筋の斜頭 ☐ Oblique head of adductor hallucis

③ ☐ 短母趾屈筋,内側頭と外側頭 ☐ Flexor hallucis brevis, medial and lateral heads

④ ☐ 長腓骨筋の腱 ☐ Fibularis longus tendon

⑤ ☐ 後脛骨筋の腱 ☐ Tibialis posterior tendon

⑥ ☐ 底側・背側骨間筋 ☐ Plantar and dorsal interossei

Anterior Foot & Ankle

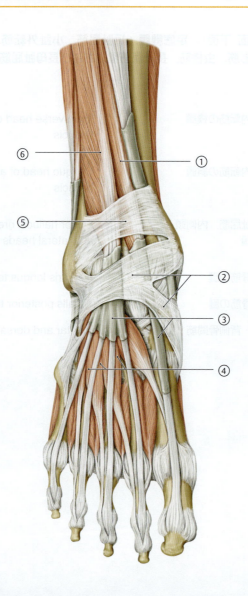

足首と足

右足，前面

① □ 長母趾伸筋 □ Extensor hallucis longus
② □ 下伸筋支帯 □ Inferior extensor retinaculum
③ □ 腱鞘 □ Tendon sheath
④ □ 短趾伸筋 □ Extensor digitorum brevis
⑤ □ 上伸筋支帯 □ Superior extensor retinaculum
⑥ □ 長趾伸筋 □ Extensor digitorum longus

 解説

支帯は腱を一定の場所に留めておく働きを持つ．伸筋支帯は長い伸筋腱を，腓骨筋支帯は腓骨筋腱を，屈筋支帯は長い屈筋腱をそれぞれ保持する．

System of the Muscles of the Foot I

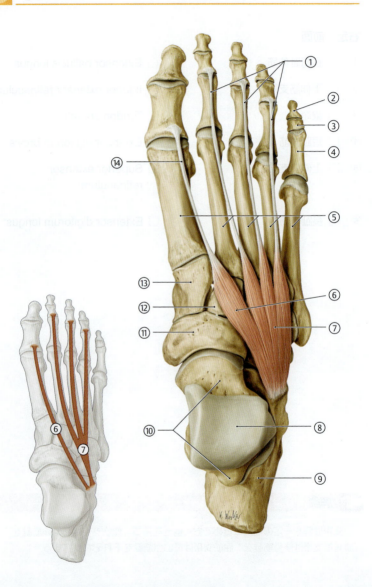

足の筋の区分 1

足背の内在筋：短趾伸筋と短母趾伸筋

①	□ 短趾伸筋の腱	□	Extensor digitorum brevis tendons
②	□ 第 5 末節骨	□	5th distal phalanx
③	□ 第 5 中節骨	□	5th middle phalanx
④	□ 第 5 基節骨	□	5th proximal phalanx
⑤	□ 第 1-5 中足骨	□	1st through 5th metatarsals
⑥	□ **短母趾伸筋**	□	**Extensor hallucis brevis**
⑦	□ **短趾伸筋**	□	**Extensor digitorum brevis**
⑧	□ 距骨滑車の上面	□	Superior trochlear surface
⑨	□ 踵骨	□	Calcaneus
⑩	□ 距骨	□	Talus
⑪	□ 舟状骨	□	Naviculare
⑫	□ 中間楔状骨	□	Intermediate cuneiform
⑬	□ 内側楔状骨	□	Medial cuneiform
⑭	□ 短母趾伸筋の腱	□	Extensor hallucis brevis tendon

筋	起始	停止	作用	神経支配
短趾伸筋	踵骨（背面）	第 2-4 趾（趾背腱膜，中節骨底）	第 2-4 趾の MTP 関節と PIP 関節：背屈	深腓骨神経 (L5-S1)
短母趾伸筋		第 1 趾（趾背腱膜，基節骨底）	第 1 趾の MTP 関節：背屈	

MTP 関節：中足趾節関節　PIP 関節：近位趾節間関節

System of the Muscles of the Foot II

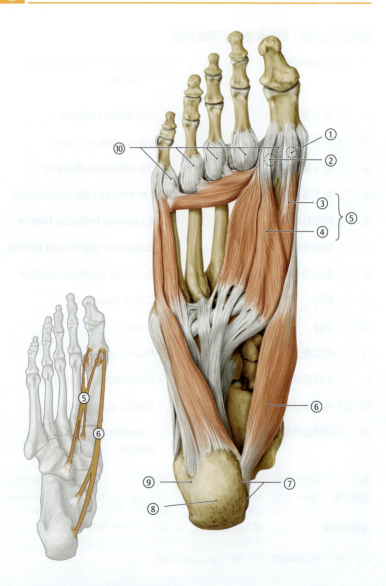

足の筋の区分 2

足底の内在筋，母趾側の部分：母趾外転筋，短母趾屈筋

① □ 内側種子骨 — □ Medial sesamoid
② □ 外側種子骨 — □ Lateral sesamoid
③ □ 短母趾屈筋の内側頭 — □ **Medial head of flexor hallucis brevis**
④ □ 短母趾屈筋の外側頭 — □ **Lateral head of flexor hallucis brevis**
⑤ □ 短母趾屈筋 — □ **Flexor hallucis brevis**
⑥ □ 母趾外転筋 — □ **Abductor hallucis**
⑦ □ 内側突起 — □ Medial process
⑧ □ 踵骨隆起 — □ Calcaneal tuberosity
⑨ □ 外側突起 — □ Lateral process
⑩ □ 中足趾節関節の関節包 — □ Metatarsophalangeal joint capsules

筋	起始	停止	作用	神経支配
母趾外転筋	・踵骨隆起(内側突起) ・足底腱膜	第1趾の基節骨底(内側種子骨を介して停止する)	・第1趾のMTP関節：第1趾の底屈・外転 ・縦足弓の保持	内側足底神経(L5-S1)
短母趾屈筋，内側頭	・内側楔状骨 ・中間楔状骨 (pp.614, 615参照) ・踵立方靱帯		・第1趾のMTP関節：底屈 ・縦足弓の保持	
短母趾屈筋，外側頭		第1趾の基節骨底(外側種子骨を介して停止する)		外側足底神経(S1-S2)

MTP関節：中足趾節関節

System of the Muscles of the Foot III

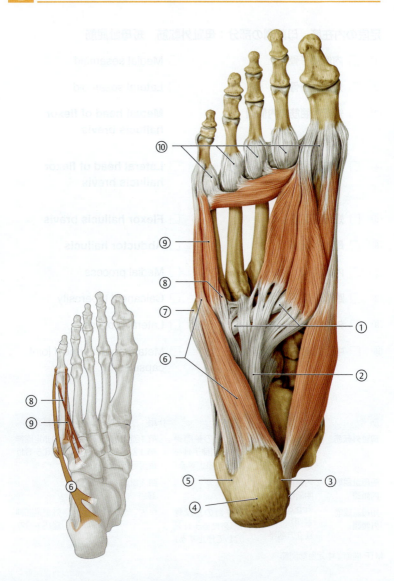

足の筋の区分 3

足底の内在筋，小趾側の部分：小趾外転筋，短小趾屈筋，小趾対立筋

① □ 長腓骨筋の腱　　　　　　　　□ Fibularis longus tendon
② □ 長足底靱帯　　　　　　　　　□ Long plantar ligament
③ □ 内側突起　　　　　　　　　　□ Medial process
④ □ 踵骨隆起　　　　　　　　　　□ Calcaneal tuberosity
⑤ □ 外側突起　　　　　　　　　　□ Lateral process
⑥ □ 小趾外転筋　　　　　　　　　□ **Abductor digiti minimi**
⑦ □ 第5中足骨粗面　　　　　　　□ Tuberosity of 5th metatarsal
⑧ □ 小趾対立筋　　　　　　　　　□ **Opponens digiti minimi**
⑨ □ 短小趾屈筋　　　　　　　　　□ **Flexor digiti minimi brevis**
⑩ □ 中足趾節関節の関節包　　　　□ Metatarsophalangeal joint capsules

筋	起始	停止	作用	神経支配
小趾外転筋	・踵骨隆起(外側突起，下面) ・足底腱膜	・第5趾(基節骨底) ・第5中足骨(粗面)	・第5趾のMTP関節：底屈・外転 ・縦足弓の保持	外側足底神経(S1-S2)
短小趾屈筋	・第5中足骨底 ・長足底靱帯	第5基節骨底	第5趾のMTP関節：底屈	
小趾対立筋	・長足底靱帯 ・長腓骨筋腱の足底腱鞘	第5中足骨	第5中足骨を足底方向および正中方向に軽く引き寄せる	

MTP関節：中足趾節関節

System of the Muscles of the Foot IV

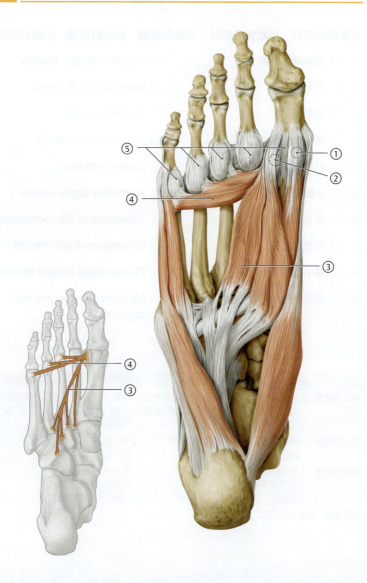

下肢 621

足の筋の区分 4

足底の内在筋，母趾側の部分：母趾内転筋

① □ 内側種子骨 　　　　　　　　□ Medial sesamoid

② □ 外側種子骨 　　　　　　　　□ Lateral sesamoid

③ □ **母趾内転筋の斜頭** 　　　　　□ **Adductor hallucis, oblique head**

④ □ **母趾内転筋の横頭** 　　　　　□ **Adductor hallucis, transverse head**

⑤ □ 中足趾節関節の関節包 　　　□ Metatarsophalangeal joint capsules

筋	起始	停止	作用	神経支配
母趾内転筋の斜頭	・第2-4中足骨底 ・立方骨 ・外側楔状骨（588, 589頁参照）	第1趾の基節骨底（共通腱が外側種子骨を介して停止する）	・第1趾のMTP関節：底屈，第1趾の内転 ・縦足弓の保持	外側足底神経（S1-S2）
母趾内転筋の横頭	第3-5趾のMTP関節，深横中足靱帯		・第1趾のMTP関節：底屈，第1趾の内転 ・横足弓の保持	

MTP関節：中足趾節関節

System of the Muscles of the Foot V

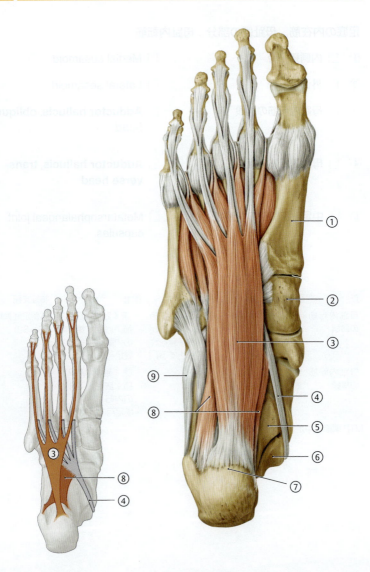

足の筋の区分 5

足底の内在筋，中央部：短趾屈筋，足底方形筋

①	□ 第 1 中足骨	□	1st metatarsal
②	□ 内側楔状骨	□	Medial cuneiform
③	□ 短趾屈筋	□	**Flexor digitorum brevis**
④	□ 長趾屈筋の腱	□	Flexor digitorum longus tendon
⑤	□ 載距突起	□	Sustentaculum tali
⑥	□ 距骨後突起	□	Posterior process of talus
⑦	□ 踵骨隆起	□	Calcaneal tuberosity
⑧	□ 足底方形筋	□	**Quadratus plantae**
⑨	□ 長腓骨筋の腱	□	Fibularis longus tendon

筋	起始	停止	作用	神経支配
短趾屈筋	・踵骨隆起(内側突起) ・足底腱膜	第 2-5 趾(中節骨の側面)	・第 2-5 趾の MTP 関節と PIP 関節：底屈 ・縦足弓の保持	内側足底神経 (L5-S1)
足底方形筋	踵骨隆起の足底面(内側縁と足底縁)		長趾屈筋の引っ張り方向の転換と増強	外側足底神経 (S1-S2)

MTP 関節：中足趾節関節　PIP 関節：近位趾節間関節

System of the Muscles of the Foot VI

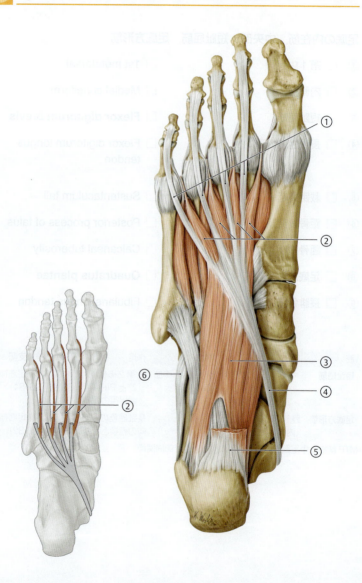

足の筋の区分 6

足底の内在筋，中央部：第1-4虫様筋

① ☐ 長趾屈筋の腱　　　　　　　☐ Flexor digitorum longus tendon

② ☐ **第1-4虫様筋**　　　　　　☐ **1st through 4th lumbricals**

③ ☐ 足底方形筋　　　　　　　　☐ Quadratus plantae

④ ☐ 長趾屈筋　　　　　　　　　☐ Flexor digitorum longus

⑤ ☐ 短趾屈筋　　　　　　　　　☐ Flexor digitorum brevis

⑥ ☐ 長腓骨筋の腱　　　　　　　☐ Fibularis longus tendon

筋	起始	停止	作用	神経支配
第1-2虫様筋	長趾屈筋腱（内側縁）*	第2-5趾（趾背腱膜）	・第2-5趾のMTP関節：底屈 ・第2-5趾のIP関節：背屈 ・趾の又を閉じる（第2-5趾の第1趾への内転）	内側足底神経（S1-S2）
第3-4虫様筋				外側足底神経（S1-S2）

IP関節：趾節間関節　MTP関節：中足趾節関節

解説

虫様筋は長趾屈筋腱の内側縁から起始している．長趾屈筋が収縮すると，虫様筋の起始が近位方向に移動し，虫様筋の筋膜が引き伸ばされる．このような状態では，虫様筋は通常よりも強い力を発生する．

System of the Muscles of the Foot VII

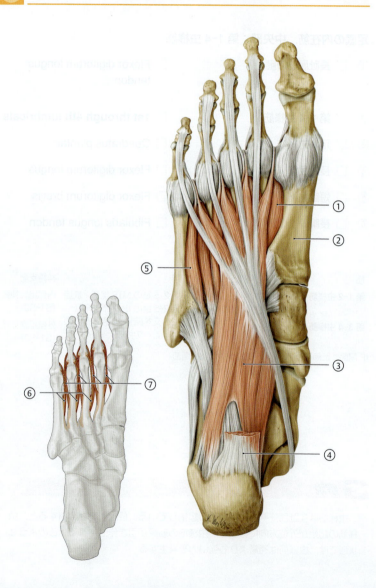

足の筋の区分 7

足底の内在筋，中央部：第 1-3 底側骨間筋と第 1-4 背側骨間筋

① ☐ 第 1 背側骨間筋　　　　　☐ 1st dorsal interosseous

② ☐ 第 1 中足骨　　　　　　　☐ 1st metatarsal

③ ☐ 足底方形筋　　　　　　　☐ Quadratus plantae

④ ☐ 短趾屈筋　　　　　　　　☐ Flexor digitorum brevis

⑤ ☐ 第 3 底側骨間筋　　　　　☐ 3rd plantar interosseous

⑥ ☐ **第 1-3 底側骨間筋**　　　☐ **1st through 3rd plantar interossei**

⑦ ☐ **第 1-4 背側骨間筋**　　　☐ **1st through 4th dorsal interossei**

筋	起始	停止	作用	神経支配
第 1-3 底側骨間筋	第 3-5 中足骨（内側縁）	第 3-5 趾（基節骨底の内側面と趾背腱膜）	・第 3-5 趾の MTP 関節：底屈 ・第 3-5 趾の IP 関節：背屈 ・趾の又を閉じる（第 3-5 趾の第 2 趾への内転）	外側足底神経（S1-S2）
第 1 背側骨間筋	第 1-5 中足骨（2 頭が隣接する中足骨の側面から起始する）	第 2 趾（基節骨底の内側面と趾背腱膜）	・第 2-4 趾の MTP 関節：底屈 ・第 2-4 趾の IP 関節：背屈 ・趾の又を広げる（第 3・4 趾の第 2 趾からの外転）	
第 2-4 背側骨間筋		第 2-4 趾（基節骨底の外側面と趾背腱膜）		

IP 関節：趾節間関節　　MTP 関節：中足趾節関節

Arteries of the Lower Limb I

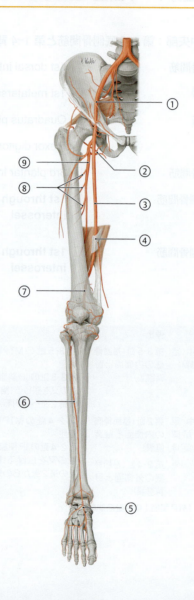

下肢の動脈 1

右下肢，前面

① ☐ 外腸骨動脈 　　　　　　　　☐ External iliac artery
② ☐ 内側大腿回旋動脈 　　　　　☐ Medial circumflex femoral artery

③ ☐ 大腿動脈 　　　　　　　　　☐ Femoral artery
④ ☐ 内転筋管と大内転筋 　　　　☐ Adductor canal (with adductor magnus)

⑤ ☐ 足背動脈 　　　　　　　　　☐ Dorsal pedal artery
⑥ ☐ 前脛骨動脈 　　　　　　　　☐ Anterior tibial artery
⑦ ☐ 膝窩動脈 　　　　　　　　　☐ Popliteal artery
⑧ ☐ 第1-3貫通動脈 　　　　　　☐ 1st through 3rd perforating arteries

⑨ ☐ 大腿深動脈 　　　　　　　　☐ Deep artery of thigh

解説

　下肢へ血液を供給する最も主要な動脈は外腸骨動脈であり，鼠径靱帯の遠位で大腿動脈となる．大腿動脈は腱裂孔を通過して膝の後方（膝窩）に入り，膝窩動脈となる．膝窩動脈は下腿に達すると，3本の主要な動脈（前脛骨動脈，後脛骨動脈，腓骨動脈）に分かれる．これらの3本の動脈は足首と足でいくつかの吻合路を形成する．

Arteries of the Lower Limb II

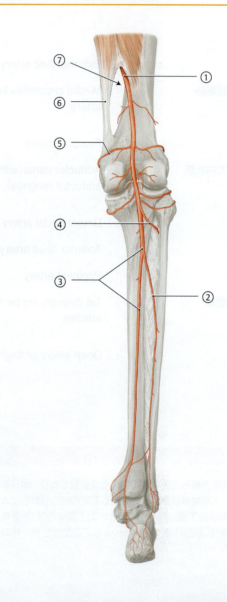

下肢の動脈 2

右下肢，後面

① □ 膝窩動脈　　　　　　　　□ Popliteal artery

② □ 腓骨動脈　　　　　　　　□ Fibular artery

③ □ 後脛骨動脈　　　　　　　□ Posterior tibial artery

④ □ 前脛骨動脈　　　　　　　□ Anterior tibial artery

⑤ □ 内側上膝動脈　　　　　　□ Superior medial genicular artery

⑥ □ 大内転筋の腱　　　　　　□ Adductor magnus tendon

⑦ □ ［内転筋］腱裂孔　　　　□ Adductor hiatus

Lumbosacral Plexus I

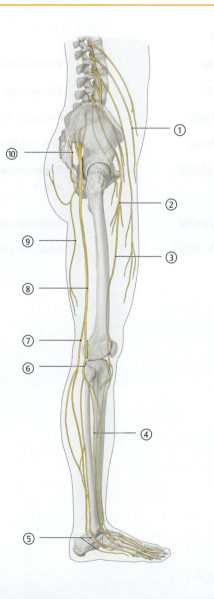

腰仙骨神経叢 1

右側,外側面

① ☐ 腸骨鼠径神経　　　　☐ Ilio-inguinal nerve
② ☐ 大腿神経　　　　　　☐ Femoral nerve
③ ☐ 伏在神経　　　　　　☐ Saphenous nerve
④ ☐ 浅腓骨神経　　　　　☐ Superficial fibular nerve
⑤ ☐ 内側・外側足底神経　☐ Medial and lateral plantar nerves
⑥ ☐ 総腓骨神経　　　　　☐ Common fibular nerve
⑦ ☐ 脛骨神経　　　　　　☐ Tibial nerve
⑧ ☐ 坐骨神経　　　　　　☐ Sciatic nerve
⑨ ☐ 後大腿皮神経　　　　☐ Posterior femoral cutaneous nerve
⑩ ☐ 陰部神経　　　　　　☐ Pudendal nerve

解説

下肢の筋の多くは仙骨神経叢に由来する神経(坐骨神経など)に支配される.ただし,下肢の前面と内側面の筋は腰神経叢に由来する神経(大腿神経と閉鎖神経)に支配される.

Lumbosacral Plexus II

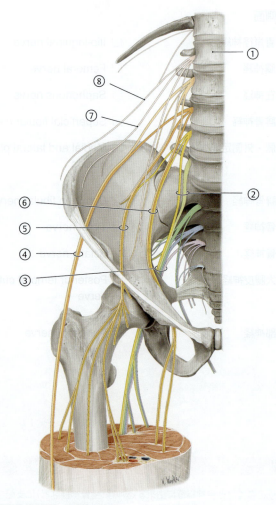

Q 腰仙骨神経幹とは何か？

腰仙骨神経叢 2

右側，前面

① □ 第1腰椎　　　　　　　□ L1 vertebra
② □ 腰仙骨神経幹　　　　　□ Lumbosacral trunk
③ □ 坐骨神経　　　　　　　□ Sciatic nerve
④ □ 外側大腿皮神経　　　　□ Lateral cutaneous nerve of thigh
⑤ □ 大腿神経　　　　　　　□ Femoral nerve
⑥ □ 閉鎖神経　　　　　　　□ Obturator nerve
⑦ □ 腸骨鼡径神経　　　　　□ Ilio-inguinal nerve
⑧ □ 腸骨下腹神経　　　　　□ Iliohypogastric nerve

A 腰仙骨神経幹は第4・5腰神経の前枝からなり，骨盤腔を下行して仙骨神経叢に加わる．

Nerves of the Lumbar Plexus I

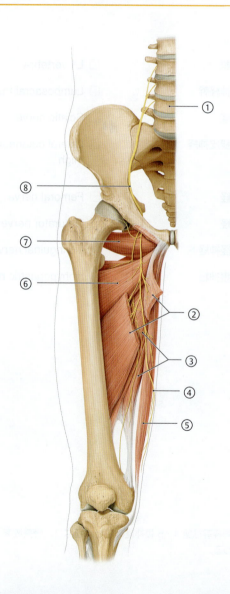

腰神経叢からの神経 1

右側，前面

① □ 第4腰椎　　□ L4 vertebra

② □ 長内転筋　　□ Adductor longus

③ □ 大内転筋　　□ Adductor magnus

④ □ 皮枝　　　　□ Cutaneous branch

⑤ □ 薄筋　　　　□ Gracilis

⑥ □ 短内転筋　　□ Adductor brevis

⑦ □ 外閉鎖筋　　□ Obturator externus

⑧ □ 閉鎖神経　　□ Obturator nerve

Nerves of the Lumbar Plexus II

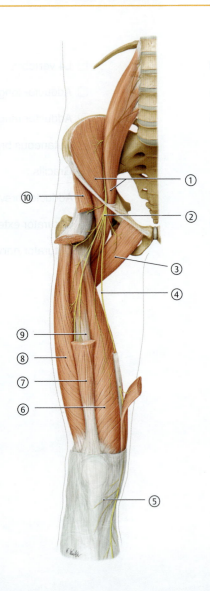

腰神経叢からの神経 2

右側，前面

① □ 腸腰筋　　　　　□ Iliopsoas
② □ 大腿神経　　　　□ Femoral nerve
③ □ 恥骨筋　　　　　□ Pectineus
④ □ 伏在神経　　　　□ Saphenous nerve
⑤ □ 膝蓋下枝　　　　□ Infrapatellar branch
⑥ □ 内側広筋　　　　□ Vastus medialis
⑦ □ 大腿直筋　　　　□ Rectus femoris
⑧ □ 外側広筋　　　　□ Vastus lateralis
⑨ □ 中間広筋　　　　□ Vastus intermedius
⑩ □ 縫工筋　　　　　□ Sartorius

臨床

　大腿四頭筋は膝関節を伸展させる唯一の筋であるため，その支配神経である大腿神経が損傷を受けると膝関節の伸展が行えなくなる．

Nerves of the Sacral Plexus I

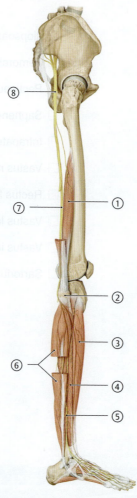

Q 深腓骨神経が損傷を受けると，どのような障害が現れるか？

仙骨神経叢からの神経 1

右下肢，外側面

① ☐ 大腿二頭筋の短頭　　☐ Short head of biceps femoris
② ☐ 腓骨頭　　☐ Head of fibula
③ ☐ 前脛骨筋　　☐ Tibialis anterior
④ ☐ 長趾伸筋　　☐ Extensor digitorum longus
⑤ ☐ 浅腓骨神経　　☐ Superficial fibular nerve
⑥ ☐ 長腓骨筋　　☐ Fibularis longus
⑦ ☐ 総腓骨神経　　☐ Common fibular nerve
⑧ ☐ 坐骨神経　　☐ Sciatic nerve

　深腓骨神経の損傷では，足首の背屈が行えなくなるとともに，第1趾間の感覚が損なわれる．

Nerves of the Sacral Plexus II

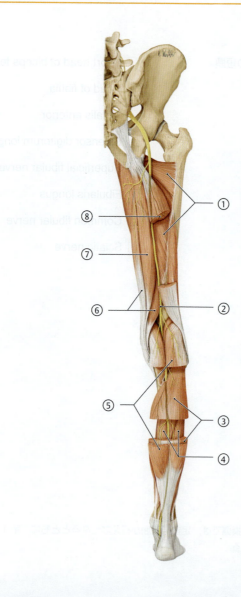

仙骨神経叢からの神経 2

右下肢，後面

① □ 大内転筋，筋性の停止部　　□ Adductor magnus, muscular insertion
② □ 脛骨神経　　□ Tibial nerve
③ □ ヒラメ筋　　□ Soleus
④ □ 深層の屈筋群　　□ Deep flexors
⑤ □ 腓腹筋　　□ Gastrocnemius
⑥ □ 半膜様筋　　□ Semimembranosus
⑦ □ 半腱様筋　　□ Semitendinosus
⑧ □ 大腿二頭筋の長頭　　□ Long head of biceps femoris

解説

脛骨神経は坐骨神経の枝であり，大腿後面の筋（大腿二頭筋の短頭を除く），下腿後面の筋，足底の筋を支配する．

Superficial Veins & Nerves

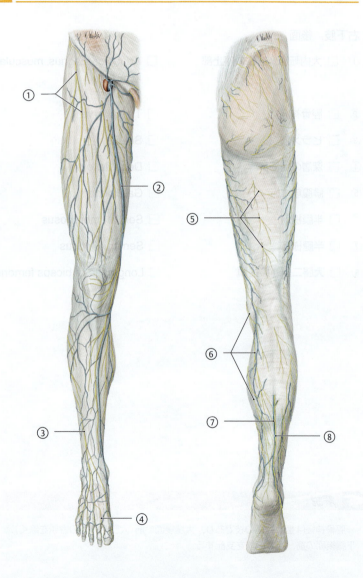

皮静脈と皮神経

右下肢．左：前面，右：後面

① ☐ 外側大腿皮神経 — ☐ Lateral cutaneous nerve of thigh
② ☐ 大伏在静脈 — ☐ Great saphenous vein
③ ☐ 浅腓骨神経 — ☐ Superficial fibular nerve
④ ☐ 深腓骨神経 — ☐ Deep fibular nerve
⑤ ☐ 後大腿皮神経 — ☐ Posterior femoral cutaneous nerve
⑥ ☐ 伏在神経（大腿神経の枝） — ☐ Saphenous nerve（femoral nerve）
⑦ ☐ 小伏在静脈 — ☐ Short saphenous vein
⑧ ☐ 腓腹神経 — ☐ Sural nerve

解説

皮静脈は深静脈（動脈に伴行する静脈）に流れ込む．皮静脈の流入部は様々な位置に見られるが，特に重要なのが大伏在静脈と小伏在静脈であり，それぞれ大腿静脈と膝窩静脈に流入する．

Inguinal Region

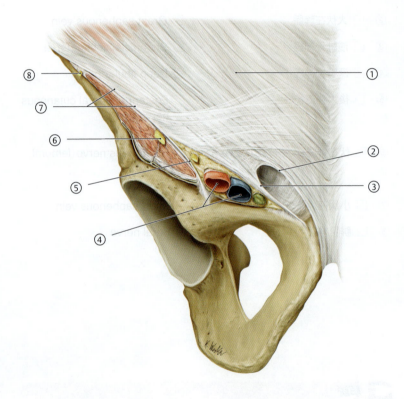

鼠径部

右側，前面

① ☐ 外腹斜筋腱膜 — ☐ External oblique aponeurosis
② ☐ 浅鼠径輪の内側脚 — ☐ Medial crus of superficial inguinal ring
③ ☐ 浅鼠径輪の外側脚 — ☐ Lateral crus of superficial inguinal ring
④ ☐ 大腿動脈・静脈 — ☐ Femoral artery and vein
⑤ ☐ 腸恥筋膜弓 — ☐ Iliopectineal arch
⑥ ☐ 大腿神経 — ☐ Femoral nerve
⑦ ☐ 鼠径靱帯 — ☐ Inguinal ligament
⑧ ☐ 外側大腿皮神経 — ☐ Lateral cutaneous nerve of thigh

解説

鼠径靱帯と鼠径管の後方には，大腿に向かう筋，神経，血管の通路が存在する．筋（腸腰筋）と神経（大腿神経）は筋裂孔を，脈管（大腿動脈・静脈，リンパ管）は血管裂孔を通過する．2つの裂孔は腸恥筋膜弓によって隔てられる．

Sciatic Foramina

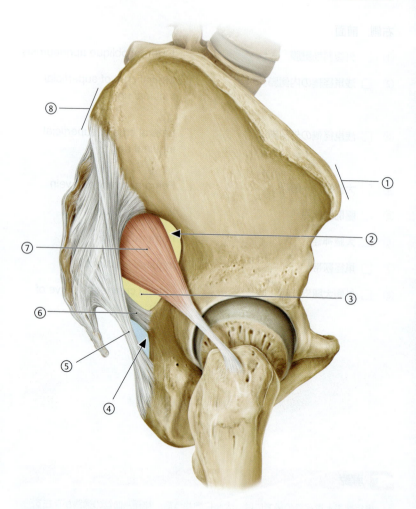

Q 小坐骨孔を通過するものは何か？

坐骨孔

右側,外側面

① ☐ 上前腸骨棘 — ☐ Anterior superior iliac spine
② ☐ 大坐骨孔の梨状筋上孔 — ☐ Suprapiriform portion of greater sciatic foramen
③ ☐ 大坐骨孔の梨状筋下孔 — ☐ Infrapiriform portion of greater sciatic foramen
④ ☐ 小坐骨孔 — ☐ Lesser sciatic foramen
⑤ ☐ 仙結節靱帯 — ☐ Sacrotuberous ligament
⑥ ☐ 仙棘靱帯 — ☐ Sacrospinous ligament
⑦ ☐ 梨状筋 — ☐ Piriformis
⑧ ☐ 上後腸骨棘 — ☐ Posterior superior iliac spine

A 陰部神経と内陰部動脈・静脈が小坐骨孔を通り,会陰に達する.

Neurovasculature of the Anterior Thigh

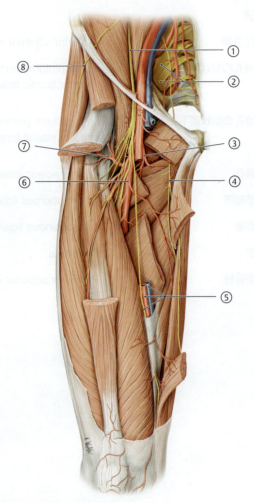

股関節に分布する動脈は何か？

大腿前面の神経・血管

右大腿,前面

① ☐ 大腿神経 ☐ Femoral nerve
② ☐ 仙骨神経叢 ☐ Sacral plexus
③ ☐ 内側大腿回旋動脈 ☐ Medial circumflex femoral artery
④ ☐ 閉鎖神経 ☐ Obturator nerve
⑤ ☐ 大腿動脈・静脈,伏在神経（広筋内転筋膜の内側にある） ☐ Femoral artery and vein, saphenous nerve (in vastoadductor membrane)
⑥ ☐ 大腿深動脈 ☐ Deep artery of thigh
⑦ ☐ 外側大腿回旋動脈,上行枝 ☐ Lateral circumflex femoral artery, ascending branch
⑧ ☐ 外側大腿皮神経 ☐ Lateral cutaneous nerve of thigh

A 股関節には内側・外側大腿回旋動脈が分布する.

Neurovasculature of the Posterior Thigh

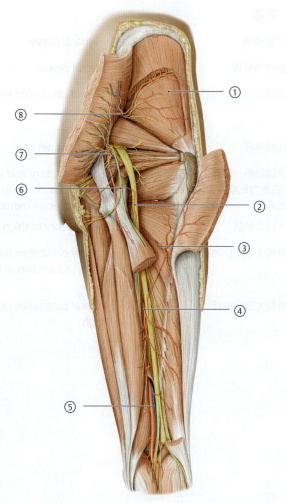

どの神経の損傷によってトレンデレンブルグ試験が陽性となるか？

大腿後面の神経・血管

右大腿, 後面

① □ 小殿筋　　　　　　　　□ Gluteus minimus
② □ 坐骨神経,　　　　　　 □ Sciatic nerve (with artery)
　　　坐骨神経伴行動脈
③ □ 第1貫通動脈　　　　　□ 1st perforating artery
④ □ 第2貫通動脈　　　　　□ 2nd perforating artery
⑤ □ 膝窩動脈・静脈　　　　□ Popliteal artery and vein
⑥ □ 後大腿皮神経　　　　　□ Posterior femoral cutaneous nerve
⑦ □ 陰部神経　　　　　　　□ Pudendal nerve
⑧ □ 上殿動脈・静脈・神経　□ Superior gluteal artery, vein, and nerve

　トレンデレンブルグ試験とは，片足立ちにより，中殿筋と小殿筋（いずれも上殿神経に支配される）の筋力を検査する方法である．上殿神経が損傷され，中殿筋と小殿筋に筋力低下（麻痺）が生じた場合，障害側で片足立ちをすると，骨盤が正常側（遊脚側）へ傾く．この状態をトレンデレンブルグ試験陽性という．

Neurovasculature of the Posterior Leg

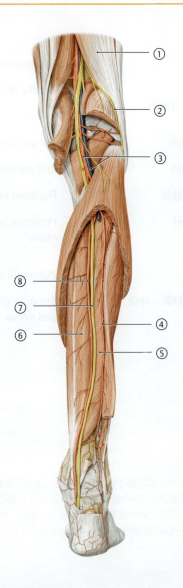

下腿後面の神経・血管

右下腿，後面

① □ 大腿二頭筋　　　　　　□ Biceps femoris
② □ 総腓骨神経　　　　　　□ Common fibular nerve
③ □ 膝窩動脈・静脈　　　　□ Popliteal artery and vein
④ □ 腓骨動脈　　　　　　　□ Fibular artery
⑤ □ 後脛骨筋　　　　　　　□ Tibialis posterior
⑥ □ 長趾屈筋　　　　　　　□ Flexor digitorum longus
⑦ □ 脛骨神経　　　　　　　□ Tibial nerve
⑧ □ 後脛骨動脈　　　　　　□ Posterior tibial artery

The Tarsal Tunnel

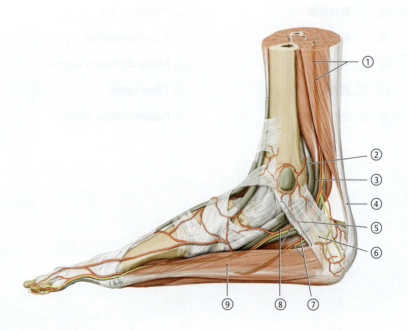

足根管

右足，内側面

① 脛骨神経，後脛骨動脈 — Tibial nerve, posterior tibial artery
② 後脛骨筋 — Tibialis posterior
③ 長趾屈筋 — Flexor digitorum longus
④ 踵骨腱（アキレス腱） — Calcaneal (Achilles') tendon
⑤ 足根管 — Tarsal tunnel
⑥ 屈筋支帯 — Flexor retinaculum
⑦ 外側足底動脈・神経 — Lateral plantar artery and nerve
⑧ 内側足底動脈・神経 — Medial plantar artery and nerve
⑨ 母趾外転筋 — Abductor hallucis

Neurovasculature of the Lateral Leg

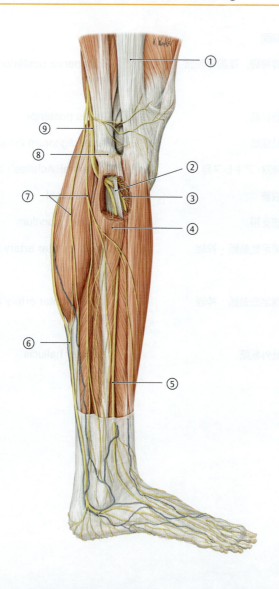

下腿外側の神経・血管

右下腿，外側面

① ☐ 腸脛靱帯　　　　　　　☐ Iliotibial tract
② ☐ 前下腿筋間中隔　　　　☐ Anterior intermuscular septum of leg
③ ☐ 深腓骨神経　　　　　　☐ Deep fibular nerve
④ ☐ 長腓骨筋　　　　　　　☐ Fibularis longus
⑤ ☐ 浅腓骨神経　　　　　　☐ Superficial fibular nerve
⑥ ☐ 腓腹神経　　　　　　　☐ Sural nerve
⑦ ☐ 外側腓腹皮神経　　　　☐ Lateral sural cutaneous nerve
⑧ ☐ 腓骨頭　　　　　　　　☐ Head of fibula
⑨ ☐ 総腓骨神経　　　　　　☐ Common fibular nerve

解説

　総腓骨神経は皮膚の直下で，腓骨頭を取り巻くように走行した後，下腿筋膜を貫いて外側区画に入る．総腓骨神経が腓骨頭の部位で圧迫されると，下腿の前区画と外側区画にある筋に筋力低下(麻痺)が生じる．これらの筋の筋力低下では，下垂足が見られ，足の外反も困難となる．

Neurovasculature of the Anterior Leg

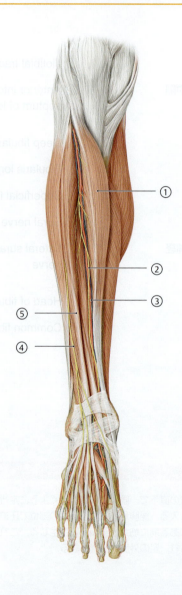

下腿前面の神経・血管

右下腿,前面

① □ 前脛骨筋　　　　　　　□ Tibialis anterior
② □ 深腓骨神経　　　　　　□ Deep fibular nerve
③ □ 前脛骨動脈・静脈　　　□ Anterior tibial artery and vein
④ □ 浅腓骨神経　　　　　　□ Superficial fibular nerve
⑤ □ 長趾伸筋　　　　　　　□ Extensor digitorum longus

臨床

　筋の浮腫や血腫によって下腿の区画(コンパートメント)内の組織圧が異常に高まると,神経や血管が圧迫される.このような状態が長時間続くと,筋や神経が虚血に陥り,不可逆的な障害が残る場合がある.下腿の前区画にこのような状態が生じると,患者は耐えがたい激痛に見舞われ,足趾の背屈が困難となる(前コンパートメント症候群と呼ばれ,コンパートメント症候群の中でも一般的なものである).このような患者では,下腿筋膜を緊急に切開し,区画内の組織圧を下げなければならない.

Neurovasculature of the Dorsum

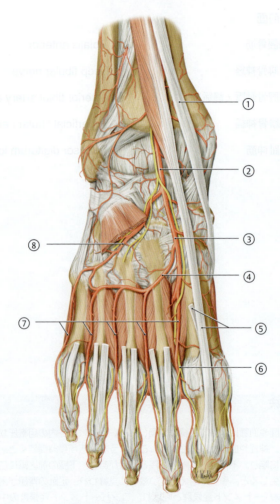

足背動脈はどの動脈から起始するか？

足背の神経・血管

右足，足背面（上面）

①	□ 前脛骨筋の腱	□ Tibialis anterior tendon
②	□ 前脛骨動脈	□ Anterior tibial artery
③	□ 足背動脈	□ Dorsal pedal artery
④	□ 弓状動脈	□ Arcuate artery
⑤	□ 長・短母趾伸筋の腱	□ Extensors hallucis longus and brevis tendons
⑥	□ 深腓骨神経の皮枝	□ Cutaneous branch of deep fibular nerve
⑦	□ 背側中足動脈	□ Dorsal metatarsal arteries
⑧	□ 外側足根動脈	□ Lateral tarsal artery

A 足背動脈は前脛骨動脈（膝窩動脈の枝）の延長である．

Neurovasculature of the Sole

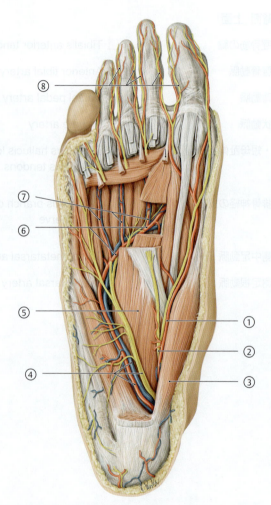

Q 下腿の神経のうち，外側・内側足底神経を出すのはどれか？

足底の神経・血管

右足，足底面（下面）

① ☐ 内側足底動脈　　　　　☐ Medial plantar artery

② ☐ 内側足底神経　　　　　☐ Medial plantar nerve

③ ☐ 母趾外転筋　　　　　　☐ Abductor hallucis

④ ☐ 外側足底動脈・静脈・神経　☐ Lateral plantar artery, vein, and nerve

⑤ ☐ 足底方形筋　　　　　　☐ Quadratus plantae

⑥ ☐ 深足底動脈弓　　　　　☐ Deep plantar arch

⑦ ☐ 底側中足動脈　　　　　☐ Plantar metatarsal arteries

⑧ ☐ 固有底側趾動脈・神経　　☐ Proper plantar digital arteries and nerves

A 　脛骨神経は足に入ると，外側・内側足底神経に分岐し，足底の筋を支配する．

Transverse Section of the Thigh

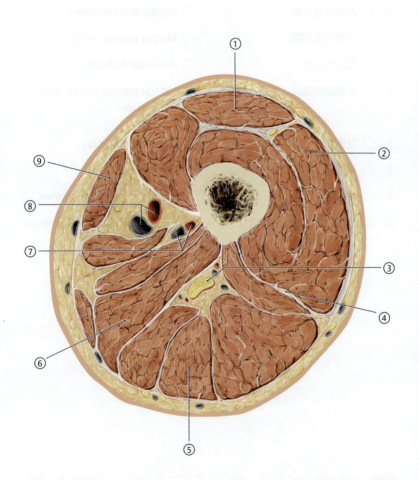

大腿の横断面

右大腿，近位方向（上方）から見たところ

① □ 大腿直筋　　　　　　□ Rectus femoris
② □ 外側広筋　　　　　　□ Vastus lateralis
③ □ 坐骨神経　　　　　　□ Sciatic nerve
④ □ 外側大腿筋間中隔　　□ Lateral femoral intermuscular septum
⑤ □ 半腱様筋　　　　　　□ Semitendinosus
⑥ □ 大内転筋　　　　　　□ Adductor magnus
⑦ □ 大腿深動脈・静脈　　□ Deep artery of thigh, deep femoral vein of thigh
⑧ □ 大腿動脈・静脈　　　□ Femoral artery and vein
⑨ □ 縫工筋　　　　　　　□ Sartorius

Transverse Section of the Leg

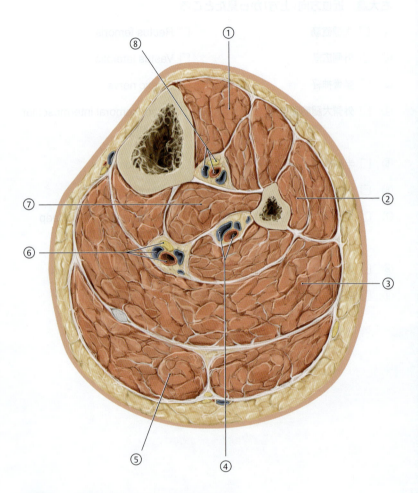

 下腿の外側区画に分布する動脈は何か？

下腿の横断面

右下腿，近位面（上面）

① □ 前脛骨筋　　　　　　　　□ Tibialis anterior
② □ 短腓骨筋　　　　　　　　□ Fibularis brevis
③ □ ヒラメ筋　　　　　　　　□ Soleus
④ □ 腓骨動脈・静脈　　　　　□ Fibular artery and vein
⑤ □ 腓腹筋の内側頭　　　　　□ Medial head of gastrocnemius
⑥ □ 脛骨神経，後脛骨動脈・静脈　□ Tibial nerve, posterior tibial artery and vein
⑦ □ 後脛骨筋　　　　　　　　□ Tibialis posterior
⑧ □ 深腓骨神経，前脛骨動脈・静脈　□ Deep fibular nerve, anterior tibial artery and vein

A 外側区画には太い動脈が通過しないため，この区画には前脛骨動脈の枝や腓骨動脈の貫通枝が分布する．

Surface Anatomy

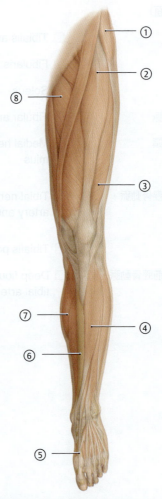

股関節の周囲で触知できる大腿骨の隆起は何か？

下肢の体表解剖

左下肢，前面

① □ 大腿筋膜張筋　　　□ Tensor fasciae latae
② □ 大腿直筋　　　　　□ Rectus femoris
③ □ 外側広筋　　　　　□ Vastus lateralis
④ □ 前脛骨筋　　　　　□ Tibialis anterior
⑤ □ 長母趾伸筋の腱　　□ Extensor hallucis longus tendon
⑥ □ 脛骨　　　　　　　□ Tibia
⑦ □ 腓腹筋　　　　　　□ Gastrocnemius
⑧ □ 長内転筋　　　　　□ Adductor longus

 大腿骨の近位部で体表から触知できるのは大転子だけである．

頭頸部 Head & Neck

頭蓋の骨 1-3 …… 674	内耳 …… 776
頭蓋底 1-3 …… 680	下顎骨 …… 778
表情筋 …… 686	口腔の三叉神経 …… 780
頭部の筋の区分 1-3 …… 688	舌背 …… 782
脳神経 1-10 …… 694	舌の筋 …… 784
感覚神経支配 …… 714	舌の感覚性神経支配と味覚神経支配 …… 786
頭蓋と顔面の動脈 1, 2 …… 716	舌の神経と血管 …… 788
頭頸部の静脈 1, 2 …… 720	口腔の区分 1, 2 …… 790
顔面浅層の神経・血管 1, 2 …… 724	唾液腺 1, 2 …… 794
耳下腺咬筋部 1, 2 …… 728	咽頭筋 1, 2 …… 798
側頭下窩 1-3 …… 732	咽頭の神経・血管 …… 802
翼口蓋窩 …… 738	頸部の筋の概観 …… 804
眼窩の骨 …… 740	頸部の筋 1-6 …… 806
眼窩の筋 …… 742	頸部の動脈 …… 818
眼窩の神経 1, 2 …… 744	頸部の神経 …… 820
眼窩の局所解剖 1, 2 …… 748	甲状腺 …… 822
眼瞼と結膜 …… 752	甲状腺の位置 …… 824
涙器 …… 754	喉頭の構造 …… 826
眼球の構造 …… 756	喉頭腔 …… 828
鼻腔の骨 1-3 …… 758	喉頭の神経・血管 1, 2 …… 830
鼻腔の神経・血管 1, 2 …… 764	頸部の部位 …… 834
外耳 …… 768	胸郭上口 1, 2 …… 836
耳介の構造 …… 770	外側頸三角部の局所解剖 1, 2 …… 840
鼓室 …… 772	頭頸部の体表解剖 …… 844
耳小骨連鎖 …… 774	

Bones of the Skull I

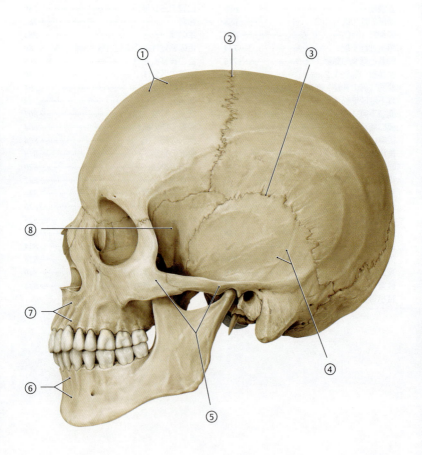

頭蓋の骨 1

左外側面

① □ 前頭骨　　　　　　　　□ Frontal bone
② □ 冠状縫合　　　　　　　□ Coronal suture
③ □ 鱗状縫合　　　　　　　□ Squamous suture
④ □ 側頭骨の鱗部　　　　　□ Squamous part of temporal bone
⑤ □ 頬骨弓　　　　　　　　□ Zygomatic arch
⑥ □ 下顎骨　　　　　　　　□ Mandible
⑦ □ 上顎骨　　　　　　　　□ Maxilla
⑧ □ 蝶形骨の大翼　　　　　□ Greater wing of sphenoid

解説

頭蓋は脳頭蓋と顔面頭蓋に分けられる．脳頭蓋は脳を保護し，顔面頭蓋は顔面の諸部分を収容して，保護する．

Bones of the Skull II

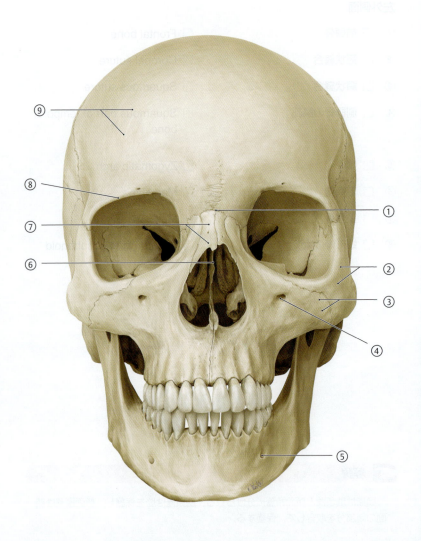

頭蓋の骨 2

前面

① □ 鼻根点　　　　　□ Nasion
② □ 頬骨　　　　　　□ Zygomatic bone
③ □ 上顎骨　　　　　□ Maxilla
④ □ 眼窩下孔　　　　□ Infra-orbital foramen
⑤ □ オトガイ孔　　　□ Mental foramen
⑥ □ 篩骨の垂直板　　□ Perpendicular plate of ethmoid bone
⑦ □ 鼻骨　　　　　　□ Nasal bone
⑧ □ 眼窩上縁　　　　□ Supra-orbital margin
⑨ □ 前頭骨　　　　　□ Frontal bone

臨床

顔面骨格は枠状の構造であるために骨折線は特徴的なパターンを示し，ル・フォールⅠ-Ⅲ型に分類される．

Bones of the Skull III

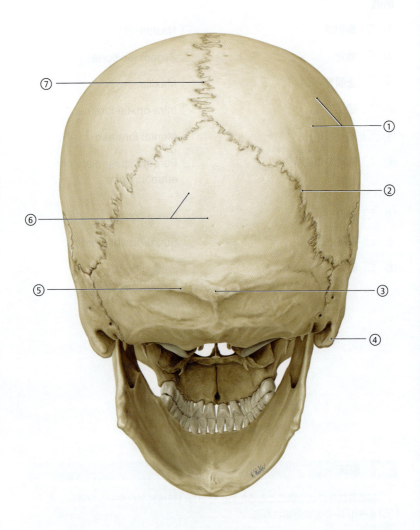

頭蓋の骨 3

後面

① ☐ 頭頂骨　　　　　　　☐ Parietal bone
② ☐ ラムダ縫合　　　　　☐ Lambdoid suture
③ ☐ 外後頭隆起　　　　　☐ External occipital protuberance
④ ☐ 乳様突起　　　　　　☐ Mastoid process
⑤ ☐ 上項線　　　　　　　☐ Superior nuchal line
⑥ ☐ 後頭骨　　　　　　　☐ Occipital bone
⑦ ☐ 矢状縫合　　　　　　☐ Sagittal suture

Base of the Skull I

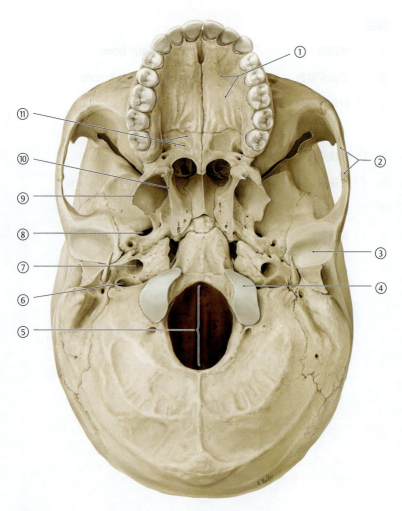

Q 外側板と内側板があるのはどの頭蓋骨か？

頭蓋底 1

下面

① ☐ 上顎骨の口蓋突起　　☐ Palatine process of maxilla
② ☐ 頬骨弓　　☐ Zygomatic arch
③ ☐ 下顎窩　　☐ Mandibular fossa
④ ☐ 後頭顆　　☐ Occipital condyle
⑤ ☐ 大後頭孔　　☐ Foramen magnum
⑥ ☐ 頸静脈孔　　☐ Jugular foramen
⑦ ☐ 頸動脈管　　☐ Carotid canal
⑧ ☐ 卵円孔　　☐ Foramen ovale
⑨ ☐ 翼状突起の外側板　　☐ Lateral plate of pterygoid process
⑩ ☐ 翼状突起の内側板　　☐ Medial plate of pterygoid process
⑪ ☐ 口蓋骨　　☐ Palatine bone

A 外側板と内側板は蝶形骨の翼状突起にある．

Base of the Skull II

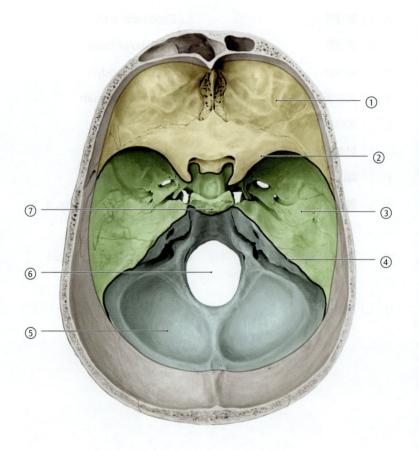

頭蓋底 2

上面

① □ 前頭蓋窩　　　□ Anterior cranial fossa
② □ 蝶形骨の小翼　□ Lesser wing of sphenoid
③ □ 中頭蓋窩　　　□ Middle cranial fossa
④ □ 錐体上縁　　　□ Petrous ridge
⑤ □ 後頭蓋窩　　　□ Posterior cranial fossa
⑥ □ 大後頭孔　　　□ Foramen magnum
⑦ □ 鞍背　　　　　□ Dorsum sellae

解説

頭蓋底の内面は連続する3つの窩からなる．これらの窩は前方から後方に向かって段階的に深くなる．

Base of the Skull III

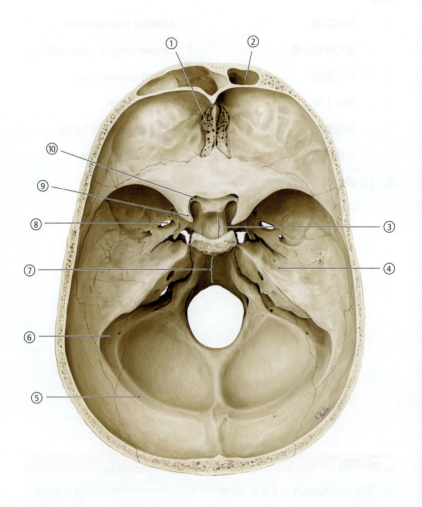

頭蓋底 3

上面

① □ 篩板　　　　　　　　□ Cribriform plate
② □ 前頭洞　　　　　　　□ Frontal sinus
③ □ 下垂体窩（トルコ鞍）　□ Hypophyseal fossa (sella turcica)
④ □ 側頭骨の岩様部　　　□ Petrous part of temporal bone
⑤ □ 横洞溝　　　　　　　□ Groove for transverse sinus
⑥ □ S状洞溝　　　　　　 □ Groove for sigmoid sinus
⑦ □ 斜台　　　　　　　　□ Clivus
⑧ □ 卵円孔　　　　　　　□ Foramen ovale
⑨ □ 前床突起　　　　　　□ Anterior clinoid process
⑩ □ 視神経管　　　　　　□ Optic canal

Muscles of Facial Expression

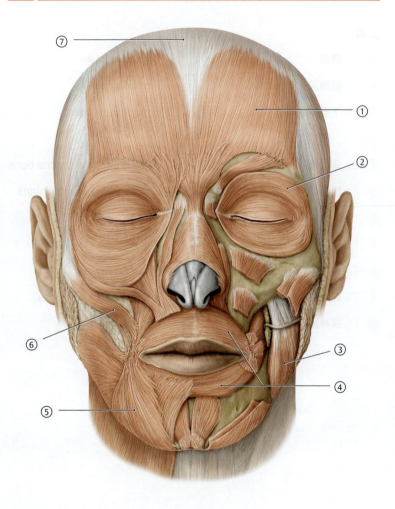

表情筋と咀嚼筋の支配神経は何か？

表情筋

前面

① □ 前頭筋(後頭前頭筋) □ Occipitofrontalis, frontal belly
② □ 眼輪筋 □ Orbicularis oculi
③ □ 咬筋 □ Masseter
④ □ 口輪筋 □ Orbicularis oris
⑤ □ 口角下制筋 □ Depressor anguli oris
⑥ □ 大頬骨筋 □ Zygomaticus major
⑦ □ 帽状腱膜 □ Galea aponeurotica (epicranial aponeurosis)

A 表情筋の運動は顔面神経に支配される．咀嚼筋は三叉神経の枝の下顎神経に支配される．

System of the Muscles of the Skull I

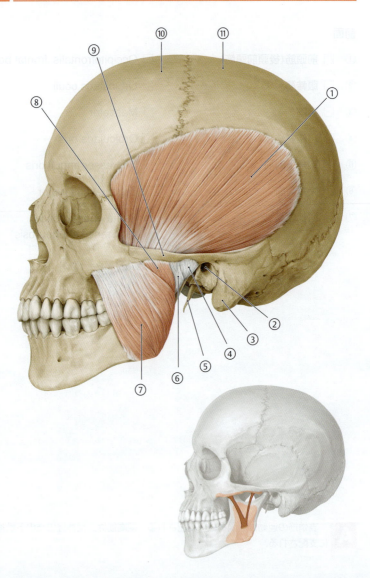

頭部の筋の区分 1

浅層の咀嚼筋:咬筋

① □ 側頭筋 　　　　　　　　　　□ Temporalis
② □ 外耳孔 　　　　　　　　　　□ External acoustic opening
③ □ 乳様突起 　　　　　　　　　□ Mastoid process
④ □ 顎関節の関節包 　　　　　　□ Joint capsule of temporo-mandiblar joint
⑤ □ 茎状突起 　　　　　　　　　□ Styloid process
⑥ □ 外側靱帯 　　　　　　　　　□ Lateral ligament
⑦ □ 咬筋の浅部 　　　　　　　　□ **Superficial part of masseter**
⑧ □ 咬筋の深部 　　　　　　　　□ **Deep part of masseter**
⑨ □ 頬骨弓 　　　　　　　　　　□ Zygomatic arch
⑩ □ 前頭骨 　　　　　　　　　　□ Frontal bone
⑪ □ 頭頂骨 　　　　　　　　　　□ Parietal bone

筋	起始	停止	作用	神経支配
咬筋の浅部	頬骨弓(前 2/3)	下顎角(咬筋粗面)	・下顎骨を引き上げる(顎を閉じる=挙上) ・下顎骨を前に出す(=前突)	下顎神経(CN V₃)の枝の咬筋神経
咬筋の深部	頬骨弓(後 1/3)			

System of the Muscles of the Skull II

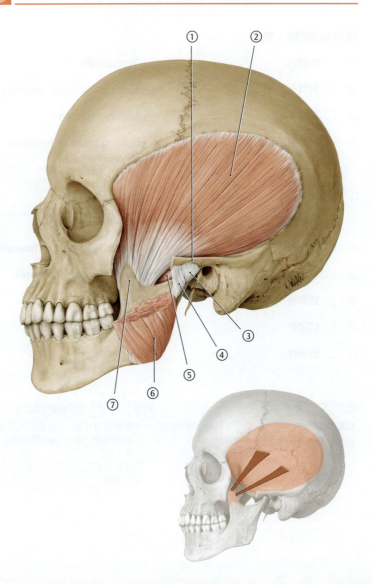

頭部の筋の区分 2

浅層の咀嚼筋：側頭筋

① □ 頬骨弓　　　　　　　　　□ Zygomatic arch

② □ 側頭筋　　　　　　　　　□ **Temporalis**

③ □ 顎関節の関節包　　　　　□ Joint capsule of temporo-mandibular joint

④ □ 外側靱帯　　　　　　　　□ Lateral ligament

⑤ □ 外側翼突筋　　　　　　　□ Lateral pterygoid

⑥ □ 咬筋　　　　　　　　　　□ Masseter

⑦ □ 筋突起　　　　　　　　　□ Coronoid process

筋	起始	停止	作用	神経支配
側頭筋	側頭窩(下側頭線)	下顎骨筋突起(先端と内側面)	・垂直線維：下顎骨を引き上げる(挙上) ・水平線維：下顎骨を後方に引く(後退) ・片側：臼磨運動(前方に移動した平衡側下顎頭を元に戻す)	下顎神経(CN V₃)の枝の深側頭神経

System of the Muscles of the Skull III

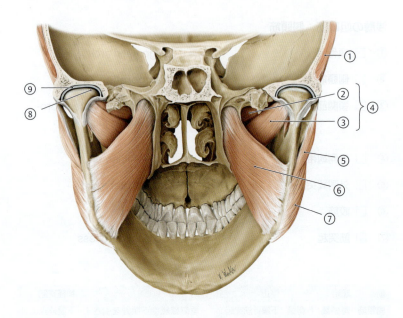

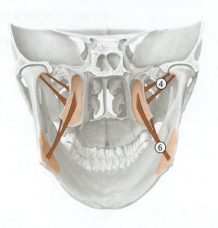

頭部の筋の区分 3

深層の咀嚼筋：内側翼突筋と外側翼突筋

① □ 側頭筋　　　　　　　　□ Temporalis

② □ 上頭　　　　　　　　　□ Superior head

③ □ 下頭　　　　　　　　　□ Inferior head

④ □ **外側翼突筋**　　　　　　□ **Lateral pterygoid**

⑤ □ 咬筋の深部　　　　　　□ Deep part of masseter

⑥ □ **内側翼突筋**　　　　　　□ **Medial pterygoid**

⑦ □ 咬筋の浅部　　　　　　□ Superficial part of masseter

⑧ □ 下顎頭，関節面　　　　□ Head of mandible, articular surface

⑨ □ 関節円板　　　　　　　□ Articular disk

筋	起始	停止	作用	神経支配
内側翼突筋	・翼突窩 ・翼状突起の外側板	下顎角内面（翼突筋粗面）	下顎骨を引き上げる（挙上）	下顎神経（CN V₃）の枝の内側翼突筋神経
外側翼突筋（上頭）	側頭下稜（蝶形骨大翼）	顎関節（関節円板）	・両側：下顎を前方に押しやり（前突），関節円板を腹側移動させることによる開口の先導 ・片側：臼磨運動の際に下顎を反対側へ動かす	下顎神経（CN V₃）の枝の外側翼突筋神経
外側翼突筋（下頭）	翼状突起の外側板（外側面）	下顎骨（関節突起）		

Cranial Nerves I

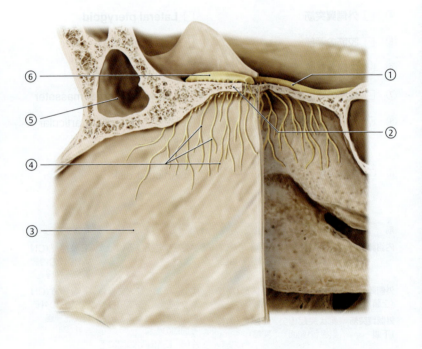

脳神経 1

左鼻中隔の一部と右鼻腔の外壁，左外側面

① □ 嗅索　　　　　　　　　　　□ Olfactory tract

② □ 篩板　　　　　　　　　　　□ Cribriform plate

③ □ 鼻中隔（篩骨の垂直板）　　　□ Nasal septum (perpendicular plate of ethmoid bone)

④ □ 嗅神経糸　　　　　　　　　□ Olfactory nerves

⑤ □ 前頭洞　　　　　　　　　　□ Frontal sinus

⑥ □ 嗅球　　　　　　　　　　　□ Olfactory bulb

Cranial Nerves II

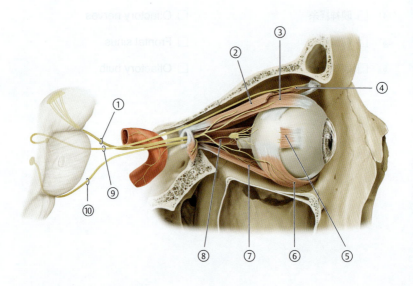

脳神経 2

右眼窩, 外側面

① □ 動眼神経　　　　　□ Oculomotor nerve (CN III)

② □ 上眼瞼挙筋　　　　□ Levator palpebrae superioris

③ □ 上直筋　　　　　　□ Superior rectus

④ □ 上斜筋　　　　　　□ Superior oblique

⑤ □ 外側直筋（断端）　□ Lateral rectus (cut)

⑥ □ 下斜筋　　　　　　□ Inferior oblique

⑦ □ 下直筋　　　　　　□ Inferior rectus

⑧ □ 内側直筋　　　　　□ Medial rectus

⑨ □ 滑車神経　　　　　□ Trochlear nerve (CN IV)

⑩ □ 外転神経　　　　　□ Abducent nerve (CN VI)

 臨床

　動眼神経は内眼筋を副交感性に支配し，外眼筋の大部分と上眼瞼挙筋を体性運動性に支配する．動眼神経の副交感性線維は毛様体神経節でシナプスを形成する．動眼神経麻痺が起こると，その影響が副交感性線維だけに現れる場合や体性線維だけに現れる場合，さらに両方に現れる場合がある．

Cranial Nerves III

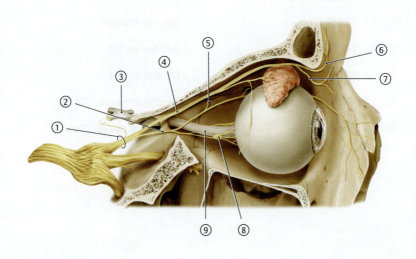

脳神経 3

右眼窩，外側面

①	□ 眼神経	□ Ophthalmic nerve (CN V₁)
②	□ 鼻毛様体神経	□ Nasociliary nerve
③	□ 視交叉	□ Optic chiasm
④	□ 前頭神経	□ Frontal nerve
⑤	□ 後篩骨神経	□ Posterior ethmoidal nerve
⑥	□ 眼窩上神経	□ Supra-orbital nerve
⑦	□ 滑車上神経	□ Supratrochlear nerve
⑧	□ 毛様体神経節	□ Ciliary ganglion
⑨	□ 視神経	□ Optic nerve (CN II)

解説

視神経は視神経管を通って眼窩に至り，他の脳神経は上眼窩裂を通って眼窩と眼球に入る．

Cranial Nerves IV

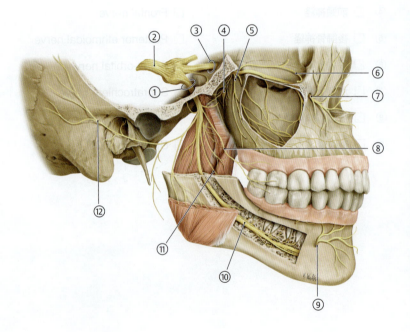

脳神経 4

右外側面

① □ 下顎神経（卵円孔を通る） □ Mandibular nerve (CN V₃, via foramen ovale)

② □ 三叉神経 □ Trigeminal nerve (CN V)

③ □ 上顎神経（正円孔を通る） □ Maxillary nerve (CN V₂, via foramen rotundum)

④ □ 翼口蓋神経節 □ Pterygopalatine ganglion

⑤ □ 上歯槽神経の後上歯槽枝 □ Posterior superior alveolar artery of superior alveolar nerves

⑥ □ 頬骨神経 □ Zygomatic nerve

⑦ □ 眼窩下神経と眼窩下孔 □ Infra-orbital nerve (and foramen)

⑧ □ 頬神経 □ Buccal nerve

⑨ □ オトガイ神経とオトガイ孔 □ Mental nerve (and foramen)

⑩ □ 下歯槽神経（下顎管にある） □ Inferior alveolar nerve (in mandibular canal)

⑪ □ 舌神経 □ Lingual nerve

⑫ □ 耳介側頭神経 □ Auriculotemporal nerve

Cranial Nerves V

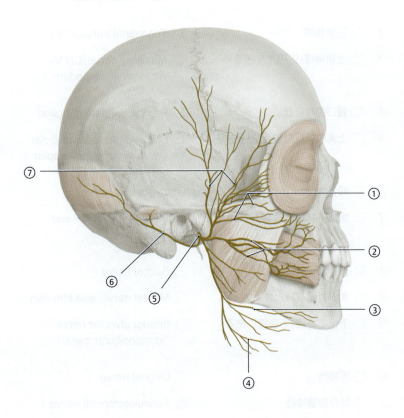

脳神経 5

右外側面

① □ 頬骨枝 □ Zygomatic branches
② □ 頬筋枝 □ Buccal branches
③ □ 下顎縁枝 □ Marginal mandibular branch
④ □ 頸枝 □ Cervical branch
⑤ □ 顔面神経 □ Facial nerve
⑥ □ 後耳介神経 □ Posterior auricular nerve
⑦ □ 側頭枝 □ Temporal branches

解説

顔面神経は表情筋を支配する．

Cranial Nerves VI

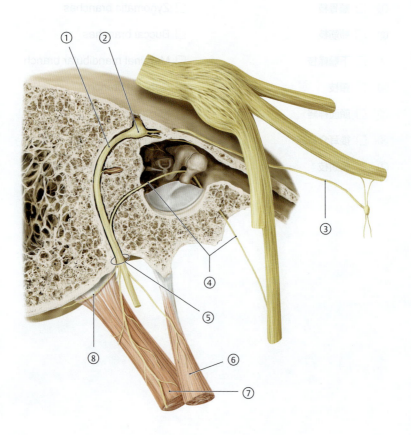

Q 鼓索神経が運ぶのはどのような線維か?

脳神経 6

右外側面

① □ 顔面神経　　　　　　□ Facial nerve (CN VII)
② □ 膝神経節　　　　　　□ Geniculate ganglion
③ □ 大錐体神経　　　　　□ Greater petrosal nerve
④ □ 鼓索神経　　　　　　□ Chorda tympani
⑤ □ 茎乳突孔　　　　　　□ Stylomastoid foramen
⑥ □ 茎突舌骨筋　　　　　□ Stylohyoid
⑦ □ 顎二腹筋の後腹　　　□ Posterior belly of digastric
⑧ □ 後耳介神経　　　　　□ Posterior auricular nerve

A 鼓索神経は，舌と軟口蓋からの味覚線維を，また顎下神経節でシナプスを形成して顎下腺と舌下腺に分布する分泌神経を運ぶ．

Cranial Nerves VII

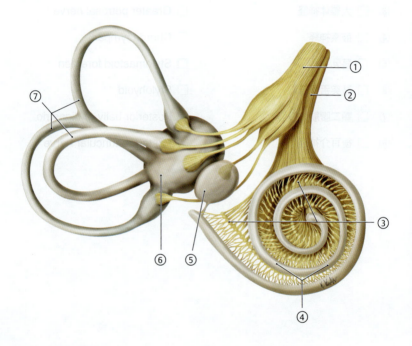

Q 内耳神経の前庭神経の損傷による影響は？

脳神経 7

前庭神経節と蝸牛神経節（ラセン神経節）
Vestibular and cochlear (spiral) ganglia

① □ 前庭神経　　　　　　　　　□ Vestibular nerve (CN VIII)

② □ 蝸牛神経　　　　　　　　　□ Cochlear nerve (CN VIII)

③ □ ラセン神経節　　　　　　　□ Spiral ganglia

④ □ 蝸牛　　　　　　　　　　　□ Cochlea

⑤ □ 球形嚢　　　　　　　　　　□ Saccule

⑥ □ 卵形嚢　　　　　　　　　　□ Utricle

⑦ □ 半規管　　　　　　　　　　□ Semicircular ducts

　内耳神経は2つの根からなる特殊体性求心性神経である．前庭神経は骨半規管，球形嚢，卵形嚢からの情報を受け取り，空間内の方向に関する情報を伝える．前庭神経が障害されると眩暈が起こる．蝸牛神経は蝸牛のコルチ器からの情報を伝える．蝸牛神経が障害されると聴覚障害が起こる．

Cranial Nerves VIII

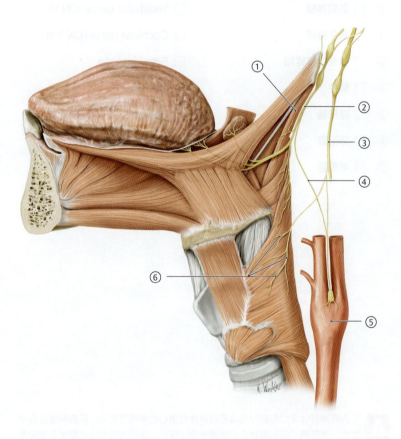

脳神経 8

左外側面

① □ 茎突咽頭筋 □ Stylopharyngeus
② □ 舌咽神経 □ Glossopharyngeal nerve (CN IX)
③ □ 迷走神経 □ Vagus nerve (CN X)
④ □ 頸動脈洞枝 □ Carotid branch
⑤ □ 頸動脈洞 □ Carotid sinus
⑥ □ 咽頭神経叢 □ Pharyngeal plexus

解説

迷走神経(CN X)の線維と舌咽神経(CN IX)の線維は合流し，咽頭神経叢を形成するとともに，頸動脈洞に分布する．

Cranial Nerves IX

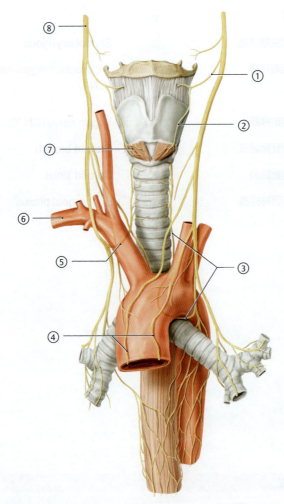

Q 甲状腺の手術の後に嗄声が起こることがあるのはなぜか？

脳神経 9

前面

① ☐ 上喉頭神経 — ☐ Superior laryngeal nerve
② ☐ 外枝 — ☐ External branch (external laryngeal nerve)
③ ☐ 左反回神経 — ☐ Left recurrent laryngeal nerve
④ ☐ 頸心臓枝 — ☐ Cervical cardiac branches
⑤ ☐ 右反回神経 — ☐ Right recurrent laryngeal nerve
⑥ ☐ 鎖骨下動脈 — ☐ Subclavian artery
⑦ ☐ 輪状甲状筋 — ☐ Cricothyroid
⑧ ☐ 迷走神経 — ☐ Vagus nerve (CN X)

A 反回神経は甲状腺の後面に接している．外科手術時に反回神経の障害によって同側の声帯と喉頭筋が麻痺することがあり，嗄声を引き起こす．

Cranial Nerves X

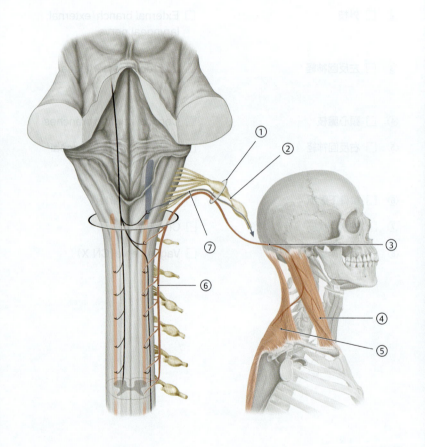

脳神経 10

脳幹の後面

① □ 頸静脈孔 □ Jugular foramen
② □ 迷走神経 □ Vagus nerve (CN X)
③ □ 副神経 □ Accessory nerve (CN XI)
④ □ 胸鎖乳突筋 □ Sternocleidomastoid
⑤ □ 僧帽筋 □ Trapezius
⑥ □ 脊髄根 □ Spinal root
⑦ □ 延髄根 □ Cranial root

解説

伝統的に副神経（CN XI）の延髄根とされてきたものは，現在では迷走神経（CN X）の一部として考えられ，脊髄根と短い距離だけ合流しているが，すぐに分離する．延髄根の線維は迷走神経を介して分配されるが，脊髄根の線維は副神経（CN XI）として伸びていく．

Sensory Innervation

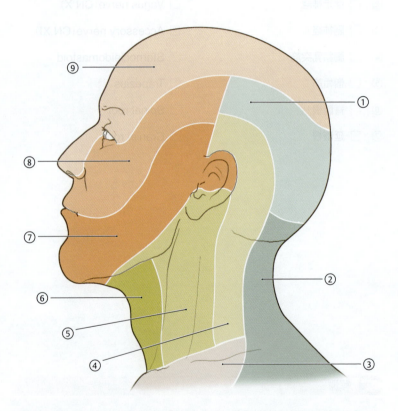

感覚神経支配

左外側面

① ☐ 大後頭神経 — ☐ Greater occipital nerve(C2)
② ☐ 脊髄神経の後枝 — ☐ Posterior dorsal ramus of spinal nerves
③ ☐ 鎖骨上神経 — ☐ Supraclavicular nerves
④ ☐ 小後頭神経 — ☐ Lesser occipital nerve
⑤ ☐ 大耳介神経 — ☐ Great auricular nerve
⑥ ☐ 頸横神経 — ☐ Transverse cervical nerve
⑦ ☐ 三叉神経の下顎神経 — ☐ Mandibular division of trigeminal nerve
⑧ ☐ 三叉神経の上顎神経 — ☐ Maxillary division of trigeminal nerve
⑨ ☐ 三叉神経の眼神経 — ☐ Ophthalmic division of trigeminal nerve

Arteries of the Skull & Face I

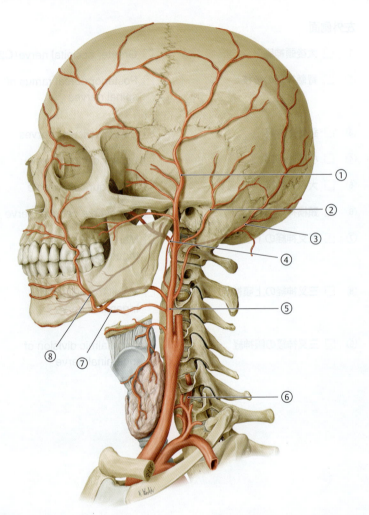

Q 左右どちらかの外頸動脈を結紮すると，顔面の組織にどのような影響が出るか？

頭蓋と顔面の動脈 1

左外側面

① □ 浅側頭動脈 □ Superficial temporal artery
② □ 後耳介動脈 □ Posterior auricular artery
③ □ 後頭動脈 □ Occipital artery
④ □ 顎動脈 □ Maxillary artery
⑤ □ 外頸動脈 □ External carotid artery
⑥ □ 椎骨動脈 □ Vertebral artery
⑦ □ 舌動脈 □ Lingual artery
⑧ □ 顔面動脈 □ Facial artery

A 　左右の外頸動脈の枝の間には吻合が多数あるため，片方の外頸動脈を結紮しても顔面の組織の血液供給にはほとんど影響はない．さらに，特に眼窩と鼻腔には外頸動脈と内頸動脈の間の吻合路がある．

Arteries of the Skull & Face II

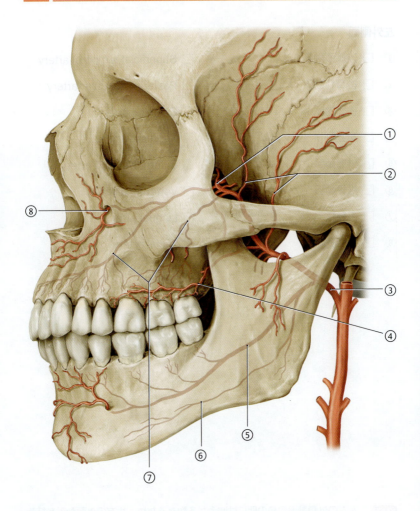

頭蓋のプテリオンの外傷が特に危険であるのはなぜか？

頭蓋と顔面の動脈 2

左外側面

① □ 蝶口蓋動脈　　　　□ Sphenopalatine artery

② □ 深側頭動脈　　　　□ Deep temporal arteries

③ □ 顎動脈　　　　　　□ Maxillary artery

④ □ 頬動脈　　　　　　□ Buccal artery

⑤ □ 下歯槽動脈　　　　□ Inferior alveolar artery

⑥ □ 顎舌骨筋枝　　　　□ Mylohyoid branch

⑦ □ 前・後上歯槽動脈　□ Anterior and posterior superior alveolar arteries

⑧ □ 眼窩下動脈　　　　□ Infra-orbital artery

 顎動脈の枝の1つである中硬膜動脈は，髄膜とその上にある頭蓋冠に分布し，プテリオンの領域の内側面を通過する．一般に外傷によって動脈が破裂すると硬膜外血腫が生じる．

Veins of the Head & Neck I

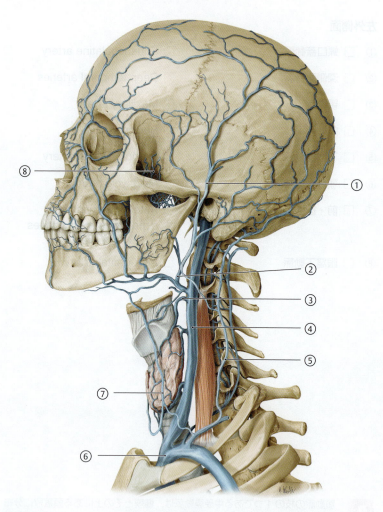

頭頸部の3本の主要な浅静脈は何か？

頭頸部 721

頭頸部の静脈 1

左外側面

① □ 浅側頭静脈　　　　　　　　□ Superficial temporal vein
② □ 下顎後静脈　　　　　　　　□ Retromandibular vein
③ □ 上甲状腺静脈　　　　　　　□ Superior thyroid vein
④ □ 内頸静脈　　　　　　　　　□ Internal jugular vein
⑤ □ 外頸静脈　　　　　　　　　□ External jugular vein
⑥ □ 左腕頭静脈　　　　　　　　□ Left brachiocephalic vein
⑦ □ 前頸静脈　　　　　　　　　□ Anterior jugular vein
⑧ □ 翼突筋静脈叢（深側頭静脈）　□ Pterygoid plexus
　　　　　　　　　　　　　　　　　　（deep temporal veins）

A　内頸静脈，外頸静脈，前頸静脈．これらの浅静脈は頭頸部から腕頭静脈へと注ぐ．

Veins of the Head & Neck II

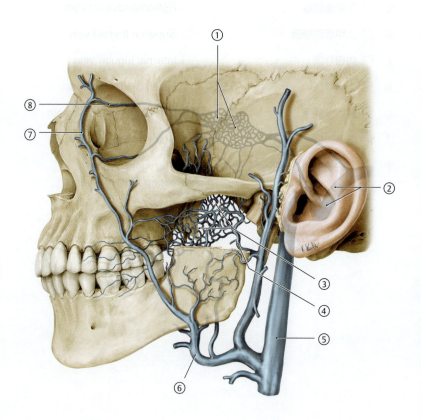

頭頸部の静脈 2

左外側面

① ☐ 海綿静脈洞　　　　　☐ Cavernous sinus
② ☐ S状静脈洞　　　　　 ☐ Sigmoid sinus
③ ☐ 翼突筋静脈叢　　　　☐ Pterygoid plexus
④ ☐ 顎静脈　　　　　　　☐ Maxillary vein
⑤ ☐ 内頸静脈　　　　　　☐ Internal jugular vein
⑥ ☐ 顔面静脈　　　　　　☐ Facial vein
⑦ ☐ 眼角静脈　　　　　　☐ Angular vein
⑧ ☐ 上眼静脈　　　　　　☐ Superior ophthalmic vein

 解説

翼突筋静脈叢は下顎枝と咀嚼筋の間にある静脈網である．海綿静脈洞は顔面静脈の枝をS状静脈洞に連絡する．

Superficial Neurovasculature I

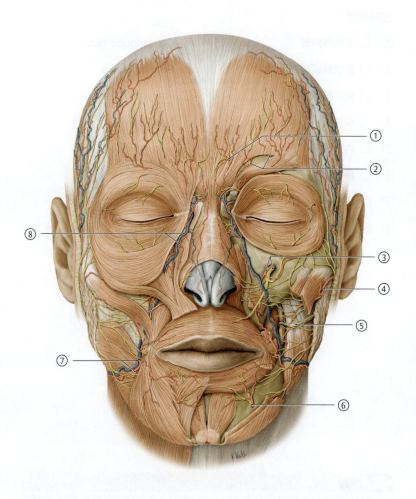

Q 鼻根と左右の唇交連によってできる三角形の領域の血管系に潜在的に存在する危険性は何か？

顔面浅層の神経・血管 1

前面

① ☐ 滑車上神経　　☐ Supratrochlear nerve

② ☐ 眼窩上神経，内・外側枝　　☐ Supra-orbital nerve, medial and lateral branches

③ ☐ 眼窩下動脈・神経（眼窩下孔にある）　　☐ Infra-orbital artery and nerve (in infra-orbital foramen)

④ ☐ 顔面横動脈　　☐ Transverse facial artery

⑤ ☐ 耳下腺管　　☐ Parotid duct

⑥ ☐ オトガイ神経（オトガイ孔にある）　　☐ Mental nerve (in mental foramen)

⑦ ☐ 顔面動脈・静脈　　☐ Facial artery and vein

⑧ ☐ 眼角動脈・静脈　　☐ Angular artery and vein

A この領域は顔面の静脈と硬膜静脈洞との連絡部位を含む．この領域の静脈には弁がないので，顔面領域の細菌感染が頭蓋腔内にまで広がる危険性が高い．

Superficial Neurovasculature II

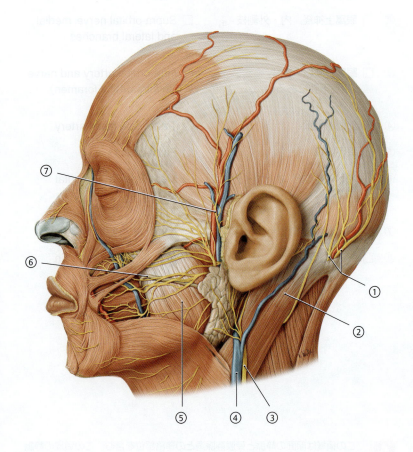

顔面浅層の神経・血管 2

左外側面

① ☐ 大後頭神経　　　☐ Greater occipital nerve
② ☐ 胸鎖乳突筋　　　☐ Sternocleidomastoid
③ ☐ 大耳介神経　　　☐ Great auricular nerve
④ ☐ 外頸静脈　　　　☐ External jugular vein
⑤ ☐ 咬筋　　　　　　☐ Masseter
⑥ ☐ 耳下腺管　　　　☐ Parotid duct
⑦ ☐ 耳介側頭神経　　☐ Auriculotemporal nerve

Parotid Region I

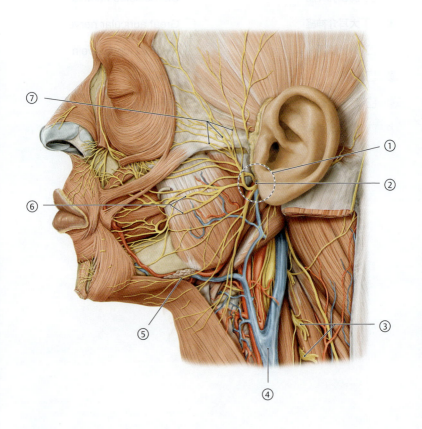

Q 顔面神経が頭蓋外に出るときに通過する孔は何か？

耳下腺咬筋部 1

左外側面

① □ 顔面神経の耳下腺神経叢 □ Parotid plexus of facial nerve (CN VII)

② □ 顔面神経 □ Facial nerve (CN VII)
③ □ 頸神経叢 □ Cervical plexus
④ □ 内頸静脈 □ Internal jugular vein
⑤ □ 顔面神経の下顎縁枝 □ Marginal mandibular branch of facial nerve

⑥ □ 顔面神経の頬筋枝 □ Buccal branches of facial nerve

⑦ □ 顔面神経の側頭枝 □ Temporal branches of facial nerve

A 顔面神経は茎乳突孔から頭蓋外に出る.

Parotid Region II

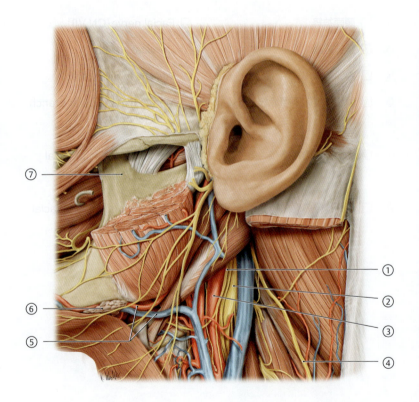

耳下腺咬筋部 2

左外側面

① □ 舌下神経 □ Hypoglossal nerve (CN XII)
② □ 上頸神経節 □ Superior cervical ganglion
③ □ 内頸動脈 □ Internal carotid artery
④ □ 副神経 □ Accessory nerve (CN XI)
⑤ □ 顔面動脈・静脈 □ Facial artery and vein
⑥ □ 顎下腺 □ Submandibular gland
⑦ □ 筋突起 □ Coronoid process

Infratemporal Fossa I

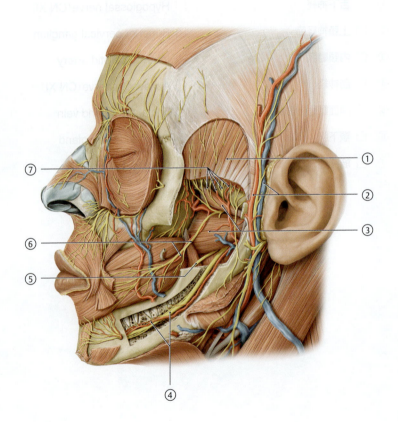

Q 外側翼突筋の機能は何か？

側頭下窩 1

左外側面

① □ 側頭筋 　　　　　　　　　□ Temporalis
② □ 浅側頭動脈・静脈 　　　　□ Superficial temporal artery and vein
③ □ 外側翼突筋 　　　　　　　□ Lateral pterygoid
④ □ 下歯槽動脈・神経（下顎管にある） 　□ Inferior alveolar artery and nerve (in mandibular canal)
⑤ □ 舌神経 　　　　　　　　　□ Lingual nerve (CN V_3)
⑥ □ 頬動脈・神経 　　　　　　□ Buccal artery and nerve
⑦ □ 深側頭動脈・神経 　　　　□ Deep temporal arteries and nerves

A 　外側翼突筋は，両側が収縮したときには下顎を前方に突き出し，片側のみが収縮したときには咀嚼時に下顎を横方向に動かす．

Infratemporal Fossa II

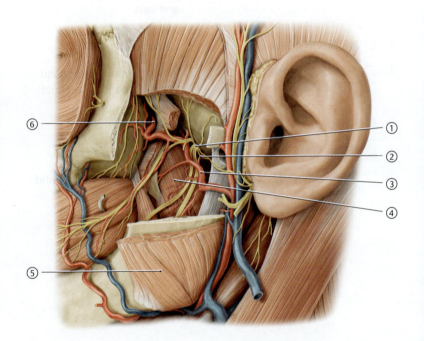

Q 側頭下窩にある主要な神経と動脈は何か？

側頭下窩 2

左外側面

① ☐ 下顎神経　　　　　　　☐ Mandibular nerve (CN V₃)

② ☐ 中硬膜動脈　　　　　　☐ Middle meningeal artery

③ ☐ 顎動脈　　　　　　　　☐ Maxillary artery

④ ☐ 内側翼突筋　　　　　　☐ Medial pterygoid

⑤ ☐ 咬筋　　　　　　　　　☐ Masseter

⑥ ☐ 蝶口蓋動脈　　　　　　☐ Sphenopalatine artery

 側頭下窩には下顎神経があり，側頭部の深部の筋と咀嚼筋に分布する．外頸動脈の枝である顎動脈は側頭下窩を横断する間に，側頭部の深部と下部の筋肉や口腔と下顎の諸構造に枝を出す．

Infratemporal Fossa III

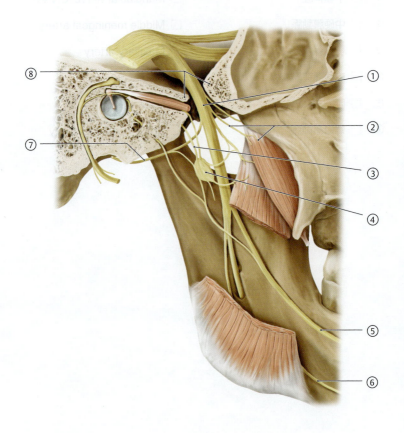

Q 耳神経節でシナプスを形成する副交感神経性の節後線維はどこに分布するか?

側頭下窩 3

内側面

① □ 下顎神経 — □ Mandibular nerve (CN V₃)
② □ 口蓋帆張筋神経と口蓋帆張筋 — □ Nerve of tensor veli palatini (with muscle)
③ □ 小錐体神経 — □ Lesser petrosal nerve
④ □ 耳神経節 — □ Otic ganglion
⑤ □ 舌神経 — □ Lingual nerve
⑥ □ 顎舌骨筋神経 — □ Mylohyoid nerve
⑦ □ 耳介側頭神経 — □ Auriculotemporal nerve
⑧ □ 卵円孔 — □ Foramen ovale

A 耳神経節でシナプスを形成した副交感神経性の節後線維は耳下腺に分布する.

Pterygopalatine Fossa

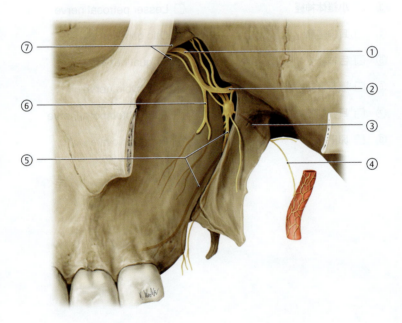

翼口蓋窩

左外側面

① □ 眼窩下神経
② □ 上顎神経
③ □ 翼突管神経（大錐体神経，深錐体神経）
④ □ 深錐体神経
⑤ □ 大口蓋神経
⑥ □ 上歯槽神経の後上歯槽枝
⑦ □ 下眼窩裂

□ Infra-orbital nerve
□ Maxillary nerve（CN V₂）
□ Nerve of pterygoid canal (greater and deep petrosal nerves)
□ Deep petrosal nerve
□ Greater palatine nerve
□ Posterior superior alveolar branches of superior alveolar nerves
□ Inferior orbital fissure

 解説

　小さなピラミッド状の翼口蓋窩は上顎神経やその枝などの中頭蓋窩，眼窩，鼻腔，口腔を進む神経・血管が交差する場所である．深錐体神経の交感性線維はシナプスを形成せずに翼口蓋窩を通過するが，大錐体神経の副交感性線維は翼口蓋神経節でシナプスを形成する．

Bones of the Orbit

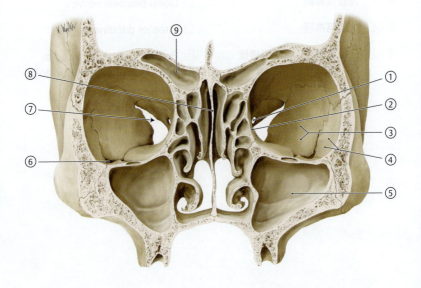

眼窩の骨

冠状断面，前面

① □ 視神経管　　　　　　　□ Optic canal
② □ 篩骨，眼窩板（紙様板）　□ Ethmoid bone, orbital plate (lamina papyracea)
③ □ 蝶形骨の大翼　　　　　□ Greater wing of sphenoid
④ □ 頬骨の眼窩面　　　　　□ Orbital surface of zygomatic bone
⑤ □ 上顎洞　　　　　　　　□ Maxillary sinus
⑥ □ 下眼窩裂　　　　　　　□ Inferior orbital fissure
⑦ □ 上眼窩裂　　　　　　　□ Superior orbital fissure
⑧ □ 篩骨の垂直板　　　　　□ Perpendicular plate of ethmoid bone
⑨ □ 前頭洞　　　　　　　　□ Frontal sinus

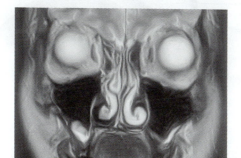

副鼻腔の MR 像

Muscles of the Orbit

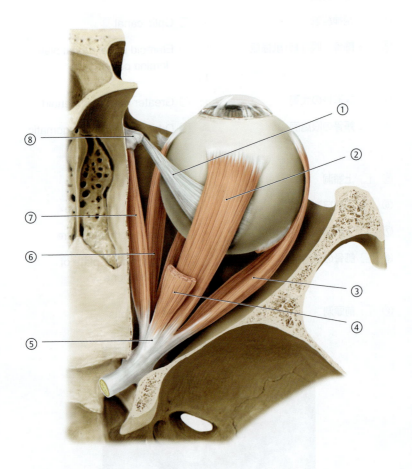

上右方の視野にある対象を見るときに，眼球を回転させる外眼筋は何か？

眼窩の筋

開かれた眼窩，上面

① □ 上斜筋の腱　　　　　□ Tendon of superior oblique
② □ 上直筋　　　　　　　□ Superior rectus
③ □ 外側直筋　　　　　　□ Lateral rectus
④ □ 上眼瞼挙筋　　　　　□ Levator palpebrae superioris
⑤ □ 総腱輪　　　　　　　□ Common tendinous ring
⑥ □ 内側直筋　　　　　　□ Medial rectus
⑦ □ 上斜筋　　　　　　　□ Superior oblique
⑧ □ 滑車　　　　　　　　□ Trochlea

A 上右方の視野を見るときには，右の下斜筋と左の上直筋が働く．

Nerves of the Orbit I

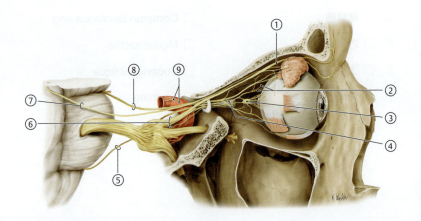

瞳孔の光反射に関わる脳神経は何か？

眼窩の神経 1

右眼窩，外側面

① □ 前頭神経 □ Frontal nerve
② □ 長毛様体神経 □ Long ciliary nerves
③ □ 毛様体神経節 □ Ciliary ganglion
④ □ 視神経 □ Optic nerve (CN II)
⑤ □ 外転神経 □ Abducent nerve (CN VI)
⑥ □ 眼神経 □ Ophthalmic nerve (CN V_1)
⑦ □ 滑車神経 □ Trochlear nerve (CN IV)
⑧ □ 動眼神経 □ Oculomotor nerve (CN III)
⑨ □ 内頸動脈と内頸動脈神経叢 □ Internal carotid artery with internal carotid plexus

A 光が入ったときに瞳孔を急速に小さくする反射には，視神経(CN II)が求心性神経，動眼神経(CN III)が遠心性神経として関与する．

Nerves of the Orbit II

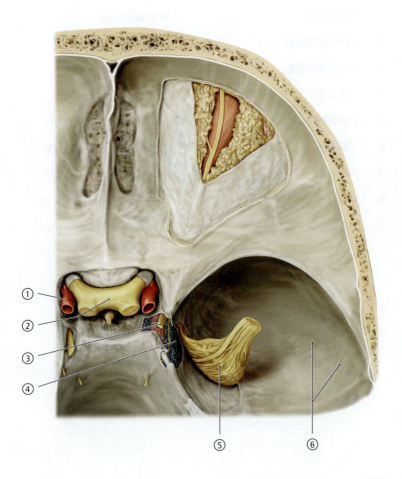

眼窩の神経 2

右側，上面

① ☐ 内頸動脈 ☐ Internal carotid artery
② ☐ 視交叉（視神経） ☐ Optic chiasm (optic nerve, CN II)
③ ☐ 動眼神経 ☐ Oculomotor nerve (CN III)
④ ☐ 海綿静脈洞 ☐ Cavernous sinus
⑤ ☐ 三叉神経節 ☐ Trigeminal ganglion
⑥ ☐ 中頭蓋窩 ☐ Middle cranial fossa

臨床

眼窩に入る視神経以外の脳神経は，海綿静脈洞を通過する．動眼神経・滑車神経・眼神経は海綿静脈洞の外壁に沿うが，外転神経は内頸動脈に接近しながら海綿静脈洞の中心を通るので，海綿静脈洞内動脈瘤の影響を受ける恐れがある．

Topography of the Orbit I

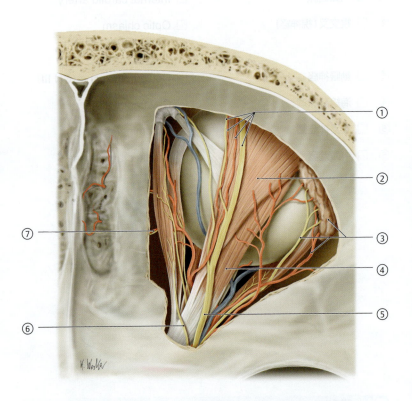

上眼瞼挙筋の機能と支配神経は何か？

眼窩の局所解剖 1

上面

① □ 眼窩上動脈・神経 □ Supra-orbital arteries and nerves

② □ 上眼瞼挙筋 □ Levator palpebrae superioris

③ □ 涙腺動脈・神経と涙腺 □ Lacrimal artery and nerve (with gland)

④ □ 上直筋 □ Superior rectus

⑤ □ 前頭神経 □ Frontal nerve

⑥ □ 滑車神経 □ Trochlear nerve (CN IV)

⑦ □ 後篩骨動脈・神経 □ Posterior ethmoidal artery and nerve

 上眼瞼挙筋は上眼瞼を挙上し，動眼神経によって支配される．下面の平滑筋線維からなる上瞼板筋は交感神経性に支配される．

Topography of the Orbit II

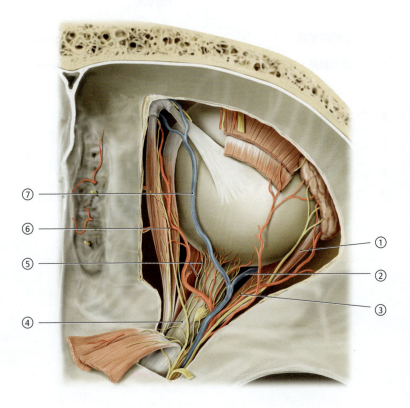

眼窩の局所解剖 2

右側，上面

① ☐ 外側直筋　　　　　　☐ Lateral rectus
② ☐ 下眼静脈　　　　　　☐ Inferior ophthalmic vein
③ ☐ 外転神経　　　　　　☐ Abducent nerve (CN VI)
④ ☐ 視神経　　　　　　　☐ Optic nerve (CN II)
⑤ ☐ 長毛様体神経　　　　☐ Long ciliary nerves
⑥ ☐ 鼻毛様体神経　　　　☐ Nasociliary nerve
⑦ ☐ 上眼静脈　　　　　　☐ Superior ophthalmic vein

Eyelid & Conjunctiva

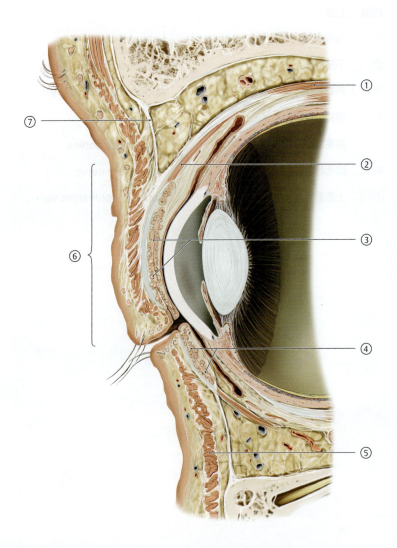

眼瞼と結膜

矢状断面

① □ 上眼瞼挙筋　　　　　　　□ Levator palpebrae superioris
② □ 上瞼板筋　　　　　　　　□ Superior tarsal muscle
③ □ 上瞼板と瞼板腺　　　　　□ Superior tarsus (with tarsal glands)
　　（マイボーム腺）
④ □ 下瞼板　　　　　　　　　□ Inferior tarsus
⑤ □ 眼輪筋の眼瞼部　　　　　□ Palpebral part of orbicularis oculi
⑥ □ 上眼瞼　　　　　　　　　□ Upper eyelid
⑦ □ 眼窩隔膜　　　　　　　　□ Orbital septum

臨床

閉経後の女性は涙腺での涙液産生不足のため，しばしば慢性的にドライアイ（乾性角結膜炎）になる．（細菌による）急性の涙腺炎症は一般的ではないが，激しい炎症を起こし，触診するときわめて柔らかいのが特徴である．上眼瞼は特徴的なＳ字カーブを描く．

Lacrimal Apparatus

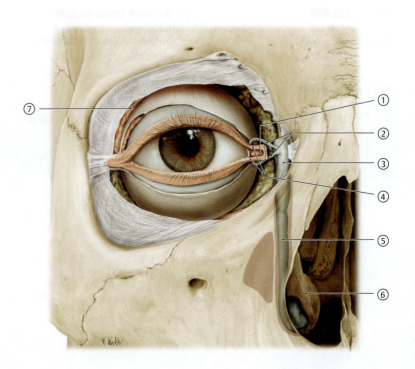

Q 涙腺の支配神経は何か？

涙器

前面

① □ 涙丘 　　　　　　　　□ Lacrimal caruncle
② □ 上・下涙小管 　　　　□ Superior and inferior lacrimal canaliculi
③ □ 涙嚢 　　　　　　　　□ Lacrimal sac
④ □ 上・下涙点 　　　　　□ Superior and inferior lacrimal punctum
⑤ □ 鼻涙管 　　　　　　　□ Nasolacrimal duct
⑥ □ 下鼻甲介 　　　　　　□ Inferior nasal concha
⑦ □ 涙腺の眼窩部 　　　　□ Lacrimal gland of orbital part

A 　節前線維は顔面神経から起こり，大錐体神経を通って翼口蓋神経節でシナプスを形成する．節後線維は上顎神経を通って涙腺に至る．

Structure of the Eyeball

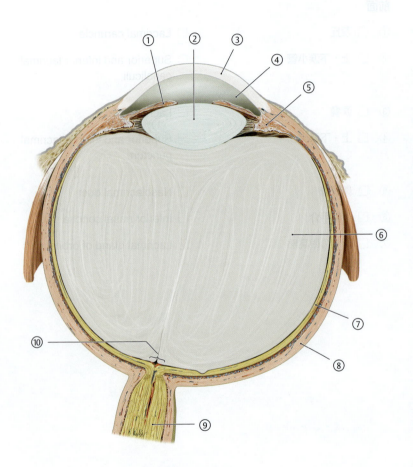

緑内障とは何か？

眼球の構造

上面

① □ 虹彩 　　　　　　　　　□ Iris
② □ 水晶体 　　　　　　　　□ Lens
③ □ 角膜 　　　　　　　　　□ Cornea
④ □ 前眼房 　　　　　　　　□ Anterior chamber
⑤ □ 毛様体, 毛様体筋 　　　□ Ciliary body, ciliary muscle
⑥ □ 硝子体 　　　　　　　　□ Vitreous body
⑦ □ 網膜 　　　　　　　　　□ Retina
⑧ □ 強膜 　　　　　　　　　□ Sclera
⑨ □ 視神経 　　　　　　　　□ Optic nerve（CN Ⅱ）
⑩ □ 視神経乳頭（視神経円板）□ Optic disc

A 　前眼房での眼房水の産生および排出の障害によって起こる眼内圧亢進状態を緑内障という．亢進した圧は眼球の強膜に付着するところで視神経を圧迫することがあり，失明する場合もある．

Bones of the Nasal Cavity I

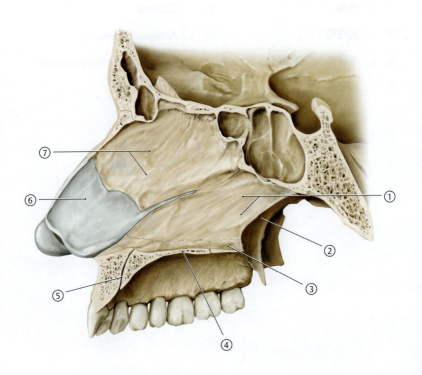

鼻腔の骨 1

傍矢状断面，左外側面

① □ 鋤骨 — □ Vomer
② □ 後鼻孔 — □ Choana
③ □ 口蓋骨の水平板 — □ Horizontal plate of palatine bone
④ □ 上顎骨の口蓋突起 — □ Palatine process of maxilla
⑤ □ 切歯管 — □ Incisive canal
⑥ □ 鼻中隔軟骨 — □ Septal nasal cartilage
⑦ □ 篩骨の垂直板 — □ Perpendicular plate of ethmoid bone

臨床

正常位の鼻中隔は鼻腔をほぼ対称に隔てている．鼻中隔が極端に外側に偏位すると鼻腔が閉塞されるが，軟骨を除去すること（鼻中隔形成術）で解消される．

Bones of the Nasal Cavity II

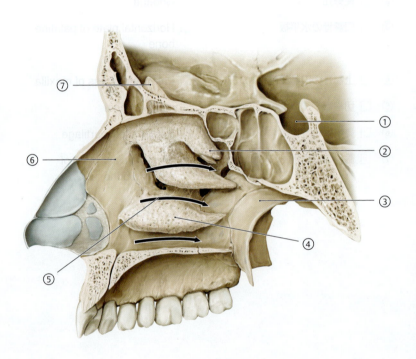

中鼻道に通じる副鼻腔はどれか？

鼻腔の骨 2

正中断面，右側内側面

① □ 下垂体窩　　　　　　　□ Hypophyseal fossa
② □ 上鼻甲介（篩骨）　　　□ Superior nasal concha (ethmoid bone)
③ □ 翼状突起の内側板　　　□ Medial plate of pterygoid process
④ □ 下鼻甲介　　　　　　　□ Inferior nasal concha
⑤ □ 中鼻道　　　　　　　　□ Middle nasal meatus
⑥ □ 上顎骨の前頭突起　　　□ Frontal process of maxilla
⑦ □ 鶏冠　　　　　　　　　□ Crista galli

A 前頭洞，上顎洞，前篩骨蜂巣と中篩骨蜂巣は中鼻道に通じる．

Bones of the Nasal Cavity III

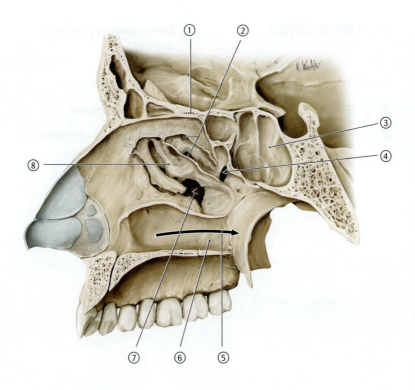

鼻腔の骨 3

正中断面，右側内側面

① □ 篩板 □ Cribriform plate
② □ 後篩骨洞の開口部 □ Orifices of posterior ethmoid sinus
③ □ 蝶形骨洞 □ Sphenoid sinus
④ □ 蝶口蓋孔 □ Sphenopalatine foramen
⑤ □ 下鼻道 □ Inferior nasal meatus
⑥ □ 口蓋骨の垂直板 □ Palatine bone, perpendicular plate
⑦ □ 上顎洞裂孔 □ Maxillary hiatus
⑧ □ 篩骨胞 □ Ethmoid bulla

解説

前頭洞，上顎洞，前篩骨蜂巣と中篩骨蜂巣は中鼻道に，蝶形骨洞は蝶篩陥凹に，後篩骨蜂巣は上鼻道に，鼻涙管は下鼻道に通じる．

Neurovasculature of the Nasal Cavity I

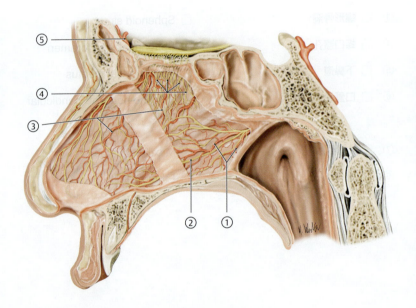

Q 通常の鼻出血に関係する鼻腔の動脈は何か？

鼻腔の神経・血管 1

左外側面

① □ 中隔後鼻枝（蝶口蓋動脈から）　　□ Posterior septal branches (from sphenopalatine artery)

② □ 鼻口蓋神経　　□ Nasopalatine nerve

③ □ 中隔前鼻枝（眼動脈から）　　□ Anterior septal branches (from ophthalmic artery)

④ □ 嗅神経糸　　□ Olfactory fibers

⑤ □ 前篩骨動脈　　□ Anterior ethmoidal artery

 通常鼻出血は鼻中隔の前部のキーゼルバッハ部位で起こり，この部位には内頸動脈の枝の前篩骨動脈と外頸動脈の枝の蝶口蓋動脈の両方からの血管が高密度で分布する．

Neurovasculature of the Nasal Cavity II

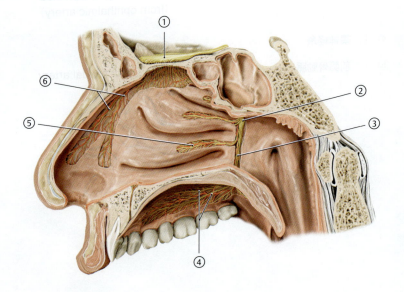

鼻腔の神経・血管 2

左外側面

① ☐ 嗅球 ☐ Olfactory bulb (CN I)

② ☐ 翼口蓋神経節 ☐ Pterygopalatine ganglion

③ ☐ 下行口蓋動脈，大・小口蓋神経 ☐ Descending palatine artery, greater and lesser palatine nerves

④ ☐ 大口蓋動脈・神経 ☐ Greater palatine artery and nerve

⑤ ☐ 下後鼻枝，外側後鼻枝 ☐ Posterior inferior nasal branches, lateral posterior nasal arteries

⑥ ☐ 前篩骨動脈 ☐ Anterior ethmoidal artery

External Ear

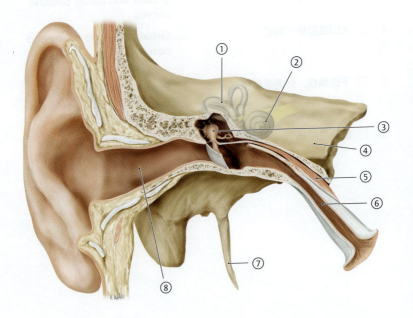

外耳

右耳の冠状断面，前面

① ☐ 外側骨半規管　　☐ Lateral semicircular canal
② ☐ 蝸牛　　☐ Cochlea
③ ☐ ツチ骨　　☐ Malleus
④ ☐ 側頭骨の岩様部　　☐ Petrous part of temporal bone
⑤ ☐ 鼓膜張筋　　☐ Tensor tympani
⑥ ☐ 耳管　　☐ Pharyngotympanic (auditory) tube
⑦ ☐ 茎状突起　　☐ Styloid process
⑧ ☐ 外耳道　　☐ External acoustic meatus

臨床

外耳道は軟骨性部で大きく弯曲している．オトスコープ(耳鏡)を挿入するときは，耳介を後上方に引くと外耳道がまっすぐになり，耳鏡を挿入することができる．

Structure of the Auricle

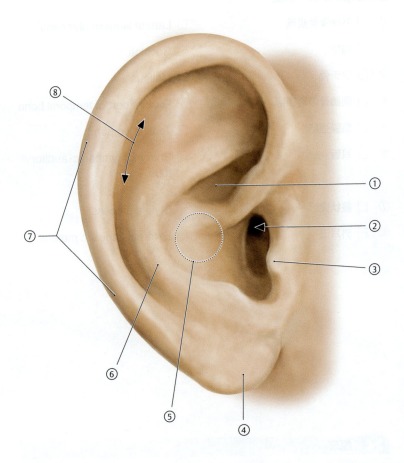

Q 耳介に分布する神経は何か？

耳介の構造

右外側面

① □ 耳甲介舟　　□ Cymba conchae

② □ 外耳道　　　□ External acoustic meatus

③ □ 耳珠　　　　□ Tragus

④ □ 耳垂　　　　□ Lobule of auricle

⑤ □ 耳甲介　　　□ Concha of auricle

⑥ □ 対輪　　　　□ Antihelix

⑦ □ 耳輪　　　　□ Helix

⑧ □ 舟状窩　　　□ Scaphoid fossa

A 耳介の神経は三叉神経(CN Ⅴ)，顔面神経(CN Ⅶ)，迷走神経(CN Ⅹ)，舌咽神経(CN Ⅸ)から起こる．頸神経叢からの小後頭神経と大耳介神経も耳介に分布する．

Tympanic Cavity

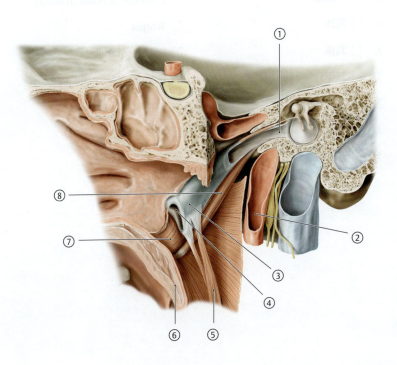

Q 嚥下や欠伸時に鼓膜の両側の圧を等しくさせるために働く筋肉は何か？

鼓室

内側面

① □ 耳管骨部　　　　　　　　□ Pharyngotympanic tube, bony part

② □ 内頸動脈　　　　　　　　□ Internal carotid artery

③ □ 耳管の軟骨部　　　　　　□ Pharyngotympanic tube, cartilaginous part

④ □ 咽頭口　　　　　　　　　□ Pharyngeal orifice

⑤ □ 耳管咽頭筋　　　　　　　□ Salpingopharyngeus

⑥ □ 口蓋垂　　　　　　　　　□ Uvula

⑦ □ 口蓋帆挙筋　　　　　　　□ Levator veli palatini

⑧ □ 口蓋帆張筋　　　　　　　□ Tensor veli palatini

軟口蓋の口蓋帆張筋と口蓋帆挙筋，および耳管咽頭筋は耳管を開口させる．

Ossicular Chain

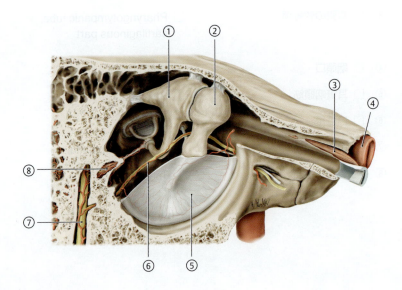

アブミ骨筋と鼓膜張筋の機能は何か？

耳小骨連鎖

外側面

① □ キヌタ骨 　　　□ Incus
② □ ツチ骨 　　　　□ Malleus
③ □ 鼓膜張筋 　　　□ Tensor tympani
④ □ 内頸動脈 　　　□ Internal carotid artery
⑤ □ 鼓膜 　　　　　□ Tympanic membrane
⑥ □ 鼓索神経 　　　□ Chorda tympani
⑦ □ 顔面神経 　　　□ Facial nerve (CN VII)
⑧ □ アブミ骨筋 　　□ Stapedius

A アブミ骨筋と鼓膜張筋は中耳の音伝導を減衰させるように働く．どちらの筋も大きな音刺激に対して反射収縮する．

Inner Ear

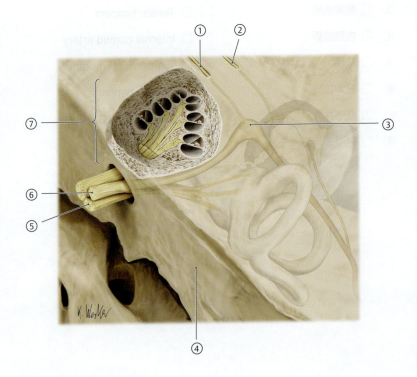

内耳

上面

① □ 大錐体神経 □ Greater petrosal nerve
② □ 小錐体神経 □ Lesser petrosal nerve
③ □ 膝神経節 □ Geniculate ganglion
④ □ 側頭骨の岩様部 □ Petrous part temporal bone
⑤ □ 前庭神経 □ Vestibular nerve (CN VIII)
⑥ □ 顔面神経 □ Facial nerve (CN VII)
⑦ □ 蝸牛 □ Cochlea

Mandible

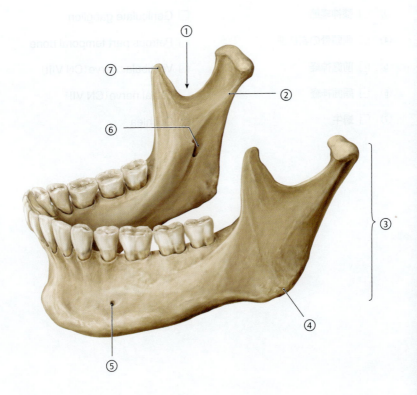

下顎骨

左斜外側面

① ☐ 下顎切痕　　　　　☐ Mandibular notch
② ☐ 関節突起　　　　　☐ Condylar process
③ ☐ 下顎枝　　　　　　☐ Ramus of mandible
④ ☐ 下顎角　　　　　　☐ Angle of mandible
⑤ ☐ オトガイ孔　　　　☐ Mental foramen
⑥ ☐ 下顎孔　　　　　　☐ Mandibular foramen
⑦ ☐ 筋突起　　　　　　☐ Coronoid process

Trigeminal Nerve in the Oral Cavity

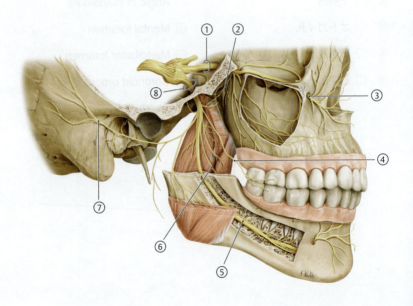

口腔の三叉神経

右外側面

① □ 上顎神経（正円孔を通る）　　□ Maxillary nerve (CN V$_2$, via foramen rotundum)

② □ 翼口蓋神経節　　□ Pterygopalatine ganglion

③ □ 眼窩下神経と眼窩下孔　　□ Infra-orbital nerve (and foramen)

④ □ 頬神経　　□ Buccal nerve

⑤ □ 下歯槽神経（下顎管にある）　　□ Inferior alveolar nerve (in mandibular canal)

⑥ □ 舌神経　　□ Lingual nerve (CN V$_3$)

⑦ □ 耳介側頭神経　　□ Auriculotemporal nerve

⑧ □ 下顎神経（卵円孔を通る）　　□ Mandibular nerve (CN V$_3$, via foramen ovale)

Dorsum of the Tongue

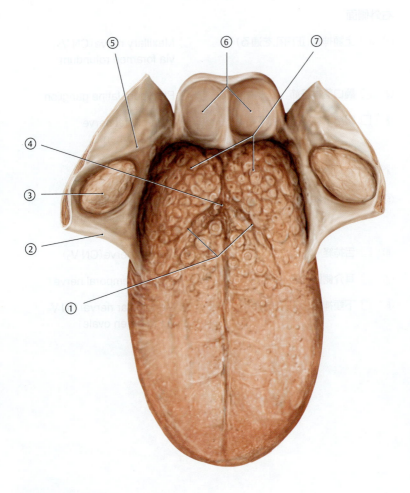

Q 舌の分界溝とは何か？

舌背

上面

① ☐ 分界溝　　　　　　　☐ Terminal sulcus

② ☐ 口蓋舌弓　　　　　　☐ Palatoglossal arch

③ ☐ 口蓋扁桃　　　　　　☐ Palatine tonsil

④ ☐ 舌盲孔　　　　　　　☐ Foramen cecum of tongue

⑤ ☐ 口蓋咽頭弓　　　　　☐ Palatopharyngeal arch

⑥ ☐ 喉頭蓋　　　　　　　☐ Epiglottis

⑦ ☐ 舌扁桃　　　　　　　☐ Lingual tonsil

A 　V字形の分界溝によって，舌は前2/3と後ろ1/3に分けられる．これは発生期に異なる鰓弓から生じたことの名残である．

Muscles of the Tongue

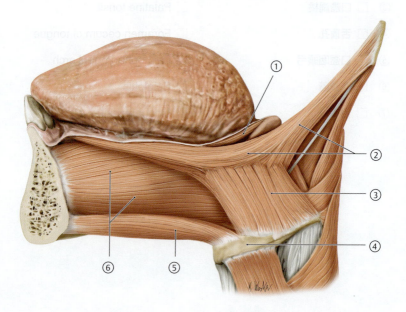

舌の筋

左外側面

① □ 口蓋舌筋　　　　　□ Palatoglossus
② □ 茎突舌筋　　　　　□ Styloglossus
③ □ 舌骨舌筋　　　　　□ Hyoglossus
④ □ 舌骨　　　　　　　□ Hyoid bone
⑤ □ オトガイ舌骨筋　　□ Geniohyoid
⑥ □ オトガイ舌筋　　　□ Genioglossus

解説

外舌筋(オトガイ舌筋，舌骨舌筋，口蓋舌筋，茎突舌筋)は骨に付着し，舌全体を動かす．内舌筋(上縦舌筋，下縦舌筋，横舌筋，垂直舌筋)は骨に付着せず，舌の形を変える．

Sensory Innervation of the Tongue

味覚
Taste

体性感覚
Somatic sensation

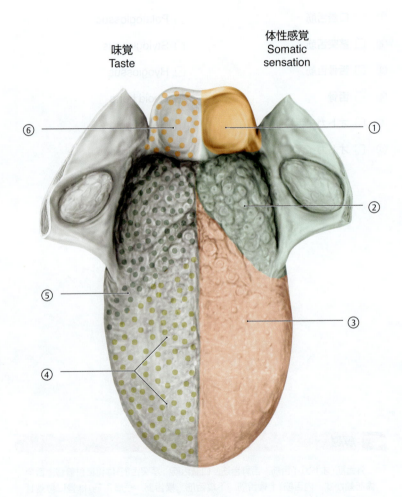

舌の感覚性神経支配と味覚神経支配

上面

① □ 迷走神経　　　　　　　□ Vagus nerve (CN X)

② □ 舌咽神経　　　　　　　□ Glossopharyngeal nerve (CN IX)

③ □ 舌神経（下顎神経）　　□ Lingual nerve (from mandibular nerve, CN V₃)

④ □ 顔面神経（鼓索神経経由）□ Facial nerve (CN VII, via chorda tympani)

⑤ □ 舌咽神経　　　　　　　□ Glossopharyngeal nerve (CN IX)

⑥ □ 迷走神経　　　　　　　□ Vagus nerve (CN X)

> **解説**
>
> ①-⑥が示しているのは舌の感覚神経支配である．口蓋舌筋は舌咽神経（CN IX）から体性運動性の神経支配を受ける．他の舌筋は舌下神経（CN XII）に支配される．

Neurovasculature of the Tongue

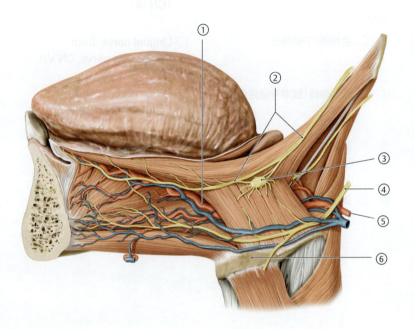

Q 片側の舌下神経の障害によって前方に突出した舌はどのような形になるか?

舌の神経と血管

左外側面

① □ 舌深動脈　　　　　　　　　□ Deep lingual artery
② □ 舌神経　　　　　　　　　　□ Lingual nerve（CN V₃）
③ □ 顎下神経節　　　　　　　　□ Submandibular ganglion
④ □ 舌下神経　　　　　　　　　□ Hypoglossal nerve（CN XII）
⑤ □ 舌動脈（外頸動脈から）　　□ Lingual artery（from external carotid artery）
⑥ □ 舌骨　　　　　　　　　　　□ Hyoid bone

片側の舌下神経が障害を受けると，障害を受けていない側のオトガイ舌筋が優位になり，舌を前方に突出させると麻痺側へ偏位する．

Boundaries of the Oral Cavity I

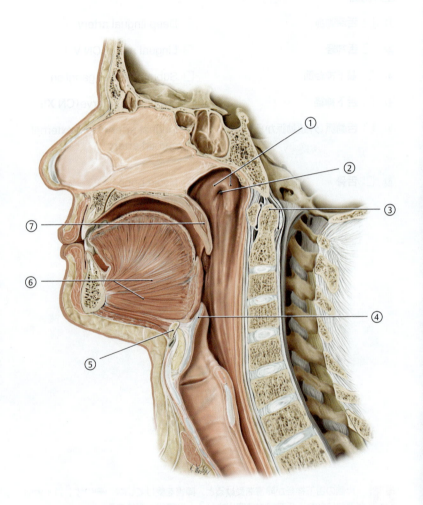

口腔の区分 1

正中断面，左外側面

① ☐ リンパ組織（耳管扁桃）を伴う耳管隆起　　☐ Torus tubarius with lymphatic tissue（tonsilla tubaria）

② ☐ 耳管咽頭口　　☐ Pharyngeal orifice of pharyngotympanic tube

③ ☐ 軸椎の歯突起　　☐ Dens of axis（C2）

④ ☐ 喉頭蓋　　☐ Epiglottis

⑤ ☐ 舌骨　　☐ Hyoid bone

⑥ ☐ オトガイ舌筋　　☐ Genioglossus

⑦ ☐ 軟口蓋（口蓋帆）　　☐ Soft palate

Boundaries of the Oral Cavity II

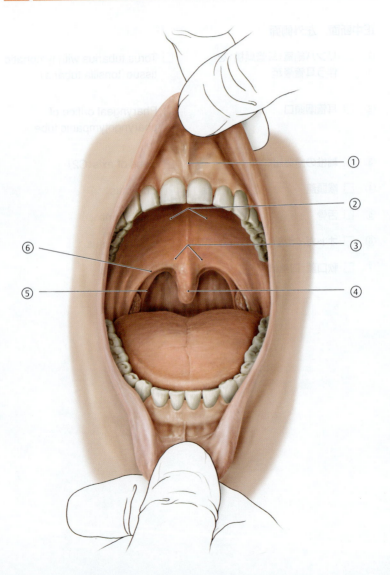

口腔の区分 2

前面

① □ 上唇小帯 □ Frenulum of upper lip
② □ 硬口蓋 □ Hard palate
③ □ 軟口蓋(口蓋帆) □ Soft palate
④ □ 口蓋垂 □ Uvula
⑤ □ 口蓋咽頭弓 □ Palatopharyngeal arch
⑥ □ 口蓋舌弓 □ Palatoglossal arch

Salivary Glands I

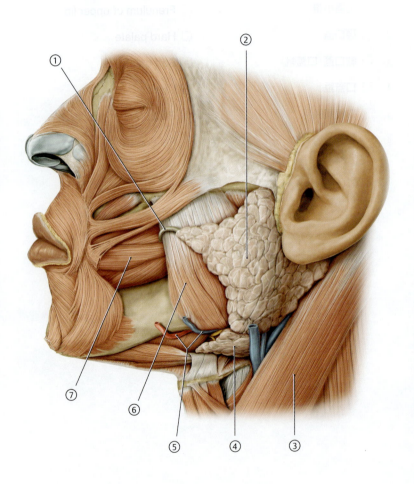

唾液腺 1

左外側面

① ☐ 耳下腺管 　　☐ Parotid duct
② ☐ 耳下腺 　　☐ Parotid gland
③ ☐ 胸鎖乳突筋 　　☐ Sternocleidomastoid
④ ☐ 顎下腺 　　☐ Submandibular gland
⑤ ☐ 顔面動脈・静脈 　　☐ Facial artery and vein
⑥ ☐ 咬筋 　　☐ Masseter
⑦ ☐ 頬筋 　　☐ Buccinator

解説

耳下腺管は頬筋を貫通して上顎第2大臼歯に対向するところに開口する.

Salivary Glands II

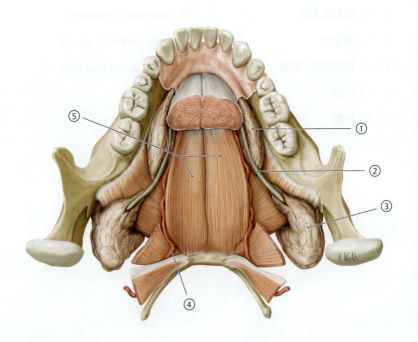

Q 三対の唾液腺それぞれからの分泌液の特徴は何か？

唾液腺 2

上面

① □ 舌下腺　　　　　　　□ Sublingual gland
② □ 顎下腺管　　　　　　□ Submandibular duct
③ □ 顎下腺　　　　　　　□ Submandibular gland
④ □ 舌動脈　　　　　　　□ Lingual artery
⑤ □ オトガイ舌骨筋　　　□ Geniohyoid

A 耳下腺の分泌液は純粋な漿液，舌下腺は主に粘液，顎下腺は混合性の漿粘液である．

Pharyngeal Muscles I

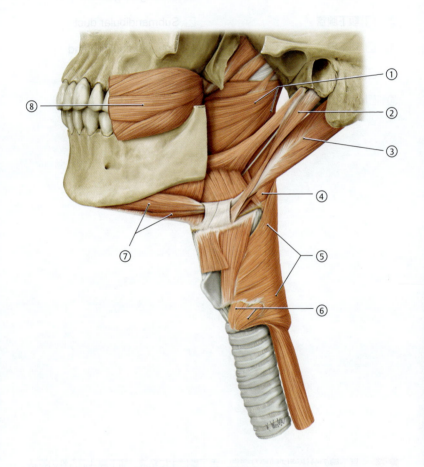

咽頭筋 1

左外側面

① □ 上咏頭収縮筋　□ Superior constrictor
② □ 茎突舌骨筋　□ Stylohyoid
③ □ 顎二腹筋（後腹）　□ Digastric (posterior belly)
④ □ 中咏頭収縮筋　□ Middle constrictor
⑤ □ 下咏頭収縮筋　□ Inferior constrictor
⑥ □ 輪状甲状筋　□ Cricothyroid
⑦ □ 顎二腹筋の前腹　□ Anterior belly of digastric
⑧ □ 頬筋　□ Buccinator

解説

咽頭の筋系は咽頭収縮筋と比較的弱い咽頭挙筋からなる．

Pharyngeal Muscles II

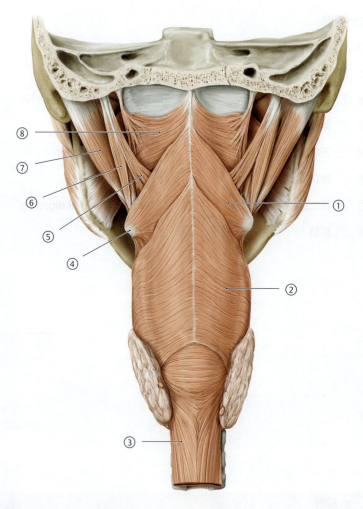

Q 咽頭収縮筋の機能は？

咽頭筋 2

後面

① ☐ 中咽頭収縮筋　　☐ Middle constrictor
② ☐ 下咽頭収縮筋　　☐ Inferior constrictor
③ ☐ 食道　　☐ Esophagus
④ ☐ 舌骨の大角　　☐ Greater horn of hyoid bone
⑤ ☐ 茎突咽頭筋　　☐ Stylopharyngeus
⑥ ☐ 茎突舌骨筋　　☐ Stylohyoid
⑦ ☐ 顎二腹筋の後腹　　☐ Posterior belly of digastric
⑧ ☐ 上咽頭収縮筋　　☐ Superior constrictor

A 　上・中・下咽頭収縮筋は，嚥下時に順に収縮して咽頭から食道への食塊の移動を助ける．

Neurovasculature of the Pharynx

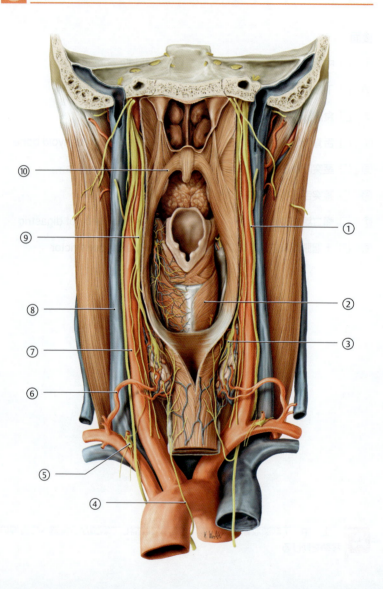

咽頭の神経・血管

後面

① □ 迷走神経 □ Vagus nerve(CN X)
② □ 後輪状披裂筋 □ Posterior crico-arytenoid
③ □ 中頸神経節 □ Middle cervical ganglion
④ □ 左反回神経 □ Left recurrent laryngeal nerve
⑤ □ 星状神経節 □ Stellate ganglion
⑥ □ 下甲状腺動脈 □ Inferior thyroid artery
⑦ □ 総頸動脈 □ Common carotid artery
⑧ □ 内頸静脈 □ Internal jugular vein
⑨ □ 交感神経幹 □ Sympathetic trunk
⑩ □ 口蓋咽頭筋 □ Palatopharyngeus

Muscles of the Neck

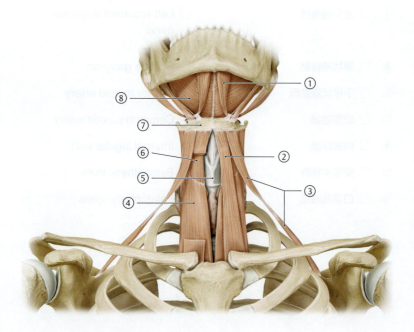

頸部の筋の概観

前面

① □ 顎二腹筋の前腹　　　□ Anterior belly of digastric
② □ 胸骨舌骨筋　　　　　□ Sternohyoid
③ □ 肩甲舌骨筋の上腹・下腹　□ Superior and inferior belly of omohyoid
④ □ 胸骨甲状筋　　　　　□ Sternothyroid
⑤ □ 甲状軟骨　　　　　　□ Thyroid cartilage
⑥ □ 甲状舌骨筋　　　　　□ Thyrohyoid
⑦ □ 舌骨　　　　　　　　□ Hyoid bone
⑧ □ 顎舌骨筋　　　　　　□ Mylohyoid

System of the Muscles of the Neck I

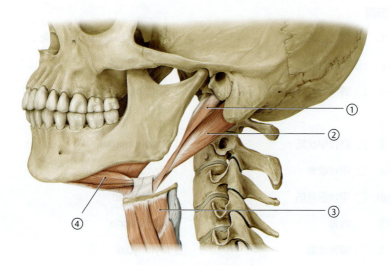

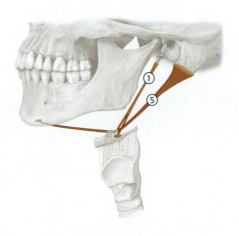

頸部の筋 1

頸部の筋，舌骨上筋群：顎二腹筋と茎突舌骨筋

① □ 茎突舌骨筋　　　　　　□ **Stylohyoid**

② □ 顎二腹筋の後腹　　　　□ **Posterior belly of digastric**

③ □ 甲状舌骨筋　　　　　　□ Thyrohyoid

④ □ 顎二腹筋の前腹　　　　□ **Anterior belly of digastric**

⑤ □ 顎二腹筋　　　　　　　□ **Digastric**

筋	起始	停止	作用	神経支配
顎二腹筋の前腹	下顎骨体	舌骨体(線維性の滑車を伴う中間腱を介して停止)	・舌骨を挙上する(嚥下時) ・下顎の開口を補助する	顎舌骨筋神経〔下顎神経(CN V₃)から分枝〕
顎二腹筋の後腹	乳様突起の内側(乳突切痕)			顔面神経(CN Ⅶ)
茎突舌骨筋	側頭骨の茎状突起	舌骨体(分岐した腱を介して停止)		

System of the Muscles of the Neck II

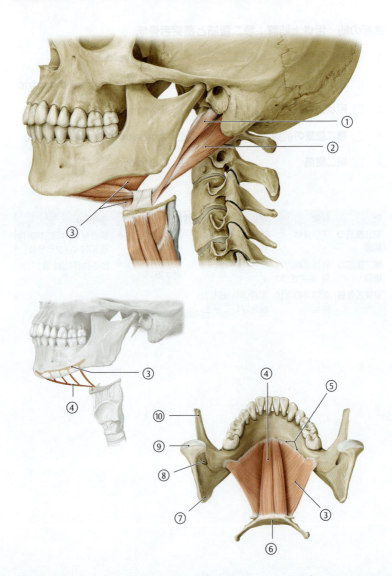

頸部の筋 2

頸部の筋，舌骨上筋群：オトガイ舌骨筋と顎舌骨筋

① ☐ 茎突舌骨筋　　　　　　☐ Stylohyoid

② ☐ 顎二腹筋の後腹　　　　☐ Posterior belly of digastric

③ ☐ 顎舌骨筋　　　　　　　☐ **Mylohyoid**

④ ☐ オトガイ舌骨筋　　　　☐ **Geniohyoid**

⑤ ☐ 顎舌骨筋線　　　　　　☐ Mylohyoid line

⑥ ☐ 舌骨体　　　　　　　　☐ Hyoid bone (body)

⑦ ☐ 下顎枝　　　　　　　　☐ Ramus of mandibular

⑧ ☐ 下顎孔　　　　　　　　☐ Mandibular foramen

⑨ ☐ 下顎頭　　　　　　　　☐ Head of mandible

⑩ ☐ 筋突起　　　　　　　　☐ Coronoid process

筋	起始	停止	作用	神経支配
オトガイ舌骨筋	下顎骨体	舌骨体	・舌骨を前方に引く（嚥下時） ・下顎の開口を補助する	第1・2頸神経(C1-C2)の前枝
顎舌骨筋	下顎骨内面（顎舌骨筋線）	舌骨体（正中に位置している腱付着部＝顎舌骨筋線の上）	・口腔底を持ち上げ，緊張させる ・舌骨を前方に引く（嚥下時） ・下顎の開口と横方向の運動（咀嚼時）を補助する	顎舌骨筋神経［下顎神経(CN V₃)から分枝］

System of the Muscles of the Neck III

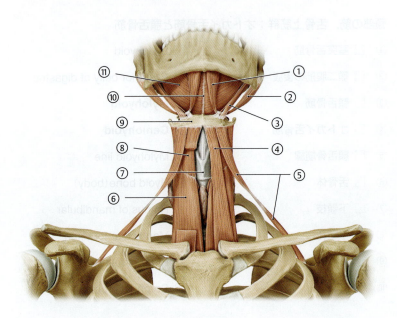

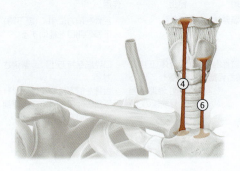

頸部の筋 3

頸部の筋，舌骨下筋群：胸骨舌骨筋と胸骨甲状筋

① □ 顎二腹筋の前腹　　　□ Anterior belly digastric

② □ 顎二腹筋の後腹　　　□ Posterior belly digastric

③ □ 茎突舌骨筋　　　　　□ Stylohyoid

④ □ **胸骨舌骨筋**　　　　□ **Sternohyoid**

⑤ □ 肩甲舌骨筋の上腹・下腹　□ Superior and inferior belly pf Omohyoid

⑥ □ **胸骨甲状筋**　　　　□ **Sternothyroid**

⑦ □ 甲状軟骨　　　　　　□ Thyroid cartilage

⑧ □ 甲状舌骨筋　　　　　□ Thyrohyoid

⑨ □ 舌骨　　　　　　　　□ Hyoid bone

⑩ □ 顎舌骨筋縫線　　　　□ Mylohyoid raphe

⑪ □ 顎舌骨筋　　　　　　□ Mylohyoid

筋	起始	停止	作用	神経支配
胸骨舌骨筋	胸骨柄および胸鎖関節の後面	舌骨体	・舌骨を押し下げる（舌骨を固定する） ・喉頭と舌骨を下げる（発声時と嚥下の最終相）	頸神経叢の頸神経ワナ（C1-C3およびC4）
胸骨甲状筋	胸骨柄の後面	甲状軟骨	・舌骨や喉頭を押し下げる ・喉頭と舌骨を下げる（発声時と嚥下の最終相）	

System of the Muscles of the Neck IV

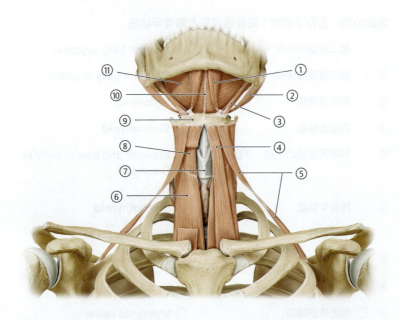

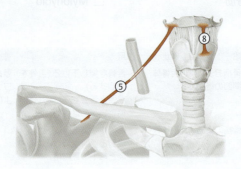

頸部の筋 4

頸部の筋，舌骨下筋群：甲状舌骨筋と肩甲舌骨筋

① □ 顎二腹筋の前腹　　　　　□ Anterior belly of digastric

② □ 顎二腹筋の後腹　　　　　□ Posterior belly of digastric

③ □ 茎突舌骨筋　　　　　　　□ Stylohyoid

④ □ 胸骨舌骨筋　　　　　　　□ Sternohyoid

⑤ □ 肩甲舌骨筋の上腹と下腹　□ **Superior and inferior belly of omohyoid**

⑥ □ 胸骨甲状筋　　　　　　　□ Sternothyroid

⑦ □ 甲状軟骨　　　　　　　　□ Thyroid cartilage

⑧ □ **甲状舌骨筋**　　　　　　□ **Thyrohyoid**

⑨ □ 舌骨　　　　　　　　　　□ Hyoid bone

⑩ □ 顎舌骨筋縫線　　　　　　□ Mylohyoid raphe

⑪ □ 顎舌骨筋　　　　　　　　□ Mylohyoid

筋	起始	停止	作用	神経支配
甲状舌骨筋	甲状軟骨	舌骨体	・舌骨を押し下げて固定する ・嚥下時に喉頭を挙上する	頸神経叢の深部の頸神経ワナ(C1-C3およびC4)
肩甲舌骨筋	肩甲骨の上縁		・舌骨を押し下げる(舌骨の固定) ・喉頭と舌骨を下げる(発声時と嚥下の最終相) ・中間腱とともに頸筋膜を引っ張り，内頸静脈を開いたままの状態にする	

System of the Muscles of the Neck V

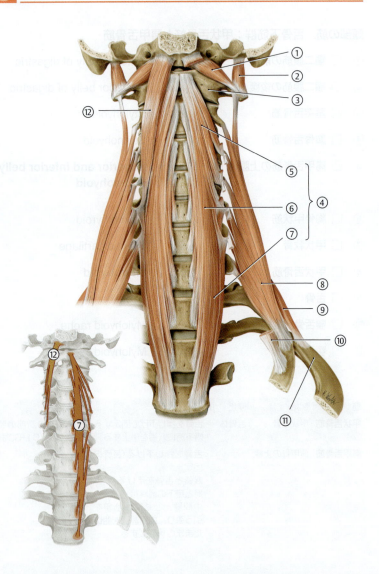

頸部の筋 5

椎骨前の頸部の筋：頭長筋と頸長筋

① □ 前頭直筋　　　　　　　□ Rectus capitis anterior
② □ 外側頭直筋　　　　　　□ Rectus capitis lateralis
③ □ 第1頸椎（環椎）　　　　□ Atlas（C1）
④ □ 頸長筋　　　　　　　　□ **Longus colli**
⑤ □ 上斜部　　　　　　　　□ **Superior oblique part**
⑥ □ 垂直部　　　　　　　　□ **Vertical part**
⑦ □ 下斜部　　　　　　　　□ **Inferior oblique part**
⑧ □ 中斜角筋　　　　　　　□ Scalenus medius（middle scalene）
⑨ □ 後斜角筋　　　　　　　□ Scalenus posterior（posterior scalene）
⑩ □ 前斜角筋　　　　　　　□ Scalenus anterior（anterior scalene）
⑪ □ 第2肋骨　　　　　　　□ 2nd rib
⑫ □ 頭長筋　　　　　　　　□ **Longus capitis**

筋	起始	停止	作用	神経支配
頭長筋	第3-6頸椎（C3-C6）の横突起の前結節	後頭骨の基底部	・片側：頭部を傾け，同側にわずかに回旋 ・両側：頭部の前方への屈曲	頸神経叢の直接の枝（C1-C4）
頸長筋，垂直部	第5頸椎 - 第3胸椎（C5-T3）の椎体の前面	第2-4頸椎（C2-C4）の前面	・片側：頸椎を傾け，同側に回旋 ・両側：頸椎の前方への屈曲	頸神経叢の直接の枝（C2-C6）
頸長筋，上斜部	第3-5頸椎（C3-C5）の横突起の前結節	環椎（C1）の前結節		
頸長筋，下斜部	第1-3胸椎（T1-T3）の椎体の前面	第5-6頸椎（C5-C6）の横突起の前結節		

System of the Muscles of the Neck VI

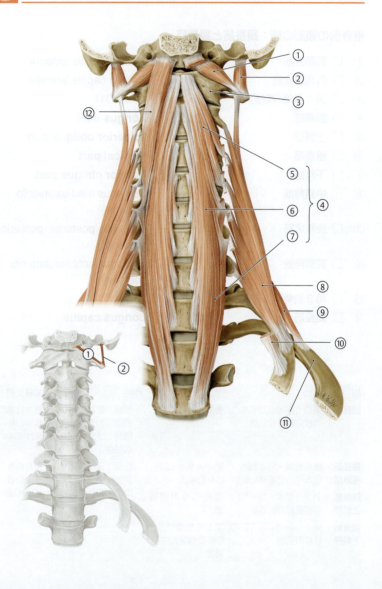

頸部の筋 6

椎骨前の頸部の筋：前頭直筋と外側頭直筋

① ☐ 前頭直筋　　　　　　☐ **Rectus capitis anterior**

② ☐ 外側頭直筋　　　　　☐ **Rectus capitis lateralis**

③ ☐ 第1頸椎（環椎）　　　☐ Atlas（C1）

④ ☐ 頸長筋　　　　　　　☐ Longus colli

⑤ ☐ 上斜部　　　　　　　☐ Superior oblique part

⑥ ☐ 垂直部　　　　　　　☐ Vertical part

⑦ ☐ 下斜部　　　　　　　☐ Inferior oblique part

⑧ ☐ 中斜角筋　　　　　　☐ Scalenus medius（middle scalene）

⑨ ☐ 後斜角筋　　　　　　☐ Scalenus posterior（posterior scalene）

⑩ ☐ 前斜角筋　　　　　　☐ Scalenus anterior（anterior scalene）

⑪ ☐ 第2肋骨　　　　　　☐ 2nd rib

⑫ ☐ 頭長筋　　　　　　　☐ Longus capitis

筋	起始	停止	作用	神経支配
前頭直筋	環椎（C1）の外側部	後頭骨の基底部	・片側：環椎後頭関節の外屈 ・両側：環椎後頭関節の前方への屈曲	第1頸神経（C1）の前枝
外側頭直筋	環椎（C1）の横突起	後頭骨の基底部（後頭顆より外側）		

Arteries of the Neck

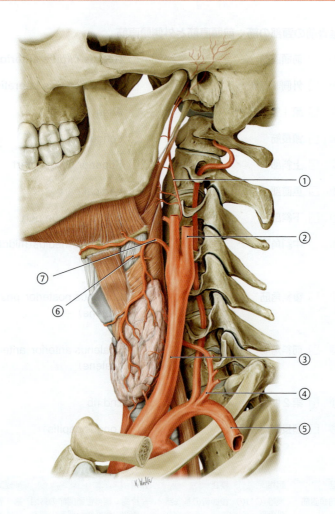

Q 内頸動脈の枝が分布する頸部の構造は何か？

頸部の動脈

左外側面

① □ 上行咽頭動脈　　□ Ascending pharyngeal artery
② □ 内頸動脈　　　　□ Internal carotid artery
③ □ 総頸動脈　　　　□ Common carotid artery
④ □ 甲状頸動脈　　　□ Thyrocervical trunk
⑤ □ 左鎖骨下動脈　　□ Left subclavian artery
⑥ □ 上喉頭動脈　　　□ Superior laryngeal artery
⑦ □ 上甲状腺動脈　　□ Superior thyroid artery

A 内頸動脈は頸部では枝を出さないため，この領域のどの構造にも分布しない．

Nerves of the Neck

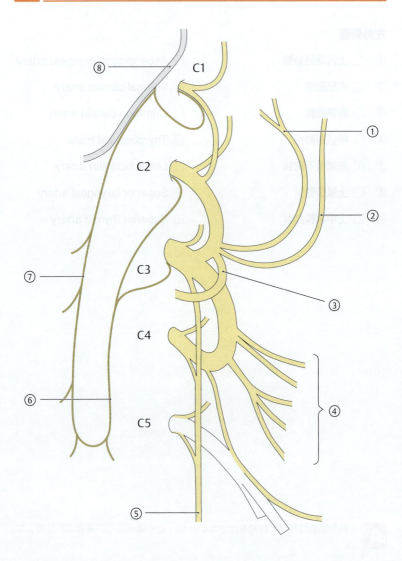

頸部の神経

① ☐ 小後頭神経 ☐ Lesser occipital nerve
② ☐ 大耳介神経 ☐ Great auricular nerve
③ ☐ 頸横神経 ☐ Transverse cervical nerve
④ ☐ 鎖骨上神経 ☐ Supraclavicular nerves
⑤ ☐ 横隔神経 ☐ Phrenic nerve
⑥ ☐ 頸神経ワナの下根 ☐ Inferior root of ansa cervicalis
⑦ ☐ 頸神経ワナの上根 ☐ Superior root of ansa cervicalis
⑧ ☐ 舌下神経 ☐ Hypoglossal nerve (CN XII)

Thyroid Gland

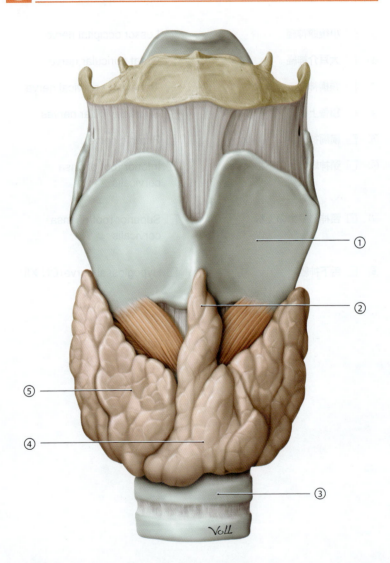

甲状腺

前面

① □ 甲状軟骨 □ Thyroid cartilage
② □ 甲状腺の錐体葉 □ Pyramidal lobe of thyroid gland
③ □ 気管 □ Trachea
④ □ 甲状腺峡部 □ Isthmus of thyroid gland
⑤ □ 甲状腺の右葉 □ Right lobe of thyroid gland

Relations of the Thyroid

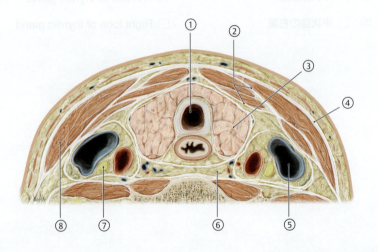

甲状腺の位置

横断面

①	☐ 気管	☐ Trachea
②	☐ 頸筋膜(筋部), 気管前葉	☐ Pretracheal layer of cervical fascia, muscular portion
③	☐ 甲状腺	☐ Thyroid gland
④	☐ 頸筋膜の浅葉	☐ Superficial (investing) layer of cervical fascia
⑤	☐ 内頸静脈	☐ Internal jugular vein
⑥	☐ 咽頭後隙	☐ Retropharyngeal space
⑦	☐ 迷走神経	☐ Vagus nerve (CN X)
⑧	☐ 胸鎖乳突筋	☐ Sternocleidomastoid

Structure of the Larynx

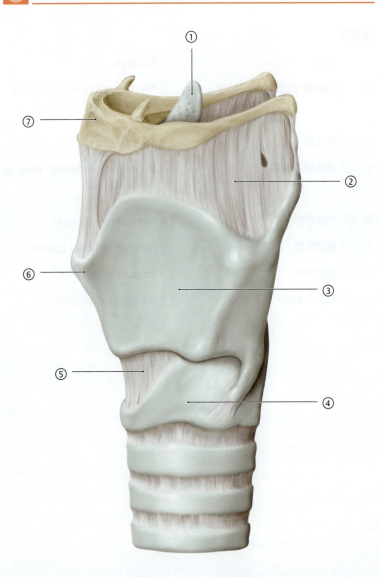

喉頭の構造

左前斜面

① □ 喉頭蓋　　　　　　　　　□ Epiglottis
② □ 甲状舌骨膜　　　　　　　□ Thyrohyoid membrane
③ □ 甲状軟骨　　　　　　　　□ Thyroid cartilage
④ □ 輪状軟骨　　　　　　　　□ Cricoid cartilage
⑤ □ 輪状甲状靱帯　　　　　　□ Cricothyroid ligament
⑥ □ 喉頭隆起　　　　　　　　□ Laryngeal prominence
⑦ □ 舌骨体　　　　　　　　　□ Hyoid bone

Cavity of the Larynx

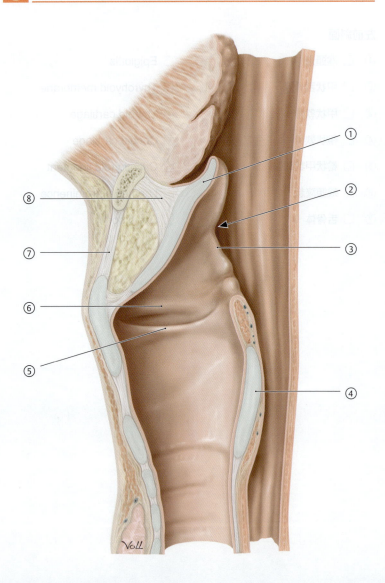

喉頭腔

正中矢状断面,右内側面

① ☐ 喉頭蓋 　　　　　　☐ Epiglottis
② ☐ 梨状陥凹 　　　　　☐ Piriform recess
③ ☐ 披裂喉頭蓋ヒダ 　　☐ Ary-epiglottic fold
④ ☐ 輪状軟骨 　　　　　☐ Cricoid cartilage
⑤ ☐ 声帯ヒダ 　　　　　☐ Vocal fold
⑥ ☐ 前庭ヒダ 　　　　　☐ Vestibular fold
⑦ ☐ 甲状舌骨靱帯 　　　☐ Thyrohyoid ligament
⑧ ☐ 舌骨喉頭蓋靱帯 　　☐ Hyo-epiglottic ligament

Neurovasculature of the Larynx I

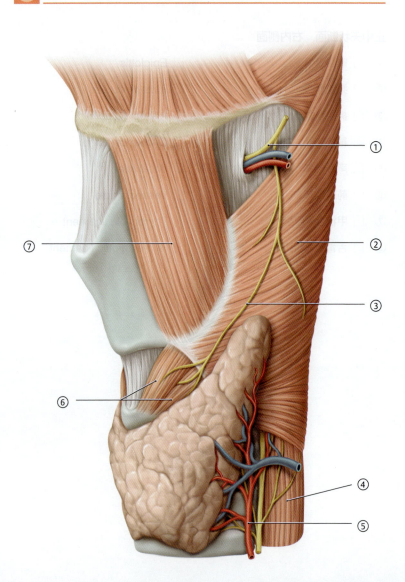

喉頭の神経・血管 1

左外側面

① ☐ 上喉頭神経の内枝　　　☐ Internal branch of superior laryngeal nerve

② ☐ 下咽頭収縮筋　　　　　☐ Inferior constrictor

③ ☐ 上喉頭神経の外枝　　　☐ External branch of superior laryngeal nerve

④ ☐ 食道　　　　　　　　　☐ Esophagus

⑤ ☐ 下甲状腺動脈　　　　　☐ Inferior thyroid artery

⑥ ☐ 輪状甲状筋　　　　　　☐ Cricothyroid

⑦ ☐ 甲状舌骨筋　　　　　　☐ Thyrohyoid

 解説

　喉頭は迷走神経の枝によって支配される．声帯ヒダより上方は上喉頭神経の内枝によって支配され，声帯ヒダより下方は反回神経に支配される．反回神経は喉頭内部の筋の運動を支配するが，唯一，喉頭の外側にある輪状甲状筋の運動神経支配は，上喉頭神経の外枝によって行われる．

Neurovasculature of the Larynx II

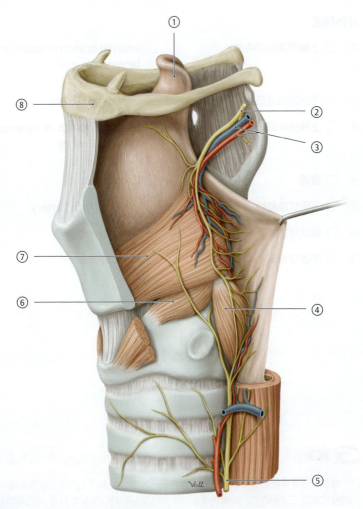

Q 声帯を外転させる喉頭筋は何か？

喉頭の神経・血管 2

左外側面

① ☐ 喉頭蓋　　　　　　　　　☐ Epiglottis
② ☐ 上喉頭神経, 内枝　　　　 ☐ Superior laryngeal nerve, internal branch
③ ☐ 上喉頭動脈・静脈　　　　 ☐ Superior laryngeal artery and vein
④ ☐ 後輪状披裂筋　　　　　　 ☐ Posterior crico-arytenoid
⑤ ☐ 下喉頭神経　　　　　　　 ☐ Inferior laryngeal nerve
⑥ ☐ 外側輪状甲状筋　　　　　 ☐ Lateral crico-thyroid
⑦ ☐ 甲状披裂筋　　　　　　　 ☐ Thyro-arytenoid
⑧ ☐ 舌骨　　　　　　　　　　 ☐ Hyoid bone

後輪状披裂筋は声帯を外転させる唯一の喉頭筋である.

Cervical Regions

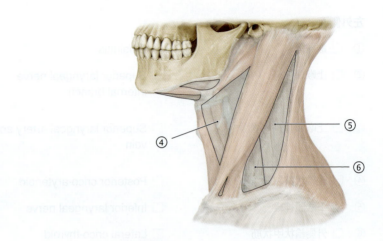

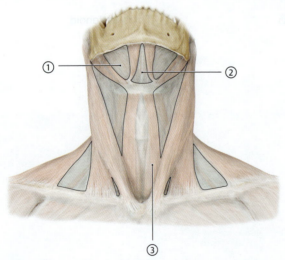

Q 頸部にある三角のうち，腕神経叢はどこにあるか，また内頸静脈はどこにあるか？

頸部の部位

上：左外側面，下：前面

① □ 顎下三角　　　　　　　□ Submandibular (digastric) triangle

② □ オトガイ下三角　　　　□ Submental triangle

③ □ 筋三角　　　　　　　　□ Muscular triangle

④ □ 頸動脈三角　　　　　　□ Carotid triangle

⑤ □ 外側頸三角部　　　　　□ Lateral cervical region

⑥ □ 肩甲鎖骨三角　　　　　□ Omoclavicular triangle

A 腕神経叢は外側頸三角部にあり，内頸静脈は総頸動脈とともに頸動脈三角を通過する．

Thoracic Inlet I

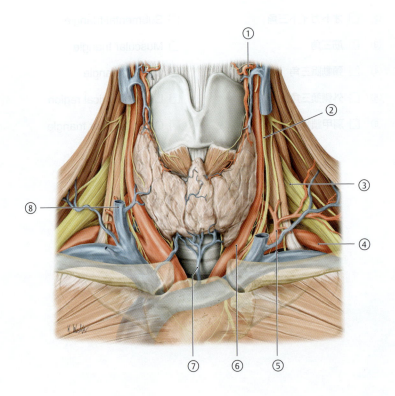

胸郭上口 1

前面

① □ 上甲状腺動脈 　　□ Superior thyroid artery
② □ 迷走神経 　　□ Vagus nerve（CN Ⅹ）
③ □ 腕神経叢 　　□ Brachial plexus
④ □ 鎖骨下動脈 　　□ Subclavian artery
⑤ □ 甲状頸動脈 　　□ Thyrocervical trunk
⑥ □ 総頸動脈 　　□ Common carotid artery
⑦ □ 下甲状腺静脈 　　□ Inferior thyroid vein
⑧ □ 内頸静脈 　　□ Internal jugular vein

Thoracic Inlet II

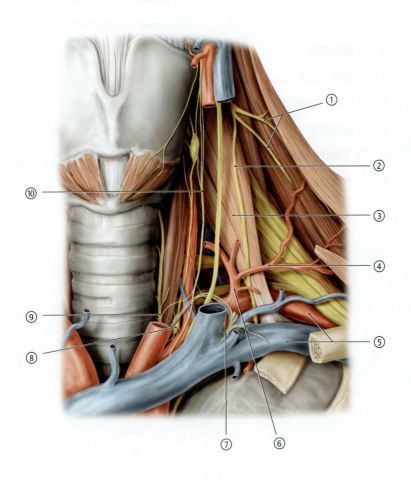

胸郭上口 2

前面

① □ 副神経 □ Accessory nerve（CN XI）
② □ 横隔神経 □ Phrenic nerve
③ □ 前斜角筋 □ Scalemus anterior（anterior scalene）
④ □ 頸横動脈 □ Transverse cervical artery
⑤ □ 鎖骨下動脈・静脈 □ Subclavian artery and vein
⑥ □ 甲状頸動脈 □ Thyrocervical trunk
⑦ □ 胸管 □ Thoracic duct
⑧ □ 星状神経節 □ Stellate ganglion
⑨ □ 反回神経 □ Recurrent laryngeal nerve
⑩ □ 交感神経幹 □ Sympathetic trunk

Lateral Cervical Topography I

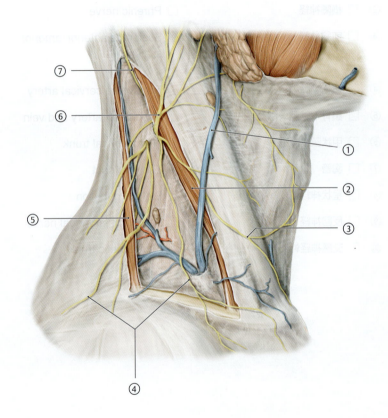

Q 神経点(エルプ点)として知られている頸の標識構造は何か？

外側頸三角部の局所解剖 1

右外側面

① □ 外頸静脈 　　　　　　　□ External jugular vein
② □ 胸鎖乳突筋 　　　　　　□ Sternocleidomastoid
③ □ 頸横神経 　　　　　　　□ Transverse cervical nerve
④ □ 鎖骨上神経 　　　　　　□ Supraclavicular nerves
⑤ □ 僧帽筋 　　　　　　　　□ Trapezius
⑥ □ 大耳介神経 　　　　　　□ Great auricular nerve
⑦ □ 小後頭神経 　　　　　　□ Lesser occipital nerve

A 頸部の神経点（エルプ点）は，胸鎖乳突筋後縁のほぼ中点にある標識構造で，頸筋膜を貫いてくる頸神経叢の皮枝がある．

Lateral Cervical Topography II

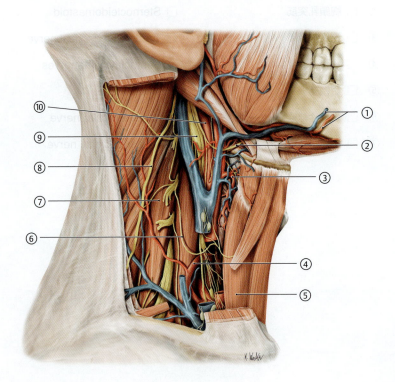

斜角筋隙の重要性は何か？

外側頸三角部の局所解剖 2

右外側面

①	□ 顔面動脈・静脈	□ Facial artery and vein
②	□ 舌下神経	□ Hypoglossal nerve (CN XII)
③	□ 上甲状腺動脈	□ Superior thyroid artery
④	□ 下甲状腺動脈	□ Inferior thyroid artery
⑤	□ 胸骨甲状筋	□ Sternothyroid
⑥	□ 頸神経ワナ	□ Ansa cervicalis
⑦	□ 中斜角筋	□ Scalenus medius (middle scalene)
⑧	□ 副神経の外枝	□ External branch of accessory nerve (CN XI)
⑨	□ 上頸神経節	□ Superior cervical ganglion
⑩	□ 内頸動脈	□ Internal carotid artery

 斜角筋隙は，頸神経叢と腕神経叢の前枝が脊柱から出て，前斜角筋と中斜角筋の間を通過する冠状断面と一致している．斜角筋隙の底部では鎖骨下動脈が腕神経叢の根部とともにある．

Surface Anatomy

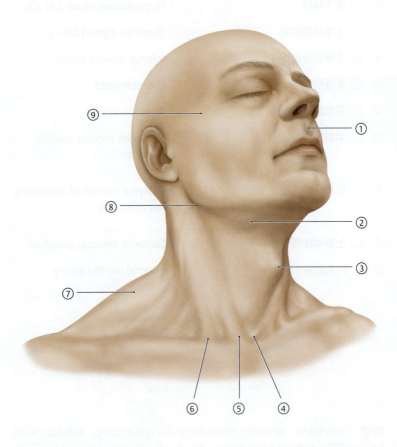

頭頸部の体表解剖

右前外側面

① □ 人中　　　　　　　　　□ Philtrum
② □ 顎下腺　　　　　　　　□ Submandibular gland
③ □ 甲状軟骨　　　　　　　□ Thyroid cartilage
④ □ 頸切痕　　　　　　　　□ Jugular notch
⑤ □ 胸鎖乳突筋の胸骨頭　　□ Sternal head of sternocleidomastoid
⑥ □ 胸鎖乳突筋の鎖骨頭　　□ Clavicular head of sternocleidomastoid
⑦ □ 僧帽筋　　　　　　　　□ Trapezius
⑧ □ 下顎角　　　　　　　　□ Angle of mandibular
⑨ □ 頬骨　　　　　　　　　□ Zygomatic bone

神経解剖 Neuroanatomy

成人の脳 1-3 ············· 848	脳の内部構造 1-3 ············· 886
髄膜 1, 2 ············· 854	脳幹 1-4 ············· 892
硬膜中隔 ············· 858	小脳 1, 2 ············· 900
脳脊髄液の循環 ············· 860	脊髄 1-10 ············· 904
脳室系 ············· 862	脊髄の動脈 ············· 924
脳の動脈 ············· 864	脊髄の静脈流出路 ············· 926
静脈洞交会 ············· 866	感覚系と運動系 ············· 928
頭蓋底にある硬膜静脈洞 ············· 868	視覚系 ············· 930
終脳 1-6 ············· 870	自律神経系 ············· 932
間脳 1, 2 ············· 882	

Adult Brain I

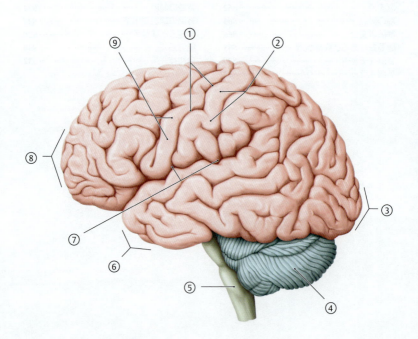

 中心溝によって分けられる2つの葉は何か？

成人の脳 1

左外側面

① ☐ 中心溝　　　　　☐ Central sulcus
② ☐ 中心後回　　　　☐ Postcentral gyrus
③ ☐ 後頭葉　　　　　☐ Occipital lobe
④ ☐ 小脳　　　　　　☐ Cerebellum
⑤ ☐ 延髄　　　　　　☐ Medulla oblongata
⑥ ☐ 側頭葉　　　　　☐ Temporal lobe
⑦ ☐ 外側溝　　　　　☐ Lateral sulcus
⑧ ☐ 前頭葉　　　　　☐ Frontal lobe
⑨ ☐ 中心前回　　　　☐ Precentralis gyrus

A 前頭葉と頭頂葉が中心溝によって分けられる．

Adult Brain II

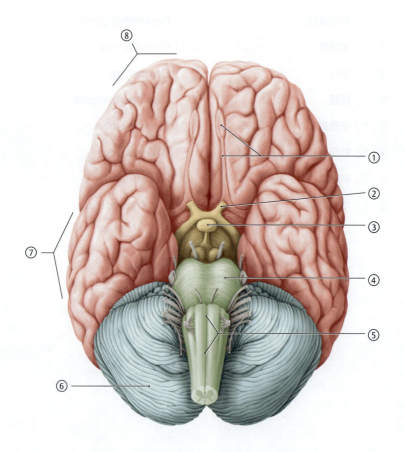

成人の脳 2

底面

①	□ 嗅球,嗅索	□ Olfactory bulb and tract
②	□ 視神経	□ Optic nerve（CN II）
③	□ 下垂体	□ Pituitary gland
④	□ 橋	□ Pons
⑤	□ 延髄	□ Medulla oblongata
⑥	□ 小脳	□ Cerebellum
⑦	□ 側頭葉	□ Temporal lobe
⑧	□ 前頭葉	□ Frontal lobe

Adult Brain III

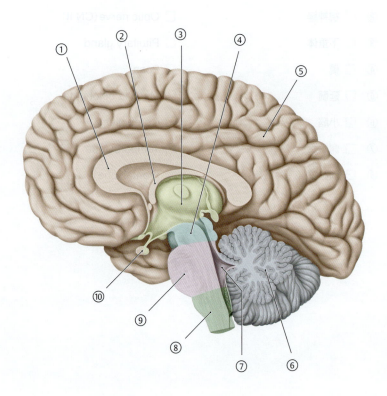

Q 第4脳室はどの脳領域間に位置しているか？

成人の脳 3

正中矢状断面．右半球の内側表面図

① □ 脳梁　　　　　□ Corpus callosum
② □ 脳弓　　　　　□ Fornix
③ □ 間脳　　　　　□ Diencephalon
④ □ 中脳　　　　　□ Mesencephalon
⑤ □ 終脳　　　　　□ Telencephalon
⑥ □ 小脳　　　　　□ Cerebellum
⑦ □ 第4脳室　　　□ Fourth ventricle
⑧ □ 延髄　　　　　□ Medulla oblongata
⑨ □ 橋　　　　　　□ Pons
⑩ □ 下垂体　　　　□ Pituitary gland

A 第4脳室は，小脳の腹側と橋の背側に位置している．

Meninges I

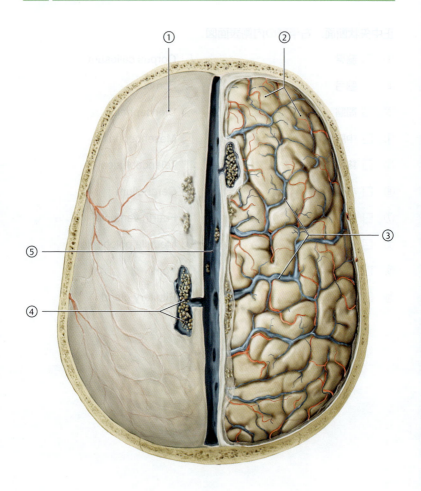

髄膜 1

上面

① □ 硬膜　　　　　　　　　　□ Dura mater
② □ 軟膜（大脳表面にある）　　□ Pia mater (on cerebral surface)
③ □ 上大脳静脈　　　　　　　□ Superior cerebral veins
④ □ クモ膜顆粒　　　　　　　□ Arachnoid granulations
　　　（クモ膜絨毛）　　　　　　　（arachnoid villi）
⑤ □ 上矢状静脈洞　　　　　　□ Superior sagittal sinus

Meninges II

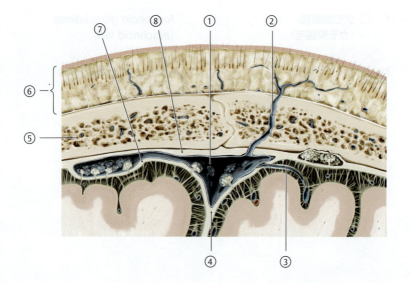

髄膜 2

冠状断面，前面

① □ 上矢状静脈洞　　　　　　□ Superior sagittal sinus
② □ 導出静脈　　　　　　　　□ Emissary vein
③ □ 架橋静脈　　　　　　　　□ Bridging vein
④ □ 大脳鎌　　　　　　　　　□ Falx cerebri
⑤ □ 板間層　　　　　　　　　□ Diploe of cranial bone
⑥ □ 頭皮　　　　　　　　　　□ Scalp
⑦ □ 硬膜，髄膜性の内層　　　□ Meningeal layer of dura mater
⑧ □ 硬膜，骨膜性の外層　　　□ Periosteal layer of dura mater

臨床

　頭蓋内出血は脳硬膜との位置関係により3つのタイプ(硬膜外出血，硬膜下出血，クモ膜下出血)に分けられる．硬膜外出血や硬膜下出血は，放置すると大きくなった血腫により脳が圧迫を受ける．血腫がさらに大きくなると，頭蓋内圧が上昇し，血腫により直接圧迫を受けている部位だけでなく，離れた部位にも損傷が及ぶ．

Dural Septa

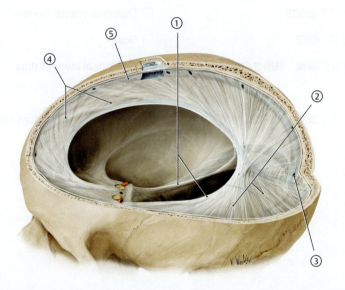

硬膜中隔

左前上外側面

① □ テント切痕　　　　□ Tentorial notch
② □ 小脳テント　　　　□ Tentorium cerebelli
③ □ 静脈洞交会　　　　□ Confluence of sinuses
④ □ 大脳鎌　　　　　　□ Falx cerebri
⑤ □ 上矢状静脈洞　　　□ Superior sagittal sinus

解説

硬膜によってできる中隔のうち，主要なものには大脳鎌，小脳テント，小脳鎌がある．このような中隔は脳の特定の部位に入り込み，脳のいくつかの部位を隔てている．

CSF Circulation

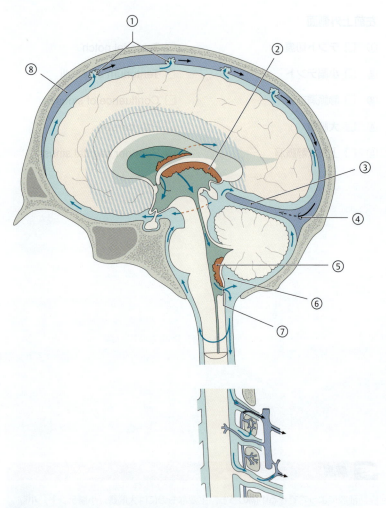

第3脳室と第4脳室を連結する構造は何か？

脳脊髄液の循環

左外側面

① ☐ クモ膜顆粒　　　　　　　　☐ Arachnoid granulations
② ☐ 第3脳室脈絡叢　　　　　　☐ Choroid plexus of third ventricle
③ ☐ 直静脈洞　　　　　　　　　☐ Straight sinus
④ ☐ 静脈洞交会　　　　　　　　☐ Confluence of the sinuses
⑤ ☐ 第4脳室脈絡叢　　　　　　☐ Choroid plexus of fourth ventricle
⑥ ☐ 小脳延髄槽（大槽）　　　　☐ Cerebellomedullary cistern (cisterna magna)
⑦ ☐ 第4脳室正中口　　　　　　☐ Median aperture (fourth ventricle)
⑧ ☐ 上矢状静脈洞　　　　　　　☐ Superior sagittal sinus

A 中脳水道が第3脳室と第4脳室を連結する．

Ventricular System

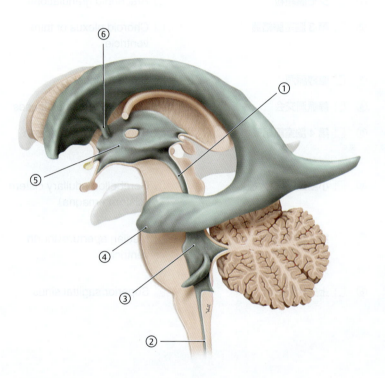

水頭症とは何か？

脳室系

左外側面

① □ 中脳水道　　　　　　□ Cerebral aqueduct
② □ 中心管　　　　　　　□ Central canal
③ □ 第4脳室　　　　　　 □ Fourth ventricle
④ □ 側脳室（下角）　　　 □ Lateral ventricle (inferior horn)
⑤ □ 第3脳室　　　　　　 □ Third ventricle
⑥ □ 室間孔　　　　　　　□ Interventricular foramen

A 水頭症は脳脊髄液が異常に溜まった状態を指す．

Arteries of the Brain

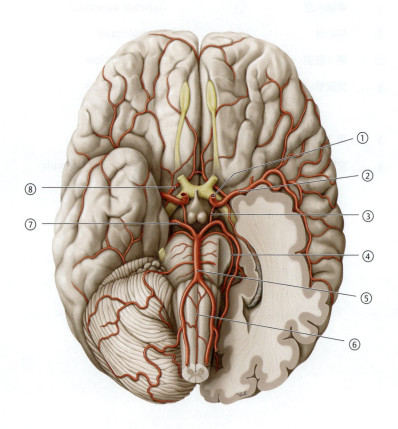

Q 前大脳動脈が分布する構造は何か？

脳の動脈

下面（底面）

① ☐ 内頸動脈 ☐ Internal carotid artery
② ☐ 中大脳動脈 ☐ Middle cerebral artery
③ ☐ 後交通動脈 ☐ Posterior communicating artery
④ ☐ 上小脳動脈 ☐ Superior cerebellar artery
⑤ ☐ 脳底動脈 ☐ Basilar artery
⑥ ☐ 前脊髄動脈 ☐ Anterior spinal artery
⑦ ☐ 後大脳動脈 ☐ Posterior cerebral artery
⑧ ☐ 前大脳動脈 ☐ Anterior cerebral artery

A 前大脳動脈は前頭葉の全体と頭頂葉の一部に分布する．

Confluence of the Sinuses

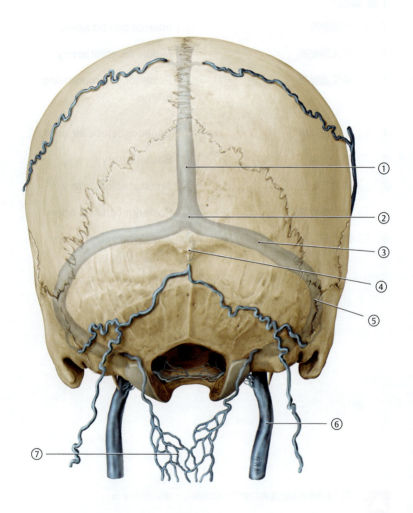

静脈洞交会

後面

① □ 上矢状静脈洞　　　　　□ Superior sagittal sinus
② □ 静脈洞交会　　　　　　□ Confluence of sinuses
③ □ 横静脈洞　　　　　　　□ Transverse sinus
④ □ 外後頭隆起　　　　　　□ External occipital protuberance

⑤ □ S状静脈洞　　　　　　□ Sigmoid sinus
⑥ □ 内頸静脈　　　　　　　□ Internal jugular vein
⑦ □ 外椎骨静脈叢　　　　　□ External vertebral venous plexus

Dural Sinuses in the Skull Base

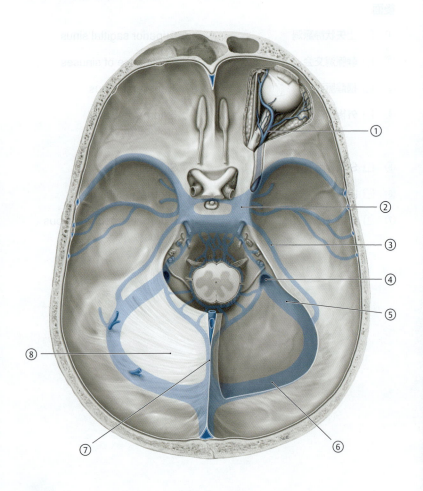

Q 小脳と大脳半球を隔てる構造は何か？

頭蓋底にある硬膜静脈洞

上面

① ☐ 上眼静脈　　　　　　　☐ Superior ophthalmic vein
② ☐ 海綿静脈洞　　　　　　☐ Cavernous sinus
③ ☐ 上錐体静脈洞　　　　　☐ Superior petrosal sinus
④ ☐ 頸静脈孔　　　　　　　☐ Jugular foramen
⑤ ☐ S状静脈洞　　　　　　☐ Sigmoid sinus
⑥ ☐ 横静脈洞　　　　　　　☐ Transverse sinus
⑦ ☐ 直静脈洞　　　　　　　☐ Straight sinus
⑧ ☐ 小脳テント　　　　　　☐ Tentorium cerebelli

　小脳と大脳半球は小脳テントによって隔てられる．小脳テントは，小脳が入っている後頭蓋窩を覆う屋根を形成する．また，小脳テントは大脳鎌に連なっている．

Telencephalon I

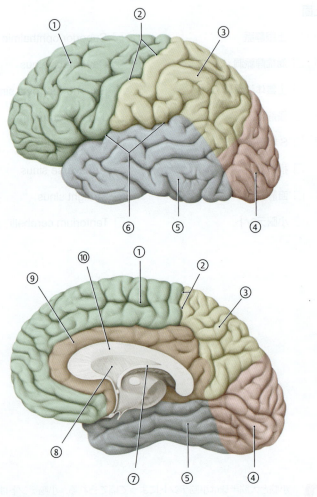

前頭葉と頭頂葉はどのような溝によって相互に分け隔てられているか？

終脳 1

上：左大脳半球の外側面，下：右大脳半球の内側面

①	□ 前頭葉	□ Frontal lobe
②	□ 中心溝	□ Central sulcus
③	□ 頭頂葉	□ Parietal lobe
④	□ 後頭葉	□ Occipital lobe
⑤	□ 側頭葉	□ Temporal lobe
⑥	□ 外側溝	□ Lateral sulcus
⑦	□ 脳弓	□ Fornix
⑧	□ 透明中隔	□ Septum pellucidum
⑨	□ 辺縁葉	□ Limbic lobe
⑩	□ 脳梁	□ Corpus callosum

前頭葉と頭頂葉は中心溝によって相互に分け隔てられている．

Telencephalon II

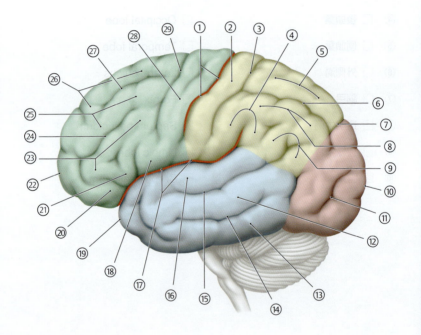

終脳 2

左大脳半球の外側面

① □ 中心溝　　　　　　　□ Central sulcus
② □ 中心後回　　　　　　□ Postcentral gyrus
③ □ 中心後溝　　　　　　□ Postcentral sulcus
④ □ 縁上回　　　　　　　□ Supramarginal gyrus
⑤ □ 上頭頂小葉　　　　　□ Superior parietal lobule
⑥ □ 頭頂間溝　　　　　　□ Intraparietal sulcus
⑦ □ 頭頂後頭溝　　　　　□ Parieto-occipital sulcus
⑧ □ 下頭頂小葉　　　　　□ Inferior parietal lobule
⑨ □ 角回　　　　　　　　□ Angular gyrus
⑩ □ 後頭極　　　　　　　□ Occipital pole
⑪ □ 月状溝　　　　　　　□ Lunate sulcus
⑫ □ 中側頭回　　　　　　□ Middle temporal gyrus
⑬ □ 下側頭回　　　　　　□ Inferior temporal gyrus
⑭ □ 下側頭溝　　　　　　□ Inferior temporal sulcus
⑮ □ 上側頭溝　　　　　　□ Superior temporal sulcus
⑯ □ 上側頭回　　　　　　□ Superior temporal gyrus
⑰ □ 外側溝　　　　　　　□ Lateral sulcus
⑱ □ (下前頭回の)弁蓋部　□ Opercular part (of inferior frontal gyrus)
⑲ □ 側頭極　　　　　　　□ Temporal pole
⑳ □ (下前頭回の)眼窩部　□ Orbital part (of inferior frontal gyrus)
㉑ □ (下前頭回の)三角部　□ Triangular part (of inferior frontal gyrus)
㉒ □ 前頭極　　　　　　　□ Frontal pole
㉓ □ 下前頭回　　　　　　□ Inferior frontal gyrus
㉔ □ 下前頭溝　　　　　　□ Inferior frontal sulcus
㉕ □ 中前頭回　　　　　　□ Middle frontal gyrus
㉖ □ 上前頭回　　　　　　□ Superior frontal gyrus
㉗ □ 上前頭溝　　　　　　□ Superior frontal sulcus
㉘ □ 中心前回　　　　　　□ Precentral gyrus
㉙ □ 中心前溝　　　　　　□ Precentral sulcus

Telencephalon III

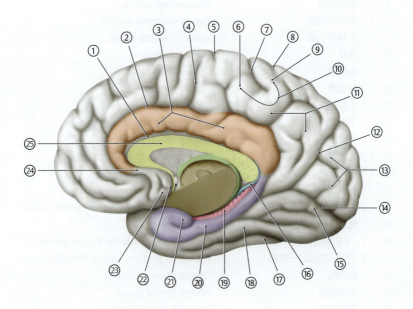

終脳 3

右大脳半球の内側面

① ☐ 脳梁溝 ☐ Sulcus of corpus callosum
② ☐ 帯状溝 ☐ Cingulate sulcus
③ ☐ 帯状回 ☐ Cingulate gyrus
④ ☐ 中心傍溝 ☐ Paracentral sulcus
⑤ ☐ 中心前溝 ☐ Precentral sulcus
⑥ ☐ 前中心傍回 ☐ Anterior paracentral gyrus
⑦ ☐ 中心溝 ☐ Central sulcus
⑧ ☐ 中心後溝 ☐ Postcentral sulcus
⑨ ☐ 後中心傍回 ☐ Posterior paracentral gyrus
⑩ ☐ 中心傍小葉 ☐ Paracentral lobule
⑪ ☐ 楔前部 ☐ Precuneus
⑫ ☐ 頭頂後頭溝 ☐ Parieto-occipital sulcus
⑬ ☐ 楔部 ☐ Cuneus
⑭ ☐ 鳥距溝 ☐ Calcarine sulcus
⑮ ☐ 舌状回 ☐ Lingual gyrus
⑯ ☐ 小帯回 ☐ Fasciolar gyrus
⑰ ☐ 外側後頭側頭回 ☐ Lateral occipitotemporal gyrus
⑱ ☐ 内側後頭側頭回 ☐ Medial occipitotemporal gyrus
⑲ ☐ 歯状回 ☐ Dentate gyrus
⑳ ☐ 海馬傍回 ☐ Parahippocampal gyrus
㉑ ☐ (海馬傍回の)鉤 ☐ Uncus (of parahippocampal gyrus)
㉒ ☐ 終板傍回 ☐ Paraterminal gyrus
㉓ ☐ 嗅傍野 ☐ Paraolfactory area
㉔ ☐ 梁下野 ☐ Subcallosal area
㉕ ☐ 脳梁 ☐ Corpus callosum

Telencephalon IV

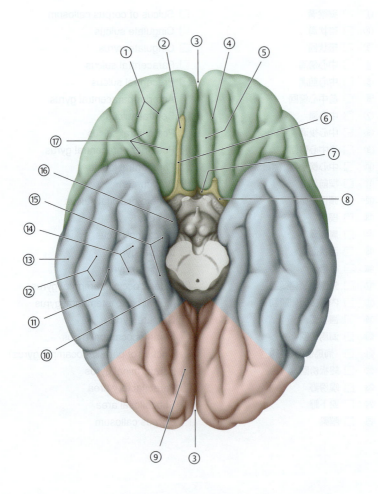

終脳 4

下面

①	□ 眼窩溝	□ Orbital sulci
②	□ 嗅球	□ Olfactory bulb
③	□ 大脳縦裂	□ Longitudinal fissure of cerebrum
④	□ 嗅溝	□ Olfactory sulcus
⑤	□ 直回	□ Gyrus rectus
⑥	□ 嗅索	□ Olfactory tract
⑦	□ 内側嗅条	□ Medial stria
⑧	□ 外側嗅条	□ Lateral stria
⑨	□ 舌状回	□ Lingual gyrus
⑩	□ 側副溝	□ Collateral sulcus
⑪	□ 後頭側頭溝	□ Occipitotemporal sulcus
⑫	□ 外側後頭側頭回	□ Lateral occipitotemporal gyrus
⑬	□ 下側頭回	□ Inferior temporal gyrus
⑭	□ 内側後頭側頭回	□ Medial occipitotemporal gyrus
⑮	□ 海馬傍回	□ Parahippocampal gyrus
⑯	□ 鉤（海馬傍回の）	□ Uncus (of parahippocampal gyrus)
⑰	□ 眼窩回	□ Orbital gyri

Telencephalon V

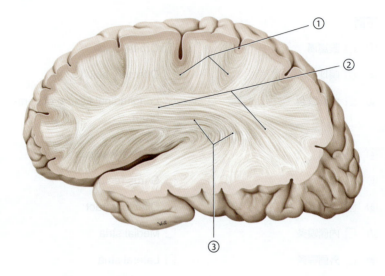

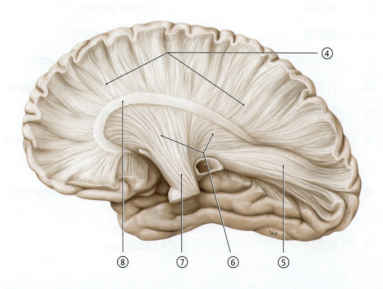

終脳 5

上：左大脳半球の外側面，下：右大脳半球の内側面

① □ 大脳弓状線維（U字線維）　□ Cerebral arcuate fibers (U fibers)

② □ 上縦束　□ Superior longitudinal fasciculus

③ □ 前頭側頭束　□ Frontotemporal fasciculus

④ □ 放線冠　□ Corona radiata

⑤ □ 視放線　□ Optic radiation

⑥ □ 内包　□ Internal capsule

⑦ □ 大脳脚　□ Cerebral peduncle

⑧ □ 脳梁　□ Corpus callosum

 解説

　肉眼では，神経細胞の細胞体が集まった部位は灰白色に，軸索（髄鞘が取り巻いている）が集まった部位は白色に見える．

Telencephalon VI : Hippocampal Formation

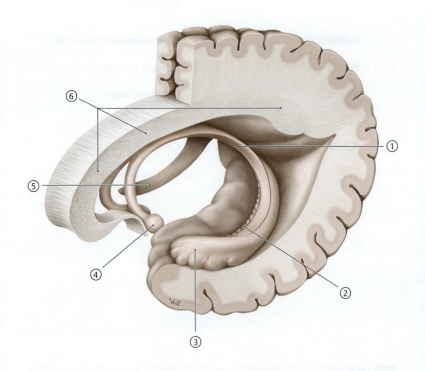

終脳6：海馬とその関連構造

左前上面

① □ 脳弓体　　　　　□ Body of fornix

② □ 歯状回　　　　　□ Dentate gyrus

③ □ 海馬　　　　　　□ Hippocampus

④ □ 乳頭体　　　　　□ Mammillary body

⑤ □ 脳弓脚　　　　　□ Crus of fornix

⑥ □ 脳梁　　　　　　□ Corpus callosum

解説

海馬，脳弓，扁桃体は辺縁系の主要な構成要素である．

Diencephalon I

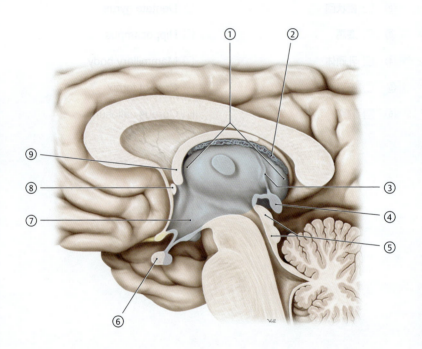

Q 下垂体前葉(腺下垂体)は胎児期にどこから形成されるか？

間脳 1

正中矢状断面

① □ 視床 □ Thalamus
② □ 脈絡叢 □ Choroid plexus
③ □ 視床髄条 □ Stria medullaris thalami
④ □ 松果体 □ Pineal gland
⑤ □ 四丘体板 □ Quadrigeminal plate
⑥ □ 下垂体の前葉（腺下垂体） □ Pituitary gland, anterior lobe (adenohypophysis)
⑦ □ 視床下部 □ Hypothalamus
⑧ □ 前交連 □ Anterior commissure
⑨ □ 脳弓 □ Fornix

　下垂体前葉（腺下垂体）は，口咽頭の上皮の突出部であるラトケ嚢に由来する．

Diencephalon II

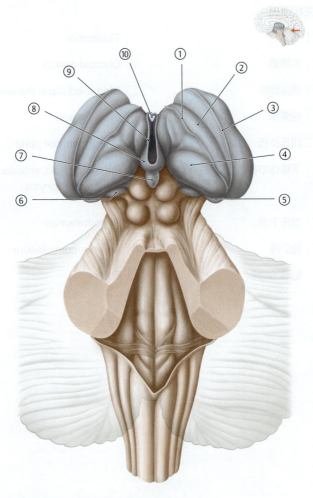

Q 視床のどの核領域で視覚路や聴覚路の中継が行われるか？

間脳 2

背側面. 小脳と終脳を取り除いてある

① □ 脈絡ヒモ　　　　　□ Choroid line
② □ 付着板　　　　　　□ Lamina affixa
③ □ 分界条　　　　　　□ Stria terminalis
④ □ 視床枕　　　　　　□ Pulvinar
⑤ □ 外側膝状体　　　　□ Lateral geniculate body
⑥ □ 内側膝状体　　　　□ Medial geniculate body
⑦ □ 松果体　　　　　　□ Pineal gland
⑧ □ 手綱　　　　　　　□ Habenula
⑨ □ 視床ヒモ　　　　　□ Tenia thalami
⑩ □ 第3脳室　　　　　□ Third ventricle

視覚路は外側膝状体で，聴覚路は内側膝状体で中継が行われる．

Internal Structures I

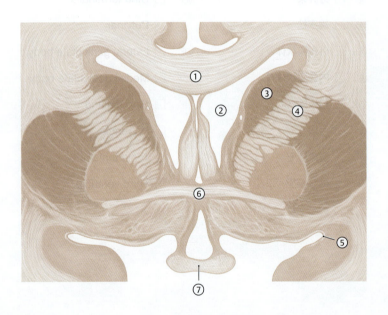

Q 左右の大脳半球をつなぐ2つの構造は何か？

脳の内部構造 1

冠状断面（視神経交叉を通る断面）

① □ 脳梁　　　　　□ Corpus callosum
② □ 側脳室　　　　□ Lateral ventricle
③ □ 尾状核　　　　□ Caudate nucleus
④ □ 内包　　　　　□ Internal capsule
⑤ □ 外側嗅条　　　□ Lateral stria
⑥ □ 前交連　　　　□ Anterior commissure
⑦ □ 視交叉　　　　□ Optic chiasm (CN II)

A 左右の大脳半球は，脳梁と前交連によって連結している．

Internal Structures II

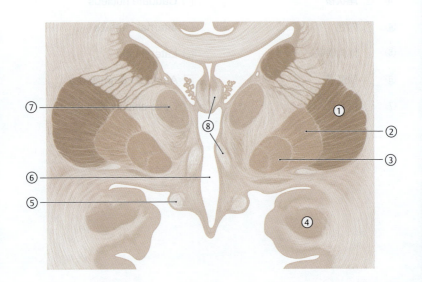

Q 扁桃体が属する機能系は何か？

脳の内部構造 2

冠状断面（灰白隆起を通る断面）

① □ 被殻　　　　　　　　　□ Putamen

② □ 淡蒼球の外節　　　　　□ Lateral segment of globus pallidus

③ □ 淡蒼球の内節　　　　　□ Medial segment of globus pallidus

④ □ 扁桃体　　　　　　　　□ Amygdaloid body

⑤ □ 視索　　　　　　　　　□ Optic tract

⑥ □ 第3脳室　　　　　　　□ Third ventricle

⑦ □ 視床（視床核）　　　　□ Thalamus

⑧ □ 脳弓　　　　　　　　　□ Fornix

A 扁桃体は辺縁系の構成要素である．

Internal Structures III

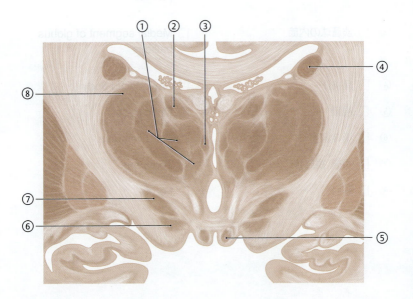

Q 視床核のうち，意識にのぼる固有覚（位置覚や運動覚）を中継するのはどれか？

脳の内部構造 3

冠状断面（乳頭体を通る断面）

① □ 視床内側核群　　　　　□ Medial thalamic nuclei

② □ 視床前核群　　　　　　□ Anterior thalamic nuclei

③ □ 視床室傍核群　　　　　□ Paraventricular nuclei

④ □ 尾状核　　　　　　　　□ Caudate nucleus

⑤ □ 乳頭体　　　　　　　　□ Mammillary body

⑥ □ 黒質　　　　　　　　　□ Substantia nigra

⑦ □ 視床下核　　　　　　　□ Subthalamic nucleus

⑧ □ 視床外側腹側核群　　　□ Ventrolateral thalamic nuclei

A 意識にのぼる固有覚は後外側腹側核を中継し，大脳皮質へ伝えられる．

Brainstem I

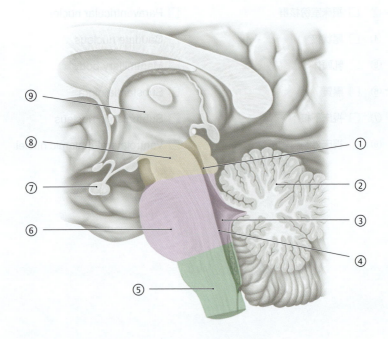

Q 脳幹は頭部から尾部に向けて，どのような部分によって構成されているか？

脳幹 1

正中矢状断面

① □ 中脳水道　　□ Cerebral aqueduct
② □ 小脳　　　　□ Cerebellum
③ □ 第4脳室　　 □ Fourth ventricle
④ □ 菱形窩　　　□ Rhomboid fossa
⑤ □ 延髄　　　　□ Medulla oblongata
⑥ □ 橋　　　　　□ Pons
⑦ □ 下垂体　　　□ Pituitary gland
⑧ □ 中脳　　　　□ Mesencephalon
⑨ □ 間脳　　　　□ Diencephalon

中脳，橋，延髄の順に連なっている．

Brainstem II

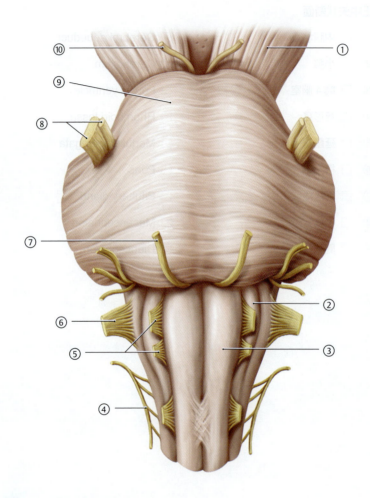

Q 橋に存在する脳神経核は何か？

脳幹 2

前面

① ☐ 大脳脚　　　　　　　　☐ Cerebral peduncle
② ☐ オリーブ　　　　　　　☐ Olive
③ ☐ 延髄の錐体　　　　　　☐ Pyramid of medulla oblongata
④ ☐ 副神経　　　　　　　　☐ Accessory nerve（CN XI）
⑤ ☐ 舌下神経　　　　　　　☐ Hypoglossal nerve（CN XII）
⑥ ☐ 迷走神経　　　　　　　☐ Vagus nerve（CN X）
⑦ ☐ 外転神経　　　　　　　☐ Abducent nerve（CN VI）
⑧ ☐ 三叉神経　　　　　　　☐ Trigeminal nerve（CN V）
⑨ ☐ 橋　　　　　　　　　　☐ Pons
⑩ ☐ 動眼神経　　　　　　　☐ Oculomotor nerve（CN III）

　三叉神経（V），外転神経（VI），顔面神経（VII），内耳神経（VIII）に関する神経核が橋に存在する．ただし，前庭神経核は延髄にまで，三叉神経脊髄路核は脊髄にまで伸び出している．

Brainstem III

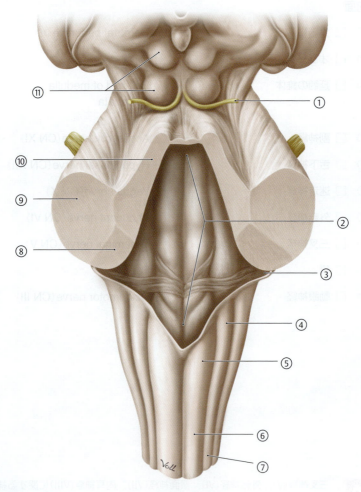

Q 脳幹の後方から出る唯一の脳神経はどれか？

脳幹 3

後面

① □ 滑車神経 　　　　　　　　□ Trochlear nerve (CN IV)

② □ 菱形窩 　　　　　　　　　□ Rhomboid fossa

③ □ 第4脳室外側陥凹 　　　　　□ Lateral recess of fourth ventricle

④ □ 楔状束結節（楔状束核） 　　□ Cuneate tubercle (cuneate nucleus)

⑤ □ 薄束結節（薄束核） 　　　　□ Gracile tubercle (gracile nucleus)

⑥ □ 薄束 　　　　　　　　　　□ Gracile fasciculus

⑦ □ 楔状束 　　　　　　　　　□ Cuneate fasciculus

⑧ □ 下小脳脚 　　　　　　　　□ Inferior cerebellar peduncle

⑨ □ 中小脳脚 　　　　　　　　□ Middle cerebellar peduncle

⑩ □ 上小脳脚 　　　　　　　　□ Superior cerebellar peduncle

⑪ □ 蓋板（四丘体板）の上丘と下丘 □ Superior and inferior colliculi of tectal (quadrigeminal) plate

滑車神経（IV）は，脳幹（中脳）の後面にある下丘の遠位から現れる．脳幹から出るその他の脳神経は，すべてが脳幹の前面から現れる．

Brainstem IV

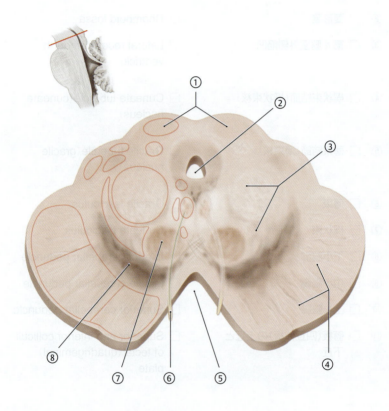

Q 中脳の背側と腹側の境界にある構造は何か？

脳幹 4

中脳の横断面．上方から見た図

① ☐ 中脳蓋　　　　　☐ Tectum
② ☐ 中脳水道　　　　☐ Cerebral aqueduct
③ ☐ 中脳被蓋　　　　☐ Tegmentum
④ ☐ 大脳脚　　　　　☐ Cerebral peduncle
⑤ ☐ 脚間窩　　　　　☐ Interpeduncular fossa
⑥ ☐ 動眼神経　　　　☐ Oculomotorius nerve (CN III)
⑦ ☐ 赤核　　　　　　☐ Red nucleus
⑧ ☐ 黒質　　　　　　☐ Substantia nigra

A 中脳水道が中脳の腹側と背側の境界に位置する．

Cerebellum I

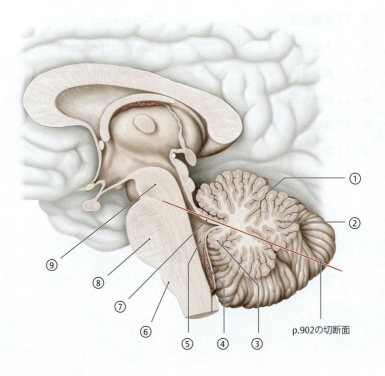

Q 小脳は頭蓋窩のうちのどこに位置しているか？

小脳 1

正中矢状断面

① □ 第一裂　　　　□ Primary fissure
② □ 水平裂　　　　□ Horizontal fissure
③ □ 小節　　　　　□ Nodule
④ □ 脈絡叢　　　　□ Choroid plexus
⑤ □ 第4脳室　　　□ Fourth ventricle
⑥ □ オリーブ　　　□ Olive
⑦ □ 上髄帆　　　　□ Superior medullary velum
⑧ □ 橋　　　　　　□ Pons
⑨ □ 中脳　　　　　□ Mesencephalon

A 小脳は後頭蓋窩に位置している．

Cerebellum II

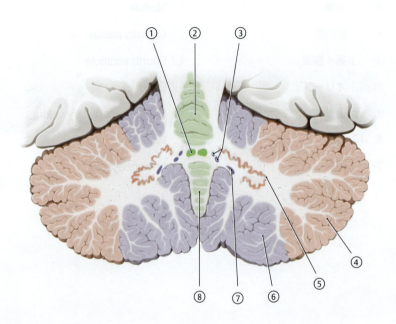

どの皮質部分がどの小脳核に投射されるか？

小脳 2

上小脳脚での断面(切断の方向については pp.900, 901 を参照). **背側面**

① □ 室頂核　　　　　□ Fastigial nucleus
② □ 小脳虫部　　　　□ Vermis
③ □ 球状核　　　　　□ Globose nuclei
④ □ 外側部　　　　　□ Lateral part
⑤ □ 歯状核　　　　　□ Dentate nucleus
⑥ □ 中間部　　　　　□ Intermediate part
⑦ □ 栓状核　　　　　□ Emboliform nucleus
⑧ □ 正中部　　　　　□ Median part

A 　脳半球，外側部は歯状核に，脳半球，中間部は栓状核に，小脳虫部，正中部は室頂核に投射される．

Spinal Cord I

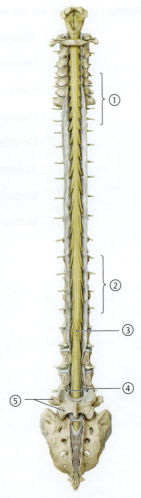

①
②
③
④
⑤

Q 成人では脊髄の下端はおよそどの高さに位置するか？

脊髄 1

後面

① □ 頸膨大　　　　　　　□ Cervical enlargement
② □ 腰膨大　　　　　　　□ Lumbosacral enlargement
③ □ 脊髄円錐　　　　　　□ Conus medullaris
④ □ 馬尾　　　　　　　　□ Cauda equina
⑤ □ 第5腰椎　　　　　　□ L5 vertebra

A 　成人では，脊髄の下端はL1の高さに位置する．これは，脊髄の成長が停止した後も，脊柱の成長が進行することによる．第1腰神経よりも下位の脊髄神経は，脊柱管内を馬尾となって下行する．

Spinal Cord II

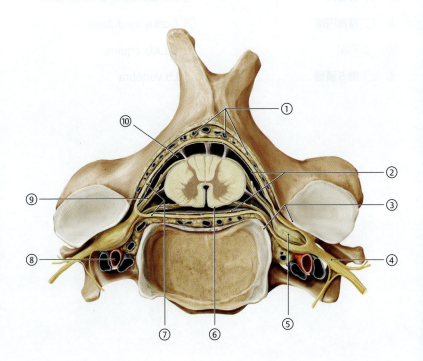

脳脊髄液によって満たされるのはどこか？

脊髄 2

横断面，上面

① ☐ 後内椎骨静脈叢　　　　☐ Posterior internal vertebral venous plexus
② ☐ 脊髄クモ膜　　　　　　☐ Spinal arachnoid mater
③ ☐ 椎間孔　　　　　　　　☐ Intervertebral foramen
④ ☐ 脊髄神経　　　　　　　☐ Spinal nerve
⑤ ☐ 脊髄神経節　　　　　　☐ Spinal ganglion
⑥ ☐ 脊髄軟膜　　　　　　　☐ Spinal pia mater
⑦ ☐ 脊髄硬膜　　　　　　　☐ Spinal dura mater
⑧ ☐ 椎骨動脈　　　　　　　☐ Vertebral artery
⑨ ☐ 後根　　　　　　　　　☐ Dorsal root
⑩ ☐ クモ膜下腔　　　　　　☐ Subarachnoid space

A 脳脊髄液はクモ膜下腔を満たしている．

Spinal Cord III

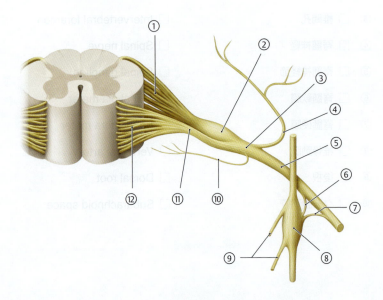

脊髄神経4枝の名称は？

脊髄 3

脊髄分節. 横断面

① □ 後根糸　　　　　□ Posterior rootlets
② □ 脊髄神経節　　　□ Spinal ganglion
③ □ 脊髄神経　　　　□ Spinal nerve
④ □ 後枝　　　　　　□ Posterior ramus
⑤ □ 前枝　　　　　　□ Anterior ramus
⑥ □ 灰白交通枝　　　□ Gray ramus communicans
⑦ □ 白交通枝　　　　□ White ramus communicans
⑧ □ 幹神経節　　　　□ Ganglion of sympathetic trunk
⑨ □ 内臓神経　　　　□ Splanchnic nerves
⑩ □ 硬膜枝　　　　　□ Meningeal branch
⑪ □ 前根　　　　　　□ Anterior root
⑫ □ 前根糸　　　　　□ Anterior rootlets

前枝, 後枝, 硬膜枝, 白交通枝.

Spinal Cord IV

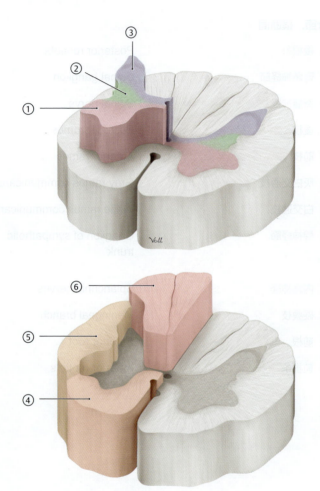

脊髄後索にはどのような上行路が走行しているか？

脊髄 4

灰白質と白質の配置（左前上方から見た図）

① □ 前柱　　　　□ Anterior column
② □ 側柱　　　　□ Lateral column
③ □ 後柱　　　　□ Posterior column
④ □ 前索　　　　□ Anterior funiculus
⑤ □ 側索　　　　□ Lateral funiculus
⑥ □ 後索　　　　□ Posterior funiculus

　後索は薄束と楔状束に分けられ、後束路が走行している。後索路は精緻に識別された機械的受容と固有受容を伝達する。後索路は脳幹で完全に交差する。

Spinal Cord V

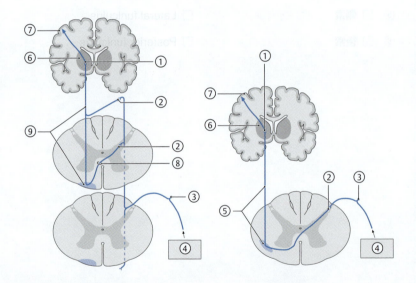

脊髄 5

上行性伝導路：前脊髄視床路および外側脊髄視床路

① □ 3次ニューロン　　　　□ 3rd neuron
② □ 2次ニューロン　　　　□ 2nd neuron
③ □ 1次ニューロン　　　　□ 1st neuron
④ □ 受容野　　　　　　　　□ Receptive field
⑤ □ 外側脊髄視床路　　　　□ Lateral spinothalamic tract
⑥ □ 視床　　　　　　　　　□ Thalamus
⑦ □ 大脳皮質感覚野　　　　□ Sensory cortex
⑧ □ 前交連　　　　　　　　□ Anterior commissure
⑨ □ 前脊髄視床路　　　　　□ Anterior spinothalamic tract

解説

前脊髄視床路と外側脊髄視床路は，疼痛，温度，大まかな機械的受容に関する情報を伝達する．これらの伝導路は脊髄で交差する．

Spinal Cord VI

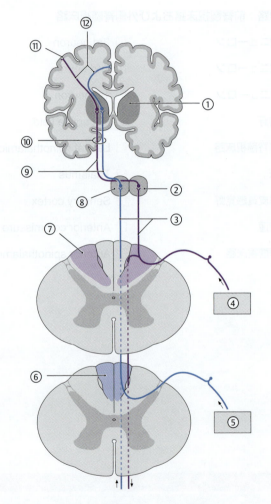

Q 後索路（薄束/楔状束）の第2ニューロンの位置は？

脊髄6

上行性伝導路：後索路（薄束，楔状束）
薄束を青色，楔状束を紫色で示してある

① □ 視床　　　　　　　　　□ Thalamus
② □ 楔状束核　　　　　　　□ Cuneate nucleus
③ □ 1次ニューロンの軸索　 □ Axon of 1st neuron
④ □ 上肢の受容野　　　　　□ Receptive field of arm
⑤ □ 下肢の受容野　　　　　□ Receptive field of leg
⑥ □ 薄束　　　　　　　　　□ Gracile fasciculus
⑦ □ 楔状束　　　　　　　　□ Cuneate fasciculus
⑧ □ 薄束核　　　　　　　　□ Gracile nucleus
⑨ □ 2次ニューロンの軸索　 □ Axon of 2nd neuron
⑩ □ 内側毛帯　　　　　　　□ Medial lemniscus
⑪ □ 中心後回　　　　　　　□ Postcentral gyrus
⑫ □ 3次ニューロンの軸索　 □ Axon of 3rd neuron

後索路（薄束/楔状束）の2次ニューロンは，延髄下部領域の薄束核/楔状束核に位置している．つまり，1次ニューロンから2次ニューロンへの中継は，脊髄では行われない．

Spinal Cord VII

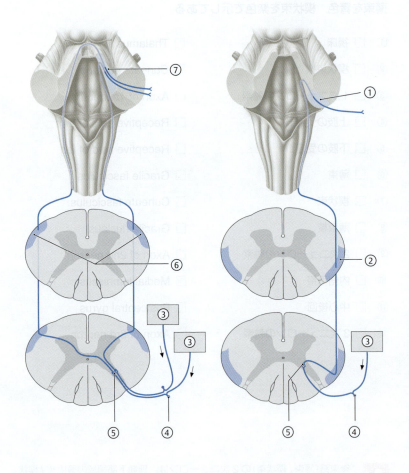

上行性伝導路の交差に関して，脊髄小脳路での特別な点は？

脊髄 7

上行性伝導路：前脊髄小脳路および後脊髄小脳路

① ☐ 下小脳脚 ☐ Inferior cerebellar peduncle
② ☐ 後脊髄小脳路 ☐ Posterior spinocerebellar tract
③ ☐ 受容野 ☐ Receptive field
④ ☐ 1次ニューロンの細胞体 ☐ Cell body of 1st neuron
⑤ ☐ 2次ニューロンの細胞体 ☐ Cell body of 2nd neuron
⑥ ☐ 前脊髄小脳路 ☐ Anterior spinocerebellar tract
⑦ ☐ 上小脳脚 ☐ Superior cerebellar peduncle

A 脊髄小脳路は同側の小脳で終わる．前脊髄小脳路の一部は脊髄でいったん交差するが，小脳で再び交差し同側性に終わる．

Spinal Cord VIII

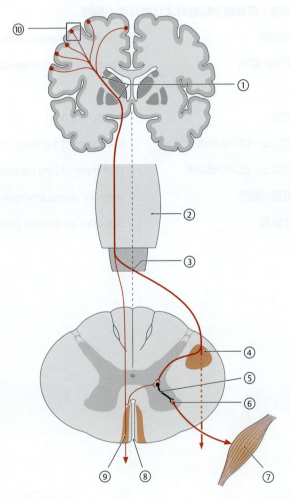

皮質脊髄線維はどこで交差するか？

脊髄 8

下行性伝導路：錐体路（前皮質脊髄路および外側皮質脊髄路）

① □ 内包　　　　　　　　□ Internal capsule
② □ 脳幹　　　　　　　　□ Brain stem
③ □ 錐体交叉　　　　　　□ Decussation of pyramids
④ □ 外側皮質脊髄路　　　□ Lateral corticospinal tract
⑤ □ 介在ニューロン　　　□ Interneuron
⑥ □ α運動ニューロン　　□ Alpha motor neuron
⑦ □ 筋　　　　　　　　　□ Muscle
⑧ □ 前正中裂　　　　　　□ Anterior median fissure
⑨ □ 前皮質脊髄路　　　　□ Anterior corticospinal tract
⑩ □ 大脳皮質運動野　　　□ Motor cortex

A 皮質脊髄線維の大半（＞80％）は錐体交叉で交差し，その先は外側皮質脊髄路として走行する．残り部分（前皮質脊髄路）は，脊髄レベルで交差する．

Spinal Cord IX

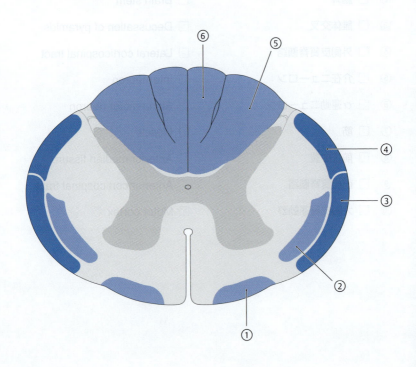

Q 温痛覚の伝導路は何か？

脊髄 9

上面

① □ 前脊髄視床路 □ Anterior spinothalamic tract
② □ 外側脊髄視床路 □ Lateral spinothalamic tract
③ □ 前脊髄小脳路 □ Anterior spinocerebellar tract
④ □ 後脊髄小脳路 □ Posterior spinocerebellar tract
⑤ □ 楔状束 □ Cuneatus fasciculus
⑥ □ 薄束 □ Gracilis fasciculus

A 温痛覚は外側脊髄視床路によって伝達される.

Spinal Cord X

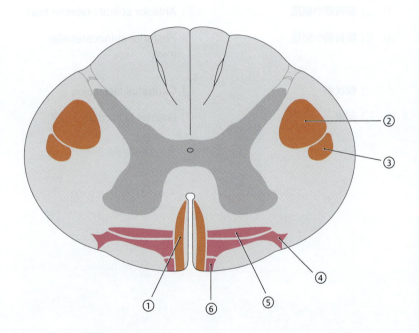

Q 脊髄に損傷を受け，障害側に痙性麻痺が出現した場合には，どの伝導路の障害が考えられるか？

脊髄 10

上面

① □ 前皮質脊髄路　　　　　□ Anterior corticospinal tract
② □ 外側皮質脊髄路　　　　□ Lateral corticospinal tract
③ □ 赤核脊髄路　　　　　　□ Rubrospinal tract
④ □ 網様体脊髄路　　　　　□ Reticulospinal tract
⑤ □ 前庭脊髄路　　　　　　□ Vestibulospinal tract
⑥ □ 視蓋脊髄路　　　　　　□ Tectospinal tract

A 　脊髄において錐体路（前・外側皮質脊髄路）が損傷されると，障害側に痙性麻痺が出現する．

Arteries of the Spinal Cord

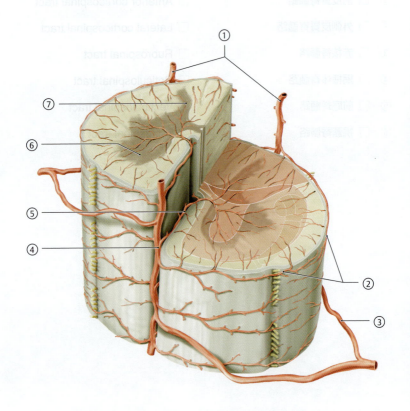

脊髄の大部分に分布する動脈は何か？

脊髄の動脈

左前上面

① □ 後脊髄動脈　　　　　　　□ Posterior spinal arteries

② □ 血管冠　　　　　　　　　□ Vasocorona

③ □ 後髄節動脈　　　　　　　□ Posterior segmental medullary artery

④ □ 前脊髄動脈　　　　　　　□ Anterior spinal artery

⑤ □ 溝動脈　　　　　　　　　□ Sulcal artery

⑥ □ 前角　　　　　　　　　　□ Anterior horn

⑦ □ 後角　　　　　　　　　　□ Posterior horn

脊髄への血流の75％は前脊髄動脈から供給される．この動脈は椎骨動脈の枝であるが、様々な高さで前髄節動脈と吻合する．

Venous Drainage of the Spinal Cord

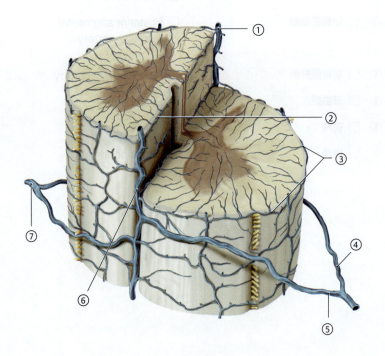

脊髄の血液は脊髄静脈を介してどの静脈に流入するのか？

脊髄の静脈流出路

左前上面

① □ 後脊髄静脈　　　□ Posterior spinal vein
② □ 溝静脈　　　　　□ Sulcal vein
③ □ 静脈輪　　　　　□ Venous ring
④ □ 後根静脈　　　　□ Posterior radicular vein
⑤ □ 前根静脈　　　　□ Anterior radicular vein
⑥ □ 前脊髄静脈　　　□ Anterior spinal vein
⑦ □ 脊髄静脈　　　　□ Spinal vein

・頸部：左右の深頸静脈
・胸郭領域：右では奇静脈，左では半奇静脈と副半奇静脈
・横隔膜下：左右の上行腰静脈

Sensory & Motor System

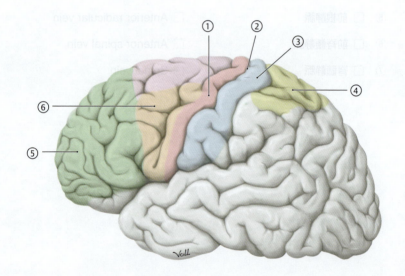

感覚系と運動系

左外側面

① □ 中心前回（一次運動野） □ Precentral gyrus（primary motor cortex）

② □ 中心溝 □ Central sulcus

③ □ 中心後回（一次体性感覚野） □ Postcentral gyrus（primary somatosensory cortex）

④ □ 後頭頂野 □ Posterior parietal cortex

⑤ □ 前頭前野 □ Prefrontal cortex

⑥ □ 運動前野 □ Premotor cortex

Visual System

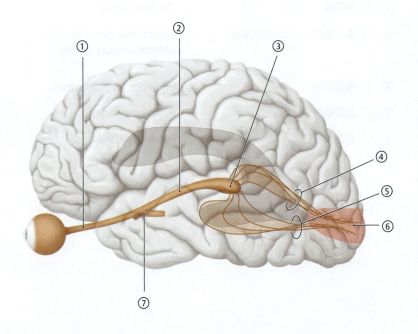

 視放線の線維のうち，視野の上半からの情報を伝達する線維はどの葉を通過するか？

視覚系

左外側面

① □ 視神経　　　　　　　　　□ Optic nerve（CN II）

② □ 視索　　　　　　　　　　□ Optic tract

③ □ 外側膝状体　　　　　　　□ Lateral geniculate body

④ □ 視放線（右視野の下半から　□ Optic radiation
　　の情報を伝える）　　　　　　（lower visual field）

⑤ □ 視放線（右視野の上半から　□ Optic radiation
　　の情報を伝える）　　　　　　（upper visual field）

⑥ □ 有線野　　　　　　　　　□ Striate area

⑦ □ 視交叉　　　　　　　　　□ Optic chiasm

　視野の上半からの情報は、視放線のうち下方の線維（側頭葉を通る線維、図の⑤）を通過する。さらに、各視放線は反対側の視野に関する情報を含む。
　したがって、ここで図示する左下の視放線が損傷されると、右上視野、いわゆる右上四分円が欠落する。

Autonomic Nervous System

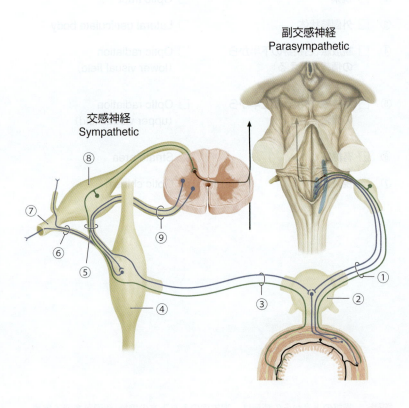

自律神経系

① □ 迷走神経　　　　　　　□ Vagus nerve (CN X)
② □ 椎前神経節　　　　　　□ Prevertebral ganglion
③ □ 内臓神経　　　　　　　□ Splanchnic nerve
④ □ 交感神経幹神経節　　　□ Sympathetic ganglion
⑤ □ 白交通枝　　　　　　　□ White ramus communicans
⑥ □ 灰白交通枝　　　　　　□ Gray ramus communicans
⑦ □ 前枝　　　　　　　　　□ Anterior ramus
⑧ □ 脊髄神経節　　　　　　□ Spinal ganglion
⑨ □ 前根　　　　　　　　　□ Anterior root

解説

　自律神経系は平滑筋，心筋，腺に分布しており，交感神経系と副交感神経系に区分される．この2つの神経系は，血流（血圧）や分泌，臓器機能を調節する際に拮抗的な作用を示すことが多い．

欧文索引

- 項目の主要掲載ページは太字で示す.
- 欧文中の a., aa. は artery, arteries を, br., brs. は branch, branches を, lig., ligs. は ligament, ligaments を, m., mm. は muscle, muscles を, n., nn. は nerve, nerves を, v., vv. は vein, veins を表す.

数字

1st
- distal phalanx　第1末節骨　445, 589
- dorsal interosseous　第1背側骨間筋　437, 443, **451**, 493, **627**
- lumbar v.　第1腰静脈　105
- lumbrical　第1虫様筋　**449**, 469
- metacarpal　第1中手骨　425, 429, 451
- metatarsal　第1中足骨　623, 627
- neuron　1次ニューロン　913
- palmar interosseous　第1掌側骨間筋　453
- perforating a.　第1貫通動脈　653
- proximal phalanx　第1基節骨　445, 591
- rib　第1肋骨　89, 93, 355, 383

2nd
- dorsal interosseous　第2背側骨間筋　451
- lumbrical　第2虫様筋　**449**, 469
- metacarpal　第2中手骨　425, 449, 453
- middle phalanx　第2中節骨　429, 449, 451, 453
- neuron　2次ニューロン　913
- palmar interosseous　第2掌側骨間筋　441, 453
- perforating a.　第2貫通動脈　653
- proximal phalanx　第2基節骨　449, 453
- rib　第2肋骨　815, 817

3rd
- dorsal interosseous　第3背側骨間筋　451
- lumbrical　第3虫様筋　449
- neuron　3次ニューロン　913
- occipital n.　第3後頭神経　73
- palmar interosseous　第3掌側骨間筋　441, 453
- plantar interosseous　第3底側骨間筋　627
- through 5th ribs　第3-5肋骨　383

4th
- distal phalanx　第4末節骨　419
- dorsal interosseous　第4背側骨間筋　451
- lumbrical　第4虫様筋　449

5th
- distal phalanx　第5末節骨　615
- metacarpal　第5中手骨　447
- metatarsal　第5中足骨　599
- middle phalanx　第5中節骨　615
- proximal phalanx　第5基節骨　615
- rib　第5肋骨　47, 55, 211, 217

10th rib　第10肋骨　99, 213
12th rib　第12肋骨　7, 99, 537

A

α-motor neuron　α運動ニューロン　919
Abdominal
- aorta　腹大動脈　307
- part
-- of pectoralis major　腹部《大胸筋の》363
-- of ureter　尿管の腹部　273
Abducent n.(CN VI)　外転神経　697, **745**, 751, 895
Abductor
- digiti minimi
-- 小指外転筋　437, **447**
-- 小趾外転筋　607, **619**
- hallucis　母趾外転筋　605, **617**, 657, 665
- pollicis
-- brevis　短母指外転筋　437, **445**

Abductor pollicis
— longus 長母指外転筋 413, **425**, 427, 443, 465, 501
— — tendon 長母指外転筋の腱 493
Accessory
− hemi-azygos v. 副半奇静脈 125
− n. (CN XI) 副神経 75, **713**, 731, 839, 895
− pancreatic duct 副膵管 271
Acetabular
− margin 寛骨臼縁 513
− roof 寛骨臼蓋 551
Acetabulum 寛骨臼 233, 509
Acromial
− end of clavicle 肩峰端《鎖骨の》 343
− facet 肩峰関節面 343
− part of deltoid 三角筋の肩峰部 391
Acromioclavicular
− joint 肩鎖関節 353
− lig. 肩鎖靱帯 353, 359
Acromion 肩峰 345, **347**, 357, 361, 377, 379, 381, 383, 385, 387, 389, 391, 397
Adductor
− brevis 短内転筋 523, 525, **549**, 637
− canal 内転筋管 629
− hallucis 母趾内転筋 621
− hiatus [内転筋]腱裂孔 525, 549, 631
− longus 長内転筋 523, **549**, 637, 671
− magnus 大内転筋 525, 527, 533, **547**, 549, 629, 637, 667
− pollicis 拇指内転筋 445
− − tendon 大内転筋の腱 631
− −, muscular insertion 大内転筋の筋性の停止部 643
− −, tendon of insertion 大内転筋の腱性の停止部 547
− minimus 小内転筋 547
− tubercle 内転筋結節 511
Ala of sacrum 仙骨翼 23, 199
Alveolar sac 肺胞嚢 187
Alveolus 肺胞 187
Ampulla 卵管膨大部 281
Amygdaloid body 扁桃体 889
Anal
− aperture 肛門裂孔 231
− columns 肛門柱 261
− pecten (white zone) 肛門櫛(白帯) 261

Anatomic snuffbox 解剖学的嗅ぎタバコ入れ 503
Anatomical neck of humerus 解剖頚《上腕骨の》 349
Anconeus 肘筋 **397**, 411
Angle
− of mandible 下顎角 779, 845
− of rib 肋骨角 83
Angular
− a. 眼角動脈 725
− gyrus 角回 873
− v. 眼角静脈 723, 725
Ankle joint 距腿関節 593, 595
Ankle mortise 足関節窩 559
Annular lig. of radius 橈骨輪状靱帯 401, 403
Anococcygeal lig. 肛門尾骨靱帯 227, 235
Ansa cervicalis 頚神経ワナ 843
Anterior
− arch of atlas (C1) 前弓《環椎(第1頚椎)の》 29
− articular facet of axis 前関節面《軸椎の》 15
− belly of digastric 顎二腹筋の前腹 799, 805, 807, 811, 813
− cerebral a. 前大脳動脈 865
− chamber of eyeball 前眼房 757
− circumflex humeral aa. 前上腕回旋動脈 455
− clinoid process 前床突起 685
− column 前柱 911
− commissure 前交連 883, 887, 913
− compartment of subtalar joint 距骨下関節, 前区(距踵舟関節) 597
− corticospinal tract 前皮質脊髄路 919, 923
− cranial fossa 前頭蓋窩 683
− cruciate lig. 前十字靱帯 567, 569
− cusp of right atrioventricular valve 前尖《右房室弁の》 149, 155
− cutaneous br. of spinal n. 前皮枝《脊髄神経の》 107
− ethmoidal a. 前篩骨動脈 765, 767
− external vertebral venous plexus 前外椎骨静脈叢 69
− funiculus of spinal cord 前索《脊髄の》 911

- horn of spinal cord　前角《脊髄の》　925
- inferior iliac spine　下前腸骨棘　201, 547, 551
- intercostal
-- brs. of internal thoracic a.　前肋間枝《内胸動脈の》　103
-- v.　前肋間静脈　69, 105
- intermuscular septum of leg　前下腿筋間中隔　659
- internal vertebral venous plexus　前内椎骨静脈叢　69
- internodal bundles　前結節間束　161
- interosseous
-- a.　前骨間動脈　491, 501
-- n.　前骨間神経　501
-- v.　前骨間静脈　501
- interventricular
-- br. of left coronary a.　前室間枝(前下行枝)　157
-- sulcus　前室間溝　145
- jugular v.　前頸静脈　721
- layer of rectus sheath　腹直筋鞘の前葉　207, 215, 221
- lobe of adenohypophysis　腺下垂体の前葉　883
- longitudinal lig.　前縦靱帯　31, **33**, 35, 201, 517
- median fissure　前正中裂　919
- mediastinum　前縦隔　119
- papillary m.　前乳頭筋　149, 153
- paracentral gyrus　前中心傍回　875
- radicular v.　前根静脈　927
- ramus/i
-- of lumbar nn.　前枝《腰神経の》　333
-- of spinal n.　前枝《脊髄神経の》　71, 909, 933
-- of thoracic aorta　前枝《胸大動脈の》　67
- root of spinal n.　前根《脊髄神経の》　909, 933
- rootlets　前根糸　909
- sacral foramina　前仙骨孔　23
- sacro-iliac lig.　前仙腸靱帯　201, 517
- septal brs.　中隔前鼻枝　765
- spinal
-- a.　前脊髄動脈　865, 925
-- v.　前脊髄静脈　927

- spinocerebellar tract　前脊髄小脳路　917, 921
- spinothalamic tract　前脊髄視床路　913, 921
- sternoclavicular lig.　前胸鎖靱帯　353, 355
- superior
-- alveolar aa.　前上歯槽動脈　719
-- iliac spine　上前腸骨棘　**197**, 207, 211, 213, 215, 337, 509, 513, 535, 541, 547, 551, 649
-- segmental a. of kidney　上前区動脈《腎臓の》　305
- talofibular lig.　前距腓靱帯　601
- thalamic nuclei　視床前核群　891
- tibial
-- a.　前脛骨動脈　**629**, 631, 661, 663, 669
-- v.　前脛骨静脈　661, 669
- tibiofibular lig.　前脛腓靱帯　601
- tubercle of atlas　前結節《環椎(第1頸椎)の》　13
- vagal trunk　前迷走神経幹　129, 331
- (ventral) ramus (intercostal n.)　前枝《肋間神経の》　107
Antihelix　対輪　771
Anulus fibrosus of intervertebral disk　線維輪《椎間円板の》　33
Aorta　大動脈　101
Aortic
- arch　大動脈弓　**123**, 133, 143, 165, 167
- hiatus of diaphragm　大動脈裂孔《横隔膜の》　97, 99
- knob　大動脈隆起　165
- valve　大動脈弁　155
Aorticorenal ganglia　大動脈腎動脈神経節　331
Apex
- of heart　心尖　143, 167
- of lung　肺尖　177, 179, 181
- of sacrum　仙骨尖　23
Apical axillary node　上腋窩リンパ節　115
Arachnoid
- granulations　クモ膜顆粒　855, 861
- villi　クモ膜絨毛　855
Arcuate
- a.　弓状動脈《足背動脈の》　663

Arcuate
- a. of kidney 弓状動脈《腎臓の》 305
- line 弓状線 197, 215
Arm 上腕 341
Articular
- br. of spinal n. 関節枝《脊髄神経の》 71
- disc
-- of distal radio-ulnar joint 関節円板《下橈尺関節の》 433
-- of sternoclavicular joint 関節円板《胸鎖関節の》 355
-- of temporomandibular joint 関節円板《顎関節の》 693
Ary-epiglottic fold 披裂喉頭蓋ヒダ 829
Ascending
- aorta 上行大動脈 121, **123**, 139, 141, 145, 165, 189
- br. of lateral circumflex femoral a. 外側大腿回旋動脈の上行枝 651
- colon 上行結腸 239, 245, 257
- lumbar v. 上行腰静脈 315
- part of trapezius 僧帽筋の上行部 371, 377
- pharyngeal a. 上行咽頭動脈 819
Atlanto-occipital joint 環椎後頭関節 27
Atlantoaxial joint 環軸関節 27
Atlas (C1) 環椎 (第1頸椎) **5**, 29, 41, 57, 63, 89, 385, 815, 817
Atrioventricular
- bundle 房室束 161
- node 房室結節 161
Auricular surface of sacrum 耳状面《仙骨の》 25
Auriculotemporal n. 耳介側頭神経 701, 727, **737**, 781
Axillary
- a. 腋窩動脈 113, 459, 463, **479**
- lymphatic plexus 腋窩リンパ叢 115
- n. 腋窩神経 459, **463**, 473, 475, 481
- recess 腋窩陥凹 359
- v. 腋窩静脈 113, 479
Axis (C2) 軸椎 (第2頸椎) **5**, 11, 29, 41, 57, 63, 89, 385
- of abduction 外転軸 539
- of adduction 内転軸 539

Axon
- of 1st neuron 1次ニューロンの軸索 915
- of 2nd neuron 2次ニューロンの軸索 915
- of 3rd neuron 3次ニューロンの軸索 915
Azygos v. 奇静脈 69, 111, **125**, 127, 135, 315

B

Bare area (diaphragmatic surface of liver) 無漿膜野 (横隔面) 263
Base
- of 1st distal phalanx 底《第1末節骨の》 419, 427
- of 1st metacarpal 底《第1中手骨の》 425
- of 1st metatarsal 底《第1中足骨の》 589
- of 1st proximal phalanx 底《第1基節骨の》 427
- of 2nd distal phalanx 底《第2末節骨の》 449
- of 2nd metacarpal 底《第2中手骨の》 417, 421
- of 3rd metacarpal 底《第3中手骨の》 421, 445
- of 5th metacarpal 底《第5中手骨の》 417, 423
- of 5th proximal phalanx 底《第5基節骨の》 423, 447
- of metacarpal 底《中手骨の》 431
Basilar a. 脳底動脈 865
Basilic v. 尺側皮静脈 457
Biceps
- brachii 上腕二頭筋 363, **395**, 405, 467, 483
-- tendon of insertion 上腕二頭筋の停止腱 395
- femoris 大腿二頭筋 **555**, 655
-- tendon 大腿二頭筋の腱 573, 575
Bicipital aponeurosis 上腕二頭筋腱膜 367, 395
Bile duct 総胆管 245, 265, 267, 269
Bochdalek's triangle ボクダレク三角 97

Body
- of bladder　膀胱体　299
- of epididymis　精巣上体体　293
- of fornix　脳弓体　881
- of pancreas　膵体　245, 271
- of sternum　胸骨体　85, 93, 167

Brachial
- a.　上腕動脈　455, 481, **483**, 485, 499
- plexus　腕神経叢　**479**, 837
- v.　上腕静脈　499

Brachialis　上腕筋　369, **395**, 407, 467, 499

Brachiocephalic trunk　腕頭動脈　143, 147

Brachioradialis　腕橈骨筋　405, **421**, 485, 501
- tendon of insertion　腕橈骨筋の停止腱　421

Brain stem　脳幹　919

Bridging v.　架橋静脈　857

Bronchiole　細気管支　185

Bronchomediastinal trunk　気管支縦隔リンパ本幹　127

Bronchopulmonary node　気管支肺リンパ節　191

Brs.
- of right pulmonary a.　右肺動脈の枝　179
- of right pulmonary vv.　右肺静脈の枝　179

Buccal
- a.　頬動脈　719, 733
- brs.　頬筋枝　703
- - of facial n.　頬筋枝《顔面神経の》　729
- n.　頬神経　701, 733, 781

Buccinator　頬筋　795, 799

Bulb
- of penis　尿道球　291
- of vestibule　前庭球　285

Bulbo-urethral gland　尿道球腺　297, 301

Bulbospongiosus　球海綿体筋　225, **235**, 285, 291, 301

C

C1-C4 transverse processes　第1-4頸椎の横突起　385

C1-C7 vertebrae　第1-7頸椎　3

C7 (vertebra prominens)　第7頸椎（隆椎）　5, 7, 11, 51, 53, 55, 57, 59, 61, 89
- spinal n.　第7頸神経　459
- spinous process　第7頸椎の棘突起　377, 385

Calcaneal
- (Achilles') tendon　踵骨腱（アキレス腱）　573, 575, 585, 657
- tuberosity　踵骨隆起　585, 605, 617, 619, 623

Calcaneofibular lig.　踵腓靱帯　603

Calcaneus　踵骨　575, 583, 591, 597, 615

Calcarine sulcus　鳥距溝　875

Capitate　有頭骨　431, 445

Capitulum of humerus　上腕骨小頭　349, 403

Cardia　噴門　253

Cardiac
- impression　心圧痕　181
- plexus　心臓神経叢　163

Carotid
- br.　頸動脈洞枝　709
- canal　頸動脈管　681
- sinus　頸動脈洞　709
- triangle　頸動脈三角　835

Carpal bones　手根骨　341

Cartilaginous part of pharyngotympanic tube　軟骨部《耳管の》　773

Cauda equina　馬尾　905

Caudate
- lobe of liver　尾状葉《肝臓の》　265
- nucleus　尾状核　887, 891

Caval opening of diaphragm　大静脈孔《横隔膜の》　95, 97, 99

Cavernous sinus　海綿静脈洞　723, 747, 869

Cecum　盲腸　257

Celiac
- ganglion　腹腔神経節　331
- node　腹腔リンパ節　329
- trunk　腹腔動脈　237, 269, 303, **309**, 321

Cell body
- of 1st neuron　1次ニューロンの細胞体　917

Cell body of 2nd neuron　2次ニューロンの細胞体　917
Central
 - axillary nodes　中心腋窩リンパ節　115
 - canal　中心管　863
 - sulcus　中心溝　849, 871, 873, 875, 929
 - tendon of diaphragm　腱中心《横隔膜の》　95, 99
Cephalic v.　橈側皮静脈　457, 477
Cerebellomedullary cistern　小脳延髄槽　861
Cerebellum　小脳　849, 851, 853, 893
Cerebral
 - aqueduct　中脳水道　863, 893, 899
 - arcuate fibers (U fibers)　大脳弓状線維　879
 - br.　頬枝《顔面神経の》　703
 - canal　子宮頸管　281
 - cardiac brs.　頸心臓枝《迷走神経の》　711
 - enlargement　頸膨大　905
 - peduncle　大脳脚　879, 895, 899
 - pleura　胸膜頂　175
 - plexus　頸神経叢　729
Cervix of uterus　子宮頸　275
Choana　後鼻孔　759
Chorda tympani　鼓索神経　705, 775
Choroid
 - line　脈絡ヒモ　885
 - plexus　脈絡叢　883, 901
 -- (third ventricle)　第3脳室脈絡叢　861
 -- (fourth ventricle)　第4脳室脈絡叢　861
Ciliary
 - body　毛様体　757
 - ganglion　毛様体神経節　699, 745
 - m.　毛様体筋　757
Cingulate
 - gyrus　帯状回　875
 - sulcus　帯状溝　875
Circumflex
 - br. of left coronary a.　回旋枝《左冠状動脈の》　157, 159
 - scapular a.　肩甲回旋動脈　475, 481
Cisterna
 - chyli　乳ビ槽　127, 329
 - magna　大槽　861

Clavicle　鎖骨　**343**, 355, 357, 379, 383, 385, 387, 391
Clavicular
 - head
 -- of pectoralis major　大胸筋の鎖骨部　387, 477
 -- of sternocleidomastoid　鎖骨頭《胸鎖乳突筋の》　379, 845
 - notch　鎖骨切痕　81, 85
 - part
 -- of deltoid　鎖骨部《三角筋の》　391
 -- of pectoralis major　鎖骨部《大胸筋の》　363
Clavipectoral fascia　鎖骨胸筋筋膜　477
Clitoris　陰核　283
Clivus　斜台　685
Coccygeus　尾骨筋　227, 229
Coccyx　尾骨　3, 25, 233, 235
Cochlea　蝸牛　707, 769, 777
Cochlear n. (CN VIII)　蝸牛神経　707
Collateral sulcus　側副溝　877
Common
 - carotid a.　総頸動脈　103, 803, **819**, 837
 - fibular n.　総腓骨神経　633, **641**, 655, 659
 - head
 -- of carpi ulnaris　共通頭《尺側手根伸筋の》　423
 -- of digiti minimi　共通頭《小指伸筋の》　423
 -- of extensor digitorum　共通頭《[総]指伸筋の》　423
 -- of flexors　共通頭《前腕屈筋の》　405, 415, 417
 -- of semitendinosus　共通頭《半腱様筋の》　555
 - hepatic
 -- a.　総肝動脈　269, 309
 -- duct　総肝管　267
 - iliac
 -- node　総腸骨リンパ節　329
 -- v.　総腸骨静脈　315
 - palmar digital aa.　総掌側指動脈　489
 - tendinous ring　総腱輪　743
Concha of auricle　耳甲介　771
Condylar process　関節突起　779

Confluence of sinuses 静脈洞交会 859, 861, 867
Conoid tubercle 円錐靱帯結節 343
Conus
 -arteriosus 動脈円錐 149
 -medullaris of spinal cord 脊髄円錐 905
Cooper's (suspensory) ligs. of breast クーパー靱帯（乳房提靱帯） 117
Coraco-acromial lig. 烏口肩峰靱帯 353, 359
Coracobrachialis 烏口腕筋 369, **387**, 467
Coracoclavicular lig. 烏口鎖骨靱帯 359
Coracoid process 烏口突起 345, 357, 365, 381, 383, 387, 389, 395, 397
Cornea 角膜 757
Corona
 -of glans 亀頭冠 291
 -radiata 放線冠 879
Coronal suture 冠状縫合 675
Coronary
 -lig. 肝冠状間膜 263
 -sinus 冠状静脈洞 147, 159
Coronoid
 -fossa 鈎突窩《上腕骨の》 403
 -process 筋突起 691, 731, 779, 809
 -process of ulna 鈎状突起《尺骨の》 399, 419
Corpus
 -callosum 脳梁 853, 871, 875, 879, 881, 887
 -cavernosum penis 陰茎海綿体 289, 291, 299
 -spongiosum penis 尿道海綿体 291
Corticonuclear fibers 皮質核線維 919
Corticospinal fibers 皮質脊髄線維 919
Costal
 -cartilage 肋軟骨 81, 83, 87, 93, 355
 -groove 肋骨溝 109
 -margin (arch) 肋骨弓 81
 -part 肋骨部（肋骨胸膜） 175
 --of diaphragm 横隔膜の肋骨部 95, 99
 --of parietal pleura 壁側胸膜の肋骨部（肋骨胸膜） 111
 --of parietal pleura 肋骨胸膜→壁側胸膜の肋骨部 111

-process/es 肋骨突起 35, 49, 53, 55, 59, 61, 99
-surface of scapula, 肩甲骨の肋骨面 395
Costoclavicular lig. 肋鎖靱帯 355
Costodiaphragmatic recess 肋骨横隔洞 109, 177
Cranial root 延髄根 713
Cremaster 精巣挙筋 293, 295
Cremasteric (cremaster) fascia 精巣挙筋膜 293, 295
Crest of greater tubercle of humerus 大結節稜《上腕骨の》 387
Cribriform plate 篩板 685, 695, 763
Cricoid cartilage 輪状軟骨 183, 827, 829
Cricothyroid 輪状甲状筋 711, 799, 831
 -lig. 輪状甲状靱帯 827
Crista
 -galli 鶏冠 761
 -terminalis 分界稜 151
Crural chiasm 下腿交叉 587
Crus
 -of fornix 脳弓脚 881
 -of penis 陰茎脚 291
Cuboid 立方骨 589, 599
Cuneate
 -fasciculus 楔状束 897, 915, 921
 -nucleus 楔状束核 897, 915
 -tubercle 楔状束結節 897
Cuneus 楔部 875
Cutaneous br.
 -of deep fibular n. 皮枝《深腓骨神経の》 663
 -of obturator n. 皮枝《閉鎖神経の》 637
Cymba conchae 耳甲介舟 771
Cystic duct 胆嚢管 267, 269

D

Decussation of pyramids 錐体交叉 919
Deep
 -a.
 --of arm 上腕深動脈 455, 475
 --of thigh 大腿深動脈 629, 651, 667
 -br.
 --of radial n. 深枝《橈骨神経の》 485
 --of ulnar n. 深枝《尺骨神経の》 471

Deep
- cervical a. 深頸動脈 73
- dorsal v. of penis 深陰茎背静脈 289
- fibular n. 深腓骨神経 **645**, 659, 661, 669
- flexors 深層の屈筋群 643
- inguinal node 深鼡径リンパ節 329
- lingual a. 舌深動脈 789
- palmar arch 深掌動脈弓 491
- part
-- of external anal sphincter 深部《外肛門括約筋の》 261
-- of masseter 咬筋の深部 **689**, 693
- penile a. 陰茎深動脈 289
- petrosal n. 深錐体神経 739
- plantar arch 深足底動脈弓 665
- temporal
-- aa. 深側頭動脈 719, 733
-- nn. 深側頭神経 733
-- vv. 深側頭静脈 721
- transverse
-- metacarpal lig. 深横中手靱帯 437
-- perineal m. 深会陰横筋 229, **233**, 285
- v. of thigh 大腿深静脈 667
Deltoid 三角筋 361, 363, 369, 371, **391**, 463, 477
- lig. 三角靱帯 603
- tuberosity of humerus 三角筋粗面《上腕骨の》 349, 391
Dens of axis(C2) 歯突起《軸椎(第 2 頸椎)の》 15, 29, 791
Dentate
- gyrus 歯状回 875, 881
- nucleus 歯状核 903
Depressor anguli oris 口角下制筋 687
Descending
- a. 後下行枝 159
- aorta 下行大動脈 121, 137, 169
- colon 下行結腸 251
- palatine a. 下行口蓋動脈 767
- part
-- of duodenum 十二指腸の下行部 255
-- of trapezius 僧帽筋の下行部 371, 377, 473
- v. 中心臓静脈 159
Detrusor 排尿筋 277

Diaphragm 横隔膜 **95**, **99**, 109, 119, 135
- leaflet 横隔膜円蓋 167
Diaphragmatic part of parietal pleura 横隔胸膜(壁側胸膜の横隔部) 109, 175
Diencephalon 間脳 853, 893
Digastric 顎二腹筋 807
Diploe of cranial bone 板間層 857
Distal
- interphalangeal joint 遠位指節間(DIP)関節 433
- radio-ulnar joint 下橈尺関節 433
- wrist crease 遠位手根線 503
Dorsal
- a. of penis 陰茎背動脈 289
- br.
-- of ulnar n. 背側枝《尺骨神経の》 497
-- of palmar digital nn. 背側枝《掌側指神経の》 497
- clitoral
-- a. 陰核背動脈 287
-- n. 陰核背神経 287
- digital
-- expansion 指背腱膜 411, 423
-- n. 背側指神経 497
- interossei of foot 背側骨間筋《足の》 611
- metatarsal aa. 背側中足動脈 663
- n. of penis 陰茎背神経 289, 301, 335
- pedal a. 足背動脈 629, 663
- root of spinal n. 後根《脊髄神経の》 107, 907
- tarsal ligs. 背側足根靱帯 601
- tubercle of radius 背側結節《橈骨の》 411, 425, 427
- venous network of hand 手背静脈網《手の》 457
Dorsum sellae 鞍背 683
Ductus
- arteriosus 動脈管 171
- deferens 精管 273, 297, 327
- venosus 静脈管 171
Duodenojejunal flexure 十二指腸空腸曲 243
Duodenum 十二指腸 253, **255**, 313
Dura mater 硬膜 855, 857

E

Ejaculatory duct　射精管　299
Emboliform nucleus　栓状核　903
Emissary v.　導出静脈　857
Endothoracic fascia　胸内筋膜　109，111
Epiglottis　喉頭蓋　783，791，827，**829**，833
Esophageal
- hiatus of diaphragm　食道裂孔《横隔膜の》　95，97，99
- plexus　食道神経叢　129
- vv.　食道静脈　319

Esophagus　食道　101，111，123，**133**，135，169，253，801，831
Ethmoid bulla　篩骨胞　763
Exclusive area of median n.　固有領域《正中神経の》　497
Extensor
- carpi
-- radialis
--- brevis　短橈側手根伸筋　413，**421**，501
--- longus　長橈側手根伸筋　411，413，**421**，501
---- tendon　長橈側手根伸筋の腱　443
-- ulnaris　尺側手根伸筋　411，**423**，443，501
- digiti
-- minimi　小指伸筋　**423**，501
- digitorum　［総］指伸筋　411，**423**，443，501
-- brevis　短趾伸筋　613，**615**
--- tendons　短趾伸筋の腱　615
-- longus　長趾伸筋　571，**581**，613，641，661
--- tendons　長趾伸筋の腱　581
-- tendon　［総］指伸筋の腱　411，465
- hallucis
-- brevis　短母趾伸筋　571，615
--- tendon　短母趾伸筋の腱　615，663
-- longus　長母趾伸筋　571，581，613
--- tendon　長母趾伸筋の腱　581，663，671
- indicis　示指伸筋　413，**427**
-- tendon　示指伸筋の腱　443
- pollicis
-- brevis　短母指伸筋　**427**，501
--- tendon　短母指伸筋の腱　493
-- longus　長母指伸筋　413，**427**，501
--- tendon　長母指伸筋の腱　443，493，503
- retinaculum of hand　伸筋支帯《手の》　443

External
- acoustic
-- meatus　外耳道　769，771
-- opening　外耳孔　689
- anal sphincter　外肛門括約筋　225，**235**，247，261
- br.
-- of accessory n.(CN XI)　外枝《副神経の》　843
-- of superior laryngeal n.　外枝《上喉頭神経の》　711，831
- carotid a.　外頸動脈　717
- iliac
-- a.　外腸骨動脈　259，629
-- node　外腸骨リンパ節　329
-- v.　外腸骨静脈　259
- intercostal mm.　外肋間筋　45，87，**91**，109，207
- jugular v.　外頸静脈　477，**721**，727，841
- oblique　外腹斜筋　77，205，**211**，337
-- aponeurosis　外腹斜筋腱膜　205，**211**，221，223，647
- occipital protuberance　外後頭隆起　377，679，867
- os of uterus　外子宮口　281
- spermatic fascia　外精筋膜　295
- urethral
-- orifice　外尿道口　283
-- sphincter　外尿道括約筋　235
- vertebral venous plexus　外椎骨静脈叢　867

F

Facet for dens　歯突起窩　13
Facial
- a.　顔面動脈　**717**，725，731，795，843
- n.(CN VII)　顔面神経　703，**705**，729，775，777，787

Facial v. 顔面静脈 **723**, 725, 731, 795, 843
Falciform lig. 肝鎌状間膜 263
Falx cerebri 大脳鎌 857, 859
Fascia lata 大腿筋膜 223
Fasciolar gyrus 小帯回 875
Fastigial nucleus 室頂核 903
Femoral
 - a. 大腿動脈 221, 303, 327, **629**, 647, 651, 667
 - n. 大腿神経 221, 633, 635, **639**, 645, 647, 651
 - v. 大腿静脈 221, 303, 327, 647, **651**, 667
Femoropatellar joint 膝蓋大腿関節 565
Femur 大腿骨 507, 547
Fibrous pericardium 線維性心膜 131, 133, 175
Fibula 腓骨 507, 539, 555, 557
Fibular
 - a. 腓骨動脈 631, 655, 669
 - v. 腓骨静脈 669
Fibularis
 - brevis 短腓骨筋 573, **583**, 669
 -- tendon 短腓骨筋の腱 583
 - longus 長腓骨筋 573, **583**, 641, 659
 -- tendon 長腓骨筋の腱 577, 583, 611, 619, 623, 625
 - tertius 第3腓骨筋 573, **583**
Flexor
 - carpi
 -- radialis 橈側手根屈筋 405, **417**, 469, 501
 --- tendon 橈側手根屈筋の腱 487
 -- ulnaris 尺側手根屈筋 405, 411, **417**, 435, 471, 501
 - digiti minimi brevis
 -- 短小指屈筋 439, **447**
 -- 短小趾屈筋 607, 619
 - digitorum
 -- brevis 短趾屈筋 607, **623**, 625, 627
 -- longus 長趾屈筋 579, **587**, 625, 655, 657
 --- tendon 長趾屈筋の腱 577, 587, 609, 623, 625
 -- profundus 深指屈筋 409, **419**, 439, 469, 471, 501
 --- tendons 深指屈筋の腱 407, 441, 449, 487
 -- superficialis 浅指屈筋 407, **417**, 469, 501
 --- tendons 浅指屈筋の腱 441, 487
 - hallucis
 -- brevis 短母趾屈筋 617
 -- longus 長母趾屈筋 579, **587**
 --- tendon 長母趾屈筋の腱 575, 587, 607
 - pollicis
 -- longus 長母指屈筋 409, **419**, 469, 501
 --- tendon 長母指屈筋の腱 407, 439, 487
 - retinaculum 屈筋支帯 435, **437**, 487, 489, 657
Foramen
 - cecum of tongue 舌盲孔 783
 - magnum 大後頭孔 681, 683
 - ovale 卵円孔 171, 173, **681**, 685, 737
 - transversarium 横突孔 11, 15, 17
Forearm 前腕 341
Fornix 脳弓 853, 871, 883, 889
Fourth ventricle 第4脳室 853, 863, 893, 901
Frenulum of upper lip 上唇小帯 793
Frontal
 - bone 前頭骨 675, 677, 689
 - lobe 前頭葉 849, 851, 871
 - n. 前頭神経 699, 745, 749
 - pole 前頭極 873
 - process of maxilla 前頭突起《上顎骨の》 761
 - sinus 前頭洞 685, 695, 741
Frontotemporal fasciculus 前頭側頭束 879
Fundus
 - of gallbladder 胆嚢底 267
 - of stomach 胃底 253
 - of uterine 子宮底 275, 279

G

Galea aponeurotica(epicranial aponeurosis) 帽状腱膜 687
Gallbladder 胆嚢 251, 265, 269

(Head of humerus) *945*

Ganglion of sympathetic trunk　幹神経節　909
Gastrocnemius　腓腹筋　**585**, 643, 671
Gastrocolic lig.　胃結腸間膜　241
Gastroduodenal a.　胃十二指腸動脈　309
Gastrosplenic lig.　胃脾間膜　241
Gemellus
 – inferior　下双子筋　541, 543, **545**
 – superior　上双子筋　541, 543, **545**
Geniculate ganglion　膝神経節　705, 777
Genioglossus　オトガイ舌筋　785, 791
Geniohyoid　オトガイ舌骨筋　785, 797, **809**
Glans
 – of clitoris　陰核亀頭　285
 – penis　陰茎亀頭　291, 293
Glenohumeral joint　肩関節(肩甲上腕関節)　353
Glenoid cavity of scapula　関節窩《肩甲骨の》　345, 357, 361, 381
Globose nuclei　球状核　903
Glossopharyngeal n.(CN IX)　舌咽神経　709, 787
Gluteal
 – surface of ilium　殿筋面《腸骨の》　543, 545
 – tuberosity of femur　殿筋粗面《大腿骨の》　541
Gluteus
 – maximus　大殿筋　77, 225, 529, 533, 535, **539**
 – medius　中殿筋　77, 529, 533, 535, 539, **541**
 – minimus　小殿筋　531, **543**, 545, 653
Gracile
 – fasciculus　薄束　897, 915, 921
 – nucleus　薄束核　897, 915
 – tubercle　薄束結節　897
Gracilis　薄筋　525, 527, 533, **549**, 637
 – tendon of insertion　薄筋の停止腱　549
Gray ramus communicans　灰白交通枝　333, 909, 933
Great
 – auricular n.　大耳介神経　73, 715, 727, **821**, 841
 – cardiac v.　大心臓静脈　157, 159
 – saphenous v.　大伏在静脈　645

Greater
 – curvature　大弯《胃の》　253
 – horn of hyoid bone　大角《舌骨の》　801
 – occipital n.　大後頭神経　73, 715, 727
 – omentum　大網　237, 239
 – palatine
 – – a.　大口蓋動脈　767
 – – n.　大口蓋神経　739, 767
 – petrosal
 – – n.　大錐体神経　705, 739, 777
 – sciatic
 – – foramen　大坐骨孔　203
 – – notch　大坐骨切痕　509
 – splanchnic n.　大内臓神経　135
 – trochanter of femur　大転子《大腿骨の》　511, 513, 515, 541, 543, 545, 549, 551, 553, 557
 – tubercle of humerus　大結節《上腕骨の》　351, 357, 387, 389, 397
 – wing of sphenoid　大翼《蝶形骨の》　675, 741
Groove
 – for fibularis longus tendon　長腓骨筋腱溝　591
 – for sigmoid sinus　S状洞溝　685
 – for spinal n.　脊髄神経溝　11
 – for subclavius　鎖骨下筋溝　343
 – for transverse sinus　横洞溝　685
 – for vertebral a.　椎骨動脈溝　13
Gyrus rectus　直回　877

H

Habenula　手綱　885
Hamate　有鈎骨　429, 447
Hard palate　硬口蓋　793
Haustra of colon　結腸膨起　257
Head
 – of 1st metacarpal　頭《第1中手骨の》　445
 – of 1st metatarsal　頭《第1中足骨の》　589
 – of 2nd distal phalanx　頭《第2末節骨の》　449
 – of femur　大腿骨頭　511, 513
 – of fibula　腓骨頭　535, 557, 559, 581, 583, 585, 587, 641, 659
 – of humerus　上腕骨頭　351, 397

Head
- of mandible 下顎頭 809
---, articular surface 下顎頭, 関節面 693
- of metacarpal 頭《中手骨の》 431
- of pancreas 膵頭 271
- of radius 橈骨頭 399, 403
- of rib 肋骨頭 83
- of talus 距骨頭 589
Helix 耳輪 771
Hemi-azygos v. 半奇静脈 125, 137, 315
Hepatic
- a. proper 固有肝動脈 245, 265, 309
- portal v. 門脈 245, 265, 319, 321
- vv. 肝静脈 269, 315
Hepatoduodenal lig. 肝十二指腸間膜 245, 253
Hepatogastric lig. 肝胃間膜 237, 253
Hepatopancreatic duct 胆膵管 269
Hilum of lung 肺門 181
Hippocampus 海馬 881
Hook of hamate 有鈎骨鈎 417, 419, 431, 447, 449
Horizontal
- fissure
-- of cerebellum 水平裂《小脳の》 901
-- of right lung 水平裂《右肺の》 167, 179
- part of duodenum 水平部《十二指腸の》 245, 255
- plate of palatine bone 水平板《口蓋骨の》 759
Humeral head of pronator teres 円回内筋の上腕頭 469
Humero-ulnar head of flexor digitorum superficialis 浅指屈筋の上腕尺骨頭 409
Humerus 上腕骨 341, 387, 393, 421, 499
Hyo-epiglottic lig. 舌骨喉頭蓋靱帯 829
Hyoglossus 舌骨舌筋 785
Hyoid bone 舌骨 379, **785**, 789, 791, 805, 809, 811, 813, 827, 833
Hypoglossal n.(CN XII) 舌下神経 731, **789**, 821, 843, 895
Hypophyseal fossa 下垂体窩 685, 761
Hypothalamus 視床下部 883
Hypothenar eminence 小指球 503

I

Ileal aa. 回腸動脈 311
Ileocecal orifice 回腸口 257
Ileocolic a. 回結腸動脈 311
Ileum 回腸 239, 243
Iliac
- crest 腸骨稜 7, 47, 49, 197, 219, 393, 509, 539, 541, 543, 545, 547
- fossa 腸骨窩 199, 217
- part
-- of latissimus dorsi 広背筋の腸骨部 393
-- of latissimus dorsi 腸骨部, 広背筋の 393
Iliacus 腸骨筋 219, 525, **537**
Ilio-inguinal n. 腸骨鼡径神経 633, 635
Iliococcygeal raphe 腸骨尾骨筋縫線 231
Iliococcygeus 腸骨尾骨筋 227, **231**
Iliocostalis 腸肋筋 43
- cervicis 頸腸肋筋 **47**, 49
- lumborum 腰腸肋筋 **47**, 49
- thoracis 胸腸肋筋 **47**, 49
Iliofemoral lig. 腸骨大腿靱帯 517, 519
Iliohypogastric n. 腸骨下腹神経 635
Iliolumbar lig. 腸腰靱帯 201, 517, 519
Iliopectineal arch 腸恥筋膜弓 537, 647
Iliopsoas 腸腰筋 219, 521, 537, 639
Iliotibial tract 腸脛靱帯 529, 535, 539, 659
Ilium 腸骨 393
Impression for costoclavicular lig. 肋鎖靱帯圧痕 343
Incisive canal 切歯管 759
Incus キヌタ骨 775
Inferior
- alveolar
-- a. 下歯槽動脈 719, 733
-- n. 下歯槽神経 701, 733, 781
- angle of scapula 下角《肩甲骨の》 347, 381, 385, 389
- articular
-- facet
--- of axis 下関節面《軸椎の》 15
--- of lumber vertebra 下関節面《腰椎の》 21

--- of thoracic vertebra 下関節面《胸椎の》 19
-- process 下関節突起 9
- belly of omohyoid 下腹《肩甲舌骨筋の》 805, 811, 813
- cerebellar peduncle 下小脳脚 897, 917
- colliculi of quadrigeminal plate 下丘《蓋板(四丘体板)の》 897
- constrictor 下咽頭収縮筋 799, 801, 831
- epigastric
-- a. 下腹壁動脈 327
-- v. 下腹壁静脈 327
- extensor retinaculum 下伸筋支帯 613
- frontal
-- gyrus 下前頭回 873
-- sulcus 下前頭溝 873
- head of lateral pterygoid 下頭《外側翼突筋の》 693
- horn of lateral ventricle 下角《側脳室の》 863
- lacrimal canaliculus 下涙小管 755
- lacrimal punctum 下涙点 755
- laryngeal n. 下喉頭神経 833
- lobar bronchi 下葉気管支 177
- lobe of left lung 下葉《左肺の》 169, 181
- mesenteric
-- a. 下腸間膜動脈 303, 313, 325
-- ganglion 下腸間膜動脈神経節 331
-- v. 下腸間膜静脈 319, 321, 325
- nasal
-- concha 下鼻甲介 755, 761
-- meatus 下鼻道 763
- nuchal line 下項線《頸神経ワナの》 63
- oblique 下斜筋 697
-- part of longus colli 下斜部《頸長筋の》 **815**, 817
- ophthalmic v. 下眼静脈 751
- orbital fissure 下眼窩裂 739, 741
- pancreaticoduodenal a. 下膵十二指腸動脈 309
- parietal lobule 下頭頂小葉 873
- part of serratus anterior 下部《前鋸筋の》 381
- pubic ramus 恥骨下肢 233, 235
- rectal
-- nn. 下直腸神経 287, 301, 335

-- plexus 下直腸動脈神経叢 335
-- rectus 下直筋 697
- root of ansa cervicalis 下根《頸神経ワナの》 821
- scapular angle 肩甲骨の下角 7
- tarsus 下瞼板 753
- temporal
-- gyrus 下側頭回 873, 877
-- sulcus 下側頭溝 873
- thoracic aperture 胸郭下口 81
- thyroid
-- a. 下甲状腺動脈 803, 831, 843
-- v. 下甲状腺静脈 131, 837
- tracheobronchial node 下気管気管支リンパ節 191
- ulnar collateral a. 下尺側側副動脈 483
- vena cava 下大静脈 101, 105, 111, 133, 141, 145, 159, 189, 245, 251, 265, 269, **307**, 321, 325
- vertebral notch 下椎切痕 21
Infra-orbital
- a. 眼窩下動脈 719, 725
- foramen 眼窩下孔 677, 701, 781
- n. 眼窩下神経 701, 725, **739**, 781
Infraglenoid tubercle 関節下結節 345, 397
Infrapatellar br. of saphenous n. 膝蓋下枝《伏在神経の》 639
Infrapiriform portion of greater sciatic foramen 大坐骨孔《梨状筋下孔の》 649
Infraspinatus 棘下筋 373, 375, **389**, 475
Infraspinous fossa 棘下窩 347
Infundibulum 卵管漏斗 281
Inguinal lig. 鼡径靱帯 **201**, 205, 211, 213, 215, 217, 221, 223, 647
Inner lip of iliac crest 内唇《腸骨稜の》 215
Innermost intercostal m. 最内肋間筋 87
Interatrial
- bundle 心房間束 161
- septum 心房中隔 151, 153
Intercondylar
- eminence of tibia 顆間隆起《脛骨の》 563
- notch of femur 顆間窩《大腿骨の》 511, 563

Intercostal n. 肋間神経 75, 109, 129
Interlobar a. 葉間動脈 305
Intermediate
 - cuneiform 中間楔状骨 615
 - part
 -- of cerebellum 中間部《小脳の》 903
 -- of serratus anterior 前鋸筋の中間部 381
 - zone of iliac crest 腸骨稜の中間線 213
Intermesenteric plexus 腸間膜動脈間神経叢 331
Internal
 - anal sphincter 内肛門括約筋 261
 - br. of superior laryngeal n. 内枝《上喉頭神経の》 831, 833
 - capsule 内包 879, 887, 919
 - carotid
 -- a. 内頸動脈 731, 745, 747, 773, 775, **819**, 843, 865
 -- plexus 内頸動脈神経叢 745
 - iliac
 -- a. 内腸骨動脈 327
 -- node 内腸骨リンパ節 329
 -- v. 内腸骨静脈 327
 - intercostal m. 内肋間筋 87, **91**, 93, 207
 - jugular v. 内頸静脈 105, 127, **721**, 723, 729, 803, 825, 837, 867
 - oblique 内腹斜筋 45, 207, **213**, 221, 223
 -- aponeurosis 内腹斜筋腱膜 213
 - os(at uterine isthmus) 内子宮口《子宮峡部の》 281
 - pudendal
 -- a. 内陰部動脈 259, 287, 301
 -- v. 内陰部静脈 259, 287, 301
 - spermatic fascia 内精筋膜 293, 295
 - thoracic
 -- a. 内胸動脈 103, 113, 131
 -- v. 内胸静脈 69, 105, 113, 131
Interneuron 介在ニューロン 919
Interossei of hand 骨間筋《手の》 471
 - membrane
 -- of forearm 前腕骨間膜 399, 419, 421, 501
 -- of leg 下腿骨間膜 539, 559, 583
 - talocalcanean lig. 骨間距踵靱帯 597
Interpeduncular fossa 脚間窩 899

Interspinales
 - cervicis 頸棘間筋 57
 - lumborum 腰棘間筋 57
Interspinous ligs. 棘間靱帯 33
Intertendinous connections of extensor digitorum 腱間結合《[総]指伸筋の》 423
Intertransversarii
 - lateralis lumborum 腰外側横突間筋 **53**, 55
 - mediales lumborum 腰外側横突間筋 **53**, 55
Intertransverse ligs. 横突間靱帯 35
Intertrochanteric
 - crest of femur 転子間稜《大腿骨の》 511, 541, 543, 545
 - line of femur 転子間線《大腿骨の》 553
Intertubercular
 - sulcus of humerus 結節間溝《上腕骨の》 349, 357, 387, 395
 - synovial sheath 結節間滑液鞘 359
Interureteral fold 尿管間ヒダ 277
Interventricular
 - foramen 室間孔 863
 - septum 心室中隔 161, 169
Intervertebral
 - disc 椎間円板 3, 5, 37
 - foramen 椎間孔 3, 37, 907
 - joint 椎体間関節 27
Intramural part of ureter 壁内部《尿管の》 277
Intraparietal sulcus 頭頂間溝 873
Iris 虹彩 757
Ischial
 - spine 坐骨棘 **197**, 199, 203, 227, 229, 235, 509, 515, 537, 543, 545
 - tuberosity 坐骨結節 197, 233, 509, **515**, 531, 541, 557
Ischio-anal fossa 坐骨肛門窩(坐骨直腸窩) 259
Ischiocavernosus 坐骨海綿体筋 225, **235**, 285, 291
Ischiofemoral lig. 坐骨大腿靱帯 519
Ischium 坐骨 555
 - of thyroid gland 甲状腺峡部 823
 - of uterine tube 卵管峡部 281

J・K

Jejunal aa. 空腸動脈 311
Joint capsule
　- of temporomandibular joint 関節包《顎関節の》 689, 691
　-, glenohumeral ligs. 関節包, 関節上腕靱帯 359
Jugular
　- foramen 頸静脈孔 681, 713, 869
　- notch 頸切痕 81, **85**, 193, 845
Kidney 腎臓 251

L

L1 第1腰椎 5, 251, 635
L1-L5 第1-5腰椎 3, 49
L3 第3腰椎 99
L4 第4腰椎 7, 637
L5 第5腰椎 237, 537, 905
Labium
　- majus 大陰唇 283
　- minus 小陰唇 283
Lacrimal
　- a. 涙腺動脈 749
　- caruncle 涙丘 755
　- gland 涙腺 749, 755
　- n. 涙腺神経 749
　- sac 涙嚢 755
Lactiferous
　- duct 乳管 117
　- sinus 乳管洞 117
Lambdoid suture ラムダ縫合 679
Lamina
　- affixa 付着板 885
　- of vertebral arch 椎弓板 9, **17**, 19, 35
Laryngeal prominence 喉頭隆起 827
Lateral
　- antebrachial cutaneous n. 外側前腕皮神経 467, 485
　- arcuate lig. 外側弓状靱帯 97
　- border of scapula 外側縁《肩甲骨の》 389, 393, 397
　- brs. of Supra-orbital n. 外側枝《眼窩上神経の》 725
　- cervical resion 外側頸三角部 835
　- collateral lig. of knee 外側側副靱帯《膝関節の》 565, 569
　- column of spinal cord 側柱《脊髄の》 911
　- condyle
　-- of femur 外側顆《大腿骨の》 511, 561, 563
　-- of tibia 外側顆《脛骨の》 581, 583
　- cord of brachial plexus 外側神経束《腕神経叢の》 459, 461, 467
　- corticospinal tract 外側皮質脊髄路 919, 923
　- crico-thyroid 外側輪状甲状筋 833
　- crus of superficial inguinal ring 外側脚《浅鼠径輪の》 647
　- cuneiform 外側楔状骨 589
　- cutaneous
　-- br.
　--- of spinal n. 外側皮枝《脊髄神経の》 107
　--- of thoracic aorta 外側皮枝《胸大動脈の》 67
　-- n. of thigh 外側大腿皮神経 635, **645**, 647, 651
　- epicondyle
　-- of femur 外側上顆《大腿骨の》 565, 585
　-- of humerus 外側上顆《上腕骨の》 351, 397, 421, 423, 425, 427
　- femoral intermuscular septum 外側大腿筋間中隔 667
　- funiculus of spinal cord 側索《脊髄の》 911
　- geniculate body 外側膝状体 885, 931
　- head
　-- of flexor hallucis brevis 外側頭《短母趾屈筋の》 611, 617
　-- of gastrocnemius 外側頭《腓腹筋の》 529, 573, 575, 585
　-- of triceps brachii 外側頭《上腕三頭筋の》 375, 397, 475, 499
　- intermuscular septum of arm 外側上腕筋間中隔 499
　- lig. 外側靱帯 689, 691
　- lip of linea aspera 外側唇《粗線の》 511
　- malleolus 外果 **559**, 573, 575, 583, 585, 595, 601

Lateral
- masses 外側塊《環椎(第1頸椎)の》 13
- meniscus 外側半月 567, 569
- occipitotemporal gyrus 外側後頭側頭回 875, 877
- part
-- of cerebellum 外側部《小脳の》《小脳の》 903
-- of vaginal fornix 外側部《腟円蓋の》 281
- patellar retinaculum 外側膝蓋支帯 551
- pectoral nn. 外側胸筋神経 477, 479
- plantar
-- a. 外側足底動脈 657, 665
-- n. 外側足底神経 633, 657, 665
-- v. 外側足底静脈 665
- plate of pterygoid process 外側板《翼状突起の》 681
- process of calcaneal tuberosity 外側突起《踵骨隆起の》 617, 619
- pterygoid 外側翼突筋 691, **693**, 733
- recess of fourth ventricle 第四脳室外側陥凹 897
- rectus 外側直筋 697, 743, 751
- segment of globus pallidus 外節《淡蒼球の》 889
- semicircular canal 外側骨半規管 769
- sesamoid 外側種子骨 617, 621
- spinothalamic tract 外側脊髄視床路 913, 921
- stria 外側嗅条 877, 887
- sulcus 外側溝 849, 871, 873
- supracondylar ridge of humerus 外側顆上稜《上腕骨の》 351
- sural cutaneous n. 外側腓腹皮神経 659
- surface of tibia 外側面《脛骨の》 583
- tarsal a. 外側足根動脈 663
- thoracic a. 外側胸動脈 113, 455, 481
- thoracic v. 外側胸静脈 113
- ventricle 側脳室 887
Latissimus dorsi 広背筋 39, 77, 367, 371, **393**, 483
Left
- anterior descending (anterior interventricular) a. 前下行枝(前室間枝) 157
- atrioventricular valve 左房室弁 153
- atrium 左心房 139, **147**, 153, 165, 169, 173
- auricle 左心耳 145
- brachiocephalic v. 左腕頭静脈 127, 143, 177, **721**
- bronchomediastinal trunk 左気管支縦隔リンパ本幹 191
- colic
-- a. 左結腸動脈 313
-- flexure 左結腸曲 257
- common carotid a. 左総頸動脈 123, 145
- coronary a. 左冠状動脈 157
- dome of diaphragm 左天蓋《横隔膜の》 99
- gastric
-- a. 左胃動脈 307, 321
-- v. 左胃静脈 319, 321
- gastro-omental
-- a. 左胃大網動脈 321
-- v. 左胃大網静脈 319, 321
- hypogastric n. 左下腹神経 335
- inferior
-- lobar bronchus 左下葉気管支 183
-- phrenic a. 左下横隔動脈 303, 317
-- rectal a. 左下直腸動脈 325
- internal
-- pudendal. 左内陰部動脈 323
-- pudendal v. 左内陰部静脈 323
- lateral aortic node 左外側大動脈リンパ節 329
- lobe of liver 肝臓の左葉 239
- lumbar trunk 左腰リンパ本幹 127
- main bronchus 左主気管支 121, 123, 137, **183**
- middle rectal a. 左中直腸動脈 325
- obturator a. 左閉鎖動脈 325
- ovarian
-- a. 左卵巣動脈 303, 317
-- v. 左卵巣静脈 317
- phrenic n. 左横隔神経 137
- pulmonary
-- a. 左肺動脈 137, 147
-- vv. 左肺静脈 133, 147
- recurrent laryngeal n. 左反回神経 129, 163, **711**, 803
- renal
-- a. 左腎動脈 303, 305, 317

(Lumbocostal enlargement)

- - v. 左腎静脈 311, 317
- semilunar cusp of aortic valve 左半月弁《大動脈弁の》 155
- subclavian
- - a. 左鎖骨下動脈 123, 129, 133, 819
- - v. 左鎖骨下静脈 133
- suprarenal v. 左副腎静脈 273, 317
- testicular
- - a. 左精巣動脈 317
- - v. 左精巣静脈 317
- vagus n. 左迷走神経 129, 137
- ventricle 左心室 143, **147**, 165

Lens 水晶体 757

Lesser
- curvature of stomach 小弯《胃の》 253
- occipital n. 小後頭神経 715, 821, 841
- omentum 小網 253
- palatine nn. 小口蓋神経 767
- petrosal n. 小錐体神経 737, 777
- sciatic foramen 小坐骨孔 203, 649
- trochanter of femur 小転子《大腿骨の》 219, 511, 513, 537, 541, 543, 545, 549, 553, 557
- tubercle of humerus 小結節《上腕骨の》 349, 357, 387
- wing of sphenoid 小翼《蝶形骨の》 683

Levator
- ani 肛門挙筋 225, 227, **231**, 249, 259, 285
- hiatus 挙筋門 231
- palpebrae superioris 上眼瞼挙筋 697, **743**, 749, 753
- scapulae 肩甲挙筋 39, 373, **385**
- veli palatini 口蓋帆挙筋 773

Levatores
- costarum 肋骨挙筋 45
- - breves 短肋骨挙筋 53, **55**
- - longi 長肋骨挙筋 53, **55**

Lig. of ovary 固有卵巣索 279

Ligamenta flava 黄色靱帯 33, 35

Ligamentum
- arteriosum 動脈管索 137, 141, 149, 173
- venosum 静脈管索 173

Limbic lobe 辺縁葉 871

Linea
- alba 白線 205, 211, 213, 215, 217, 219, 337
- aspera of femur 粗線《大腿骨の》 515

Lingual
- a. 舌動脈 717, 789, 797
- gyrus 舌状回 875, 877
- n.(CN V₃) 舌神経 701, 733, 737, 781, 787, **789**
- tonsil 舌扁桃 783

Lingula of lung 小舌《肺の》 181

Linia aspera of femur 粗線《大腿骨の》 555

Liver 肝臓 171, **263**, 265

Lobule of auricle 耳垂 771

Long
- ciliary nn. 長毛様体神経 745, 751
- head
- - of biceps brachii 長頭《上腕二頭筋の》 367, 369, 395, 499
- - of biceps femoris 長頭《大腿二頭筋の》 529, 535, 555, 557, 643
- - of triceps brachii 長頭《上腕三頭筋の》 371, 375, 397, 499
- plantar lig. 長足底靱帯 599, 619
- thoracic n. 長胸神経 461, 481

Longissimus 最長筋 43
- capitis 頭最長筋 47, **49**
- cervicis 頸最長筋 47, **49**
- thoracis 胸最長筋 47, **49**

Longitudinal cerebral fissure 大脳縦裂 877

Longus
- capitis 頭長筋 **815**, 817
- colli 頸長筋 **815**, 817

Lower
- leg 下腿 507
- trunk 下神経幹 461

Lumbar
- ganglia 腰神経節 333
- part of diaphragm 横隔膜の腰椎部 99
- splanchnic n. 腰内臓神経 333
- triangle, internal oblique 腰三角, 内腹斜筋 39
- vv. 腰静脈 125, 315

Lumbocostal
- enlargement 腰膨大 905

Lumbocostal
 −triangle 腰肋三角 97
 −trunk 腰仙骨神経幹 635
Lumbricals 虫様筋 439, 609
Lunate 月状骨 431, 447
 −sulcus 月状溝 873

M

Major
 −calyces 大腎杯 305
 −duodenal papilla 大十二指腸乳頭 255, 267
Malleus ツチ骨 769, 775
Mammillary
 −body 乳頭体 881, 891
 −process of lumbar vertebrae 乳頭突起《腰椎の》 21, 53, 55
Mandible 下顎骨 675
Mandibular
 −division of trigeminal n. 三叉神経, 下顎神経 715
 −foramen 下顎孔 779, 809
 −fossa 下顎窩 681
 −n.(CN V₃) 下顎神経 701, 735, **737**, 781
 −notch 下顎切痕 779
Manubrium of sternum 胸骨柄 85, 87, 93, 355
Marginal
 −a. 結腸辺縁動脈 311
 −mandibular br. of facial n. 下顎縁枝《顔面神経の》 703, 729
Masseter 咬筋 687, 691, 727, 735, 795
Mastoid process of temporal bone 乳様突起《側頭骨の》 49, 51, 679, 689
Maxilla 上顎骨 675, 677
Maxillary
 −a. 顎動脈 717, 719, 735
 −division of trigeminal n. 三叉神経, 上顎神経 715
 −hiatus 上顎洞裂孔 763
 −n.(CN V₂) 上顎神経 701, **739**, 781
 −sinus 上顎洞 741
 −v. 顎静脈 723

Medial
 −border
 −−of scapula 内側縁《肩甲骨の》 347, 373, 381, 385
 −brs.
 −−of spinal n. 内側枝《脊髄神経の》 71
 −−of supra-orbital n. 内側枝《眼窩上神経の》 725
 −circumflex femoral a. 内側大腿回旋動脈 629, 651
 −collateral lig. of knee 内側側副靱帯《膝関節の》 565, 567, 569
 −condyle
 −−of femur 内側顆《大腿骨の》 511, 561, 563
 −−of tibia 内側顆《脛骨の》 555, 559, 561, 563, 581
 −cord of brachial plexus 内側神経束《腕神経叢の》 459, 471
 −crus of superficial inguinal ring 内側脚《浅鼠径輪の》 647
 −cuneiform 内側楔状骨 **589**, 591, 597, 599, 615, 623
 −cutaneous br. of thoracic aorta 内側皮枝《胸大動脈の》 67
 −epicondyle
 −−of femur 内側上顆《大腿骨の》 511, 549, 561, 563, 585
 −−of humerus 内側上顆《上腕骨の》 **349**, 397, 401, 403, 405, 415, 417, 419, 421, 425, 427
 −geniculate body 内側膝状体 885
 −head
 −−of flexor hallucis brevis 内側頭《短母趾屈筋の》 611, 617
 −−of gastrocnemius 内側頭《腓腹筋の》 529, 575, 579, 585, 669
 −−of triceps brachii 内側頭《上腕三頭筋の》 375, 397, 499
 −intermuscular septum of arm 内側上腕筋間中隔 483, 499
 −lemniscus 内側毛帯 915
 −lip of linea aspera 内側唇《粗線の》 511
 −malleolus 内果 559, 571
 −meniscus 内側半月 565, 567
 −occipitotemporal gyrus 内側後頭側頭回 875, 877

- patellar retinaculum 内側膝蓋支帯 551
- pectoral nn. 内側胸筋神経 477, 479
- plantar
-- a. 内側足底動脈 657, 665
-- n. 内側足底神経 633, 657, 665
- plate of pterygoid process 内側板《翼状突起の》 681, 761
- process of calcaneal tuberosity 内側突起《踵骨隆起の》 617, 619
- pterygoid 内側翼突筋 693, 735
- rectus 内側直筋 697, 743
- segment of globus pallidus 内節《淡蒼球の》 889
- sesamoid 内側種子骨 617, 621
- stria 内側嗅条 877
- thalamic nuclei 視床内側核群 891

Median
- aperture 第四脳室正中口 861
- arcuate lig. 正中弓状靱帯 97
- cubital v. 肘正中皮静脈 457
- n. 正中神経 459, **469**, 483, 485, 487, 489, 497, 499, 501
- part of cerebellum 正中部《小脳の》 903
- sacral
-- a. 正中仙骨動脈 303
-- crest 正中仙骨稜 25
- umbilical fold 正中臍ヒダ 239

Mediastinal part of parietal pleura 縦隔胸膜（壁側胸膜の縦隔部） 131, 175
Medulla oblongata 延髄 849, 851, 853, 893
Meningeal br. of spinal n. 硬膜枝《脊髄神経の》 909
Mental foramen オトガイ孔 677, 701, 779
Mental n. オトガイ神経 701, 725
Mesencephalon 中脳 853, 893, 901
Mesentery 腸間膜 243
Mesometrium 子宮間膜 279
Mesosalpinx 卵管間膜 279
Metacarpals 中手骨 341
Metacarpophalangeal joint 中手指節（MCP）関節 433
Metatarsophalangeal joint 中足趾節関節 593
- capsules 中足趾節関節の関節包 617, 619, 621

Midcarpal joint 手根中央関節 433
Midclavicular line (MCL) 鎖骨中線 193
Middle
- cerebellar peduncle 中小脳脚 897
- cerebral a. 中大脳動脈 865
- cervical ganglion 中頸神経節 803
- cluneal nn. 中殿皮神経 75
- colic a. 中結腸動脈 311
- constrictor 中咽頭収縮筋 799, 801
- cranial fossa 中頭蓋窩 683, 747
- frontal gyrus 中前頭回 873
- internodal bundles 中結節間束 161
- lobe of right lung 中葉《右肺の》 179
- mediastinum 中縦隔 119
- meningeal a. 中硬膜動脈 735
- nasal meatus 中鼻道 761
- temporal gyri 中側頭回 873
- transverse rectal fold 中直腸横ヒダ 261

Minor duodenal papilla 小十二指腸乳頭 255
Mons pubis 恥丘 283
Motor
- cortex 大脳皮質運動野 919
- cranial n. nuclei 運動性脳神経核 919

Multifidus 多裂筋 59, **61**
Muscle 筋 919
Muscular
- coat of urinary bladder 筋層《膀胱の》 277
- triangle 筋三角 835

Musculocutaneous n. 筋皮神経 **467**, 485, 499
Musculophrenic a. 筋横隔動脈 103
Mylohyoid 顎舌骨筋 805, **809**, 811, 813
- br. of inferior alveolar a. 顎舌骨筋枝《下歯槽動脈の》 719
- line 顎舌骨筋線 809
- n. 顎舌骨筋神経 737
- raphe 顎舌骨筋縫線 811, 813

Myometrium 子宮筋層 281

N

N.
- of pterygoid canal 翼突管神経 739
- to tensor veli palatini 口蓋帆張筋神経 737

Nasal
- bone　鼻骨　677
- septum　鼻中隔　695
Nasion　鼻根点　677
Nasociliary n.　鼻毛様体神経　699, 751
Nasolacrimal duct　鼻涙管　755
Nasopalatine n.　鼻口蓋神経　765
Navicular　舟状骨《足の》　**589**, 591, 595, 597, 599, 615
Neck
- of bladder　膀胱頸　277
- of femur　大腿骨頸　511, 513
- of rib　肋骨頸　83
Nipple　乳頭　117
Nodule　小節　901
Nuchal lig.　項靱帯　29, 31, 377
Nucleus pulposus of intervertebral disk　髄核《椎間円板の》　33

O

Oblique
- fissure
  - - of left lung　斜裂《左肺の》　181
  - - of right lung　斜裂《右肺の》　167, 169, 179
- head
  - - of adductor hallucis　斜頭《母趾内転筋の》　611, 621
  - - of adductor pollicis　斜頭《母指内転筋の》　441, 445
- pericardial sinus　心膜斜洞　141
Obliquus capitis
- inferior　下頭斜筋　41, **63**, 73
- superior　上頭斜筋　41, **63**
Obliterated umbilical aa.(medial umbilical ligs.)　臍動脈の遺残(内側臍索)　173
Obturator
- canal　閉鎖管　227
- externus　外閉鎖筋　525, **547**, 637
- foramen　閉鎖孔　197, 509
- internus　内閉鎖筋　225, 231, 259, 527, 531, 541, 543, **545**
- - fascia　内閉鎖筋筋膜　229
- membrane　閉鎖膜　201, 203
- n.　閉鎖神経　635, 637, 651
Occipital
- a.　後頭動脈　73, 717
- bone　後頭骨　679
- condyle　後頭顆　681
- lobe　後頭葉　849, 871
- pole　後頭極　873
Occipitofrontalis, frontal belly　前頭筋(後頭前頭筋)　687
Occipitotemporal sulcus　後頭側頭溝　877
Oculomotor n.(CN III)　動眼神経　697, **745**, 747, 895, 899
Olecranon　肘頭　397, 399, 421, 423, 425, 427
- fossa of humerus　肘頭窩《上腕骨の》　351
Olfactory
- bulb(CN I)　嗅球　695, 767, 851, 877
- nn.　嗅神経糸　695, 765
- sulcus　嗅溝　877
- tract　嗅索　695, 851, 877
Olive　オリーブ　895, 901
Omental
- appendices　腹膜垂　257
- bursa　網嚢　251
- foramen　網嚢孔　241
Omoclavicular triangle　肩甲鎖骨三角　835
Omohyoid　肩甲舌骨筋　379, 805, 811, **813**
Opercular part of inferior frontal gyrus　弁蓋部《下前頭回の》　873
Ophthalmic
- division of trigeminal n.　三叉神経の眼神経　715
- n.(CN V₁)　眼神経　699, 745
Opponens
- digiti minimi
- - 小指対立筋　441, **447**
- - 小趾対立筋　619
- pollicis　母指対立筋　439, **445**
Optic
- canal　視神経管　685, 741
- chiasm(CN II)　視交叉　699, 747, 887, **931**
- disc　視神経乳頭(視神経円板)　757
- n.(CN II)　視神経　699, **745**, 747, 751, 757, 851, 931
- radiation　視放線　879, 931
- tract　視索　889, 931
Orbicularis
- oculi　眼輪筋　687

(Pelvic girdle) *955*

−oris 口輪筋 687
Orbital
 −gyri 眼窩回 877
 −part
 −− of inferior frontal gyrus 眼窩部《下前頭回の》 873
 −− of lacrimal gland 眼窩部《涙腺の》 755
 −plate of ethmoid bone 眼窩板《篩骨の》 741
 −septum 眼窩隔膜 753
 −sulci 眼窩溝 877
 −surface of zygomatic bone 眼窩面《頬骨の》 741
Orifices of posterior ethmoidal cells 開口部《後篩骨洞の》 763
Otic ganglion 耳神経節 737
Outer lip of iliac crest 腸骨稜の外唇 211
Oval fossa 卵円窩 151
Ovarian
 −a. 卵巣動脈 279
 −v. 卵巣静脈 279, 315
Ovary 卵巣 279

Palatine
 −bone 口蓋骨 681
 −process of maxilla 口蓋突起《上顎骨の》 681, 759
 −tonsil 口蓋扁桃 783
Palatoglossal arch 口蓋舌弓 783, 793
Palatoglossus 口蓋舌筋 785
Palatopharyngeal arch 口蓋咽頭弓 783, 793
Palatopharyngeus 口蓋咽頭筋 803
Palmar
 −aponeurosis 手掌腱膜 415, 435
 −br.
 −− of median n. 正中神経の掌枝 495
 −− of ulnar n. 掌枝《尺骨神経の》 495
 −carpal lig. 掌側手根靱帯 487, 489
 −digital nn. 掌側指神経 495
 −metacarpal aa. 掌側中手動脈 491
Palmaris
 −brevis 短掌筋 435
 −longus 長掌筋 405, **415**, 501
 −− tendon 長掌筋の腱 435

Palpebral part of orbicularis oculi 眼瞼部《眼輪筋の》 753
Pampiniform plexus 蔓状静脈叢 293, 327
Pancreas 膵臓 237, 241, 245, 251, 255, **271**, 307
Pancreatic duct 膵管 267, 271
Paracentral
 −lobule 中心傍小葉 875
 −sulcus 中心傍溝 875
Paracolic gutter 結腸傍溝 245
Parahippocampal gyrus 海馬傍回 875, 877
Paraolfactory area 嗅傍野 875
Paraterminal gyrus 終板傍回 875
Paratracheal node 気管傍リンパ節 191
Paraventricular nuclei 視床室傍核群 891
Parietal
 −bone 頭頂骨 679, 689
 −layer of serous pericardium 漿膜性心膜の壁側板 139
 −lobe 頭頂葉 871
 −peritoneum 壁側腹膜 223
Parieto-occipital sulcus 頭頂後頭溝 873, 875
Parotid
 −duct 耳下腺管 725, 727, 795
 −gland 耳下腺 795
 −plexus of facial n. (CN VII) 顔面神経の耳下腺神経叢 729
Patella 膝蓋骨 507, 547, 561, 567, 581, 583
Patellar lig. 膝蓋靱帯 523, 551, 565, 569
Pecten pubis 恥骨櫛 199
Pectinate mm. 櫛状筋 151
Pectineal line 恥骨筋線 197
Pectineus 恥骨筋 523, 547, **549**, 639
Pectoral
 −axillary node 胸筋腋窩リンパ節 115
 −fascia 胸筋筋膜 117
Pectoralis
 −major 大胸筋 117, 363, 369, **387**
 −minor 小胸筋 365, **383**, 479
Pedicle of vertebral arch 椎弓根 9, 19, 37
Pelvic
 −girdle 下肢帯 507

Pelvic
- splanchnic nn. 骨盤内臓神経 335
- ureter 尿管の骨盤部 297

Pericardiacophrenic
- a. 心膜横隔動脈 111, 131, 135
- v. 心膜横隔静脈 111, 131, 135

Pericardial cavity 心膜腔 139
Pericardium 心膜 111

Perineal
- body 会陰腱中心 233, 235
- membrane 下尿生殖隔膜筋膜(会陰膜) 225
- nn. 会陰神経 287
- raphe 会陰縫線 283
- fat capsule of kidney 脂肪被膜《腎臓の》 273

Perpendicular plate
-- of ethmoid bone 垂直板《篩骨の》 741, 759, 695, 767
-- of Palatine bone 垂直板《口蓋骨の》 763

Pes anserinus 鵞足 553, 557
Petrous part of temporal bone 岩様部《側頭骨の》 685, 769, 777
Petrous ridge 錐体上縁 683
Phalanges 指骨(指節骨) 341

Pharyngeal
- opening of auditory tube 耳管咽頭口 791
- orifice 咽頭口 773
- plexus 咽頭神経叢 709

Pharyngotympanic (auditory) tube 耳管 769
-, bony part 耳管骨部 773

Philtrum 人中 845
Phrenic n. 横隔神経 **111**, 131, 135, 461, 821, 839
Pia mater 軟膜 855
Pineal gland 松果体 883, 885
Piriform recess 梨状陥凹 829
Piriformis 梨状筋 227, 229, 527, 531, 541, **543**, 545, 649
Pisiform 豆状骨 419, 431, 447, 449, 451
Pituitary gland 下垂体 851, 853, 883, 893

Plantar
- aponeurosis 足底腱膜 605
- calcaneonavicular lig. 底側踵舟靱帯 597, 599
- chiasm 足底交叉 587
- interossei 底側骨間筋 611
- metatarsal aa. 底側中足動脈 665

Plantaris 足底筋 577, **585**
- tendon 足底筋の腱 585

Pons 橋 851, 853, 893, 895, 901

Popliteal
- a. 膝窩動脈 629, **631**, 653, 655
- v. 膝窩静脈 653, 655

Popliteus 膝窩筋 **555**, 557, 577, 579

Postcentral
- gyrus 中心後回 849, 873, 915, 929
- sulcus 中心後溝 873, 875

Posterior
- antebrachial cutaneous n. 後前腕皮神経 465
- arch of atlas 後弓《環椎(第1頸椎)の》 11, 13
- auricular
-- a. 後耳介動脈 717
-- n. 後耳介神経 703, 705
- belly of digastric 後腹《顎二腹筋の》 705, 799, 801, 807, 809, 811, 813
- border of ulna 後縁《尺骨の》 425
- cerebral a. 後大脳動脈 865
- cervical intertransversarii 頸後横突間筋 51, 53, 55
- circumflex humeral a. 後上腕回旋動脈 455, 475
- column 後柱 911
- commissure 後陰唇交連 283
- communicating a. 後交通動脈 865
- compartment of subtalar joint 距骨下関節, 後区(距踵関節) 597
- cord 後神経束 461, 463
- cranial fossa 後頭蓋窩 683
- crico-arytenoid 後輪状披裂筋 803, 833
- cruciate lig. 後十字靱帯 567, 569
- cusp of right atrioventricular valve 後尖《右房室弁の》 155
- divisions of brachial plexus 後部《腕神経叢の》 459
- ethmoidal
-- a. 後篩骨動脈 749
-- n. 後篩骨神経 699, 749

- femoral cutaneous n. 後大腿皮神経 633, 645, 653
- funiculus of spinal cord 後索《脊髄の》 911
- gluteal line 後殿筋線 543, 545
- horn of spinal cord 後角《脊髄の》 925
- inferior
-- iliac spine 下後腸骨棘 509, 515
-- nasal brs., lateral posterior nasal aa. 下後鼻枝，外側後鼻枝 767
- intercostal
-- aa. 肋間動脈 67, **103**, 109, 111
-- vv. 肋間静脈 69, **105**, 109, 111, 125
- internal vertebral venous plexus 後内椎骨静脈叢 69, 907
- internodal bundles 後結節間束 161
- interosseous
-- a. 後骨間動脈 455
-- n. 後[前腕]骨間神経 465, 501
- interventricular
-- a. 後室間枝 159
-- v. 後室間静脈 159
- labial nn. 後陰唇神経 287
- layer of rectus sheath 後葉《腹直筋鞘の》 215
- longitudinal lig. 後縦靱帯 31, 33, 35, **37**
- mediastinum 後縦隔 119
- papillary m. 後乳頭筋 153
- paracentral gyrus 後中心傍回 875
- parietal cortex 後頭頂野 929
- part of knee 膝窩 529
- process of talus 距骨後突起 623
- radicular v. 後根静脈 927
- ramus/i
-- (medial cutaneous brs.) of spinal n. 後枝《脊髄神経の》(内側皮枝) 75
-- of thoracic aorta 後枝《胸大動脈の》 67
-- of spinal n. 後枝《脊髄神経の》 71, 107, 715, 909
- rootlets 後根糸 909
- sacro-iliac ligs. 後仙腸靱帯 519
- scrotal nn. 後陰嚢神経 301
- segmental medullary a. 後節動脈 925
- semilunar cusp of aortic valve 後半月弁《大動脈弁の》 155
-- septal brs. 中隔後鼻枝 765
- spinal
-- aa. 後脊髄動脈 925
-- v. 後脊髄静脈 927
- spinocerebellar tract 後脊髄小脳路 917, 921
- superior
-- a. of superior alveolar nn. 上歯槽神経の後上歯槽枝 701
-- alveolar a. 後上歯槽動脈 719
--- brs. of superior alveolar nn. 後上歯槽枝《上歯槽神経の》 739
-- iliac spine 上後腸骨棘 515, 519, 649
- surface
-- of fibula 後面《腓骨の》 587
-- of scapula 後面《肩甲骨の》 385, 397
-- of tibia 後面《脛骨の》 587
- talofibular lig. 後距腓靱帯 603
- tibial
-- a. 後脛骨動脈 **631**, 655, 657, 669
-- v. 後脛骨静脈 669
- tibiofibular lig. 後脛腓靱帯 603
- tubercle of atlas 後結節《環椎(第1頸椎)の》 13, 63
Precentral
- gyrus 中心前回 849, 873, 929
- sulcus 中心前溝 873, 875
Precuneus 楔前部 875
Prefrontal cortex 前頭前野 929
Premotor cortex 運動前野 929
Prerectal fibers 直腸前線維 231
Pretracheal layer of cervical fascia 気管前葉《頸筋膜の》 825
Prevertebral ganglion 椎前神経節 933
Primary fissure 第一裂 901
Promontory 岬角《仙骨の》 3, **23**, 199, 203, 527, 547
Pronator quadratus 方形回内筋 409, **419**
Pronator teres 円回内筋 405, 407, **415**, 501
Proper
- palmar
-- digital aa. 固有掌側指動脈 489
-- digital nn. 固有掌側指神経 471, 489
- plantar
-- digital aa. 固有底側趾動脈 665

Proper plantar digital nn. 固有底側趾神経 665
Prostate 前立腺 247, 297, 299
Proximal
- interphalangeal joint 近位指節間(PIP)関節 433, 503
- radio-ulnar joint 上橈尺関節 399
Psoas
- arcade 腰筋弓 99
- major 大腰筋 97, 99, 219, 273, 521, **537**
Pterygoid plexus 翼突筋静脈叢 721, 723
Pterygopalatine ganglion 翼口蓋神経節 701, 767, 781
Pubic
- symphysis 恥骨結合 201, 213, 215, 217, 219, 229, 233, 235, 275
- tubercle 恥骨結節 197, 219, 509, 513
Pubococcygeus 恥骨尾骨筋 227, **231**
Pubofemoral lig. 恥骨大腿靱帯 517
Puborectalis 恥骨直腸筋 227, **231**
Pudendal n. 陰部神経 287, 335, **633**, 653
Pulmonary
- aa. 肺動脈 173
- lig. 肺間膜 179
- plexus 肺神経叢 163
- trunk 肺動脈幹 123, 141, 145, 153, 165, 177, **189**
- valve 肺動脈弁 149
Pulvinar 視床枕 885
Putamen 被殻 889
Pyloric
- antrum 幽門洞 253
- part of stomach 幽門部《胃の》 251
- sphincter 幽門括約筋 255
Pyramid of medulla oblongata 錐体《延髄の》 895
Pyramidal
- lobe of thyroid gland 錐体葉《甲状腺の》 823
- tract 錐体路 919
Pyramidalis 錐体筋 209, **217**

Q

Quadrate lobe of liver 方形葉《肝臓の》 265
Quadratus
- arcade 方形筋弓 99
- femoris 大腿方形筋 531, 541, 543, **545**
- lumborum 腰方形筋 99, **219**
- plantae 足底方形筋 609, **623**, 625, 627, 665
Quadriceps
- femoris 大腿四頭筋 553
-- tendon 大腿四頭筋の腱 521, 565
--- of insertion 停止腱《大腿四頭筋の》 551
Quadrigeminal plate 四丘体板 883

R

Radial
- a. 橈骨動脈 **455**, 485, 491, 493, 501
- collateral lig. of elbow joint 外側側副靱帯《肘関節の》 401, 403
- head of flexor digitorum superficialis 浅指屈筋の橈骨頭 409
- n. 橈骨神経 **465**, 475, 481, 499
--, dorsal digital n. 橈骨神経, 背側指神経 495, 497
--, superficial br. 橈骨神経, 浅枝 465, 497
- styloid process 茎状突起《橈骨の》 399, 421, 431
- tuberosity 橈骨粗面 395, 399, 417, 419
Radius 橈骨 341, 397, 419, 421, 423, 425, 427, 449, 451, 453, 501
Ramus
- of ischium 坐骨枝 197, 233
- of mandible 下顎枝 779, 809
Receptive field 受容野 913, 917
- 1 受容野 1 917
- 2 受容野 2 917
- of arm 上肢の受容野 915
- of leg 下肢の受容野 915
Rectal venous plexus 直腸静脈叢 261

Recto-uterine pouch 直腸子宮窩 249
Rectovesical pouch 直腸膀胱窩 247, 299
Rectum 直腸 247, 257, **259**, 275
Rectus
 −abdominis 腹直筋 209, **217**, 221, 337
 −capitis
 −−anterior 前頭直筋 815, **817**
 −−lateralis 外側頭直筋 815, **817**
 −−posterior
 −−−major 大後頭直筋 41, **63**
 −−−minor 小後頭直筋 63
 −femoris 大腿直筋 521, **551**, 553, 639, 667, 671
Recurrent laryngeal n. 反回神経 839
Red nucleus 赤核 899
Reflected head of rectus femoris 大腿直筋の反転頭 553
Renal
 −pyramids 腎錐体 305
 −v. 腎静脈 315
Respiratory bronchiole 呼吸細気管支 185, 187
Reticulospinal tract 網様体脊髄路 923
Retina 網膜 757
Retromandibular v. 下顎後静脈 721
Retropharyngeal space 咽頭後隙 825
Rhomboid
 −fossa 菱形窩 893, 897
 −major 大菱形筋 39, 373, **385**
 −minor 小菱形筋 373, **385**
Rib 肋骨 95
Right
 −ascending lumbar v. 右上行腰静脈 125
 −atrioventricular
 −−orifice 右房室口 151
 −−valve 右房室弁 151, 155
 −atrium 右心房 **147**, 149, 165, 169
 −auricle 右心耳 145
 −brachiocephalic v. 右腕頭静脈 105
 −bundle br. of atrioventricular bundle 右脚《房室束の》 161
 −colic
 −−a. 右結腸動脈 311
 −−flexure 右結腸曲 241
 −common
 −−iliac a. 右総腸骨動脈 247, 273, **303**, 325

−−iliac v. 右総腸骨静脈 247, 325
−coronary a. 右冠状動脈 157, 159
−crus of diaphragm 右脚《横隔膜の》 97
−dome of diaphragm 横隔膜の右天蓋 99
−gastric a. 右胃動脈 307
−gastro-omental a. 右胃大網動脈 307
−greater splanchnic n. 右大内臓神経 331
−hepatic duct 右肝管 267
−inferior
−−hypogastric plexus 右下下腹神経叢 333
−−lobar bronchus 右下葉気管支 183
−−suprarenal a. 右下副腎動脈 317
−internal iliac a. 右内腸骨動脈 303, 323
−internal jugular v. 右内頸静脈 125, 191
−internal pudendal v. 右内陰部静脈 325
−lobe
−−of liver, diaphragmatic surface 肝臓の右葉，横隔面 263
−−of thyroid gland 右葉《甲状腺の》 823
−lumbar trunk 右腰リンパ本幹 329
−lung (middle lobe) 右肺（中葉） 177
−main bronchus 右主気管支 121, 183
−marginal
−−br. of right coronary a. 右縁枝（鋭角縁枝）《右冠状動脈の》 157
−−v. 右辺縁静脈 157
−middle
−−rectal
−−−a. 右中直腸動脈 323
−−−v. 右中直腸静脈 323
−−suprarenal a. 右中副腎動脈 317
−obturator
−−a. 右閉鎖動脈 323
−−v. 右閉鎖静脈 323
−ovarian
−−a. 右卵巣動脈 317
−−v. 右卵巣静脈 317
−phrenic n. 右横隔神経 143, 163
−posterolateral br. 右後側壁枝 159
−pulmonary
−−a. 右肺動脈 135, 139, 149, 177, **189**
−−vv. 右肺静脈 141, 177
−recurrent laryngeal n. 右反回神経 163, 711

Right
- renal a. 右腎動脈 251
- semilunar cusp of aortic valve 右半月弁《大動脈弁の》 155
- subclavian v. 右鎖骨下静脈 191
- superior
-- lobar bronchus 右上葉気管支 183
-- suprarenal a. 右上副腎動脈 317
- testicular
-- a. 右精巣動脈 273, 317
-- v. 右精巣静脈 273, 317
- umbilical a. 右臍動脈 323
- uterine
-- a. 右子宮動脈 323
-- v. 右子宮静脈 323
- uterovaginal plexus 右子宮腟神経叢 333
- vagus n. 右迷走神経 135, 163
- ventricle 右心室 143, 157, 165
Root of mesentery 腸間膜根 245
Rotatores
- breves 短回旋筋 **59**, 61
- longi 長回旋筋 **59**, 61
Round lig. of liver 肝円索 173, 263
Rubrospinal tract 赤核脊髄路 923

S

S1-S5 vertebrae 第1-5仙椎 3
Saccule 球形囊 707
Sacral
- canal 仙骨管 25, 203
- hiatus 仙骨裂孔 25
- horn 仙骨角 25
- plexus 仙骨神経叢 331, 333, 651
Sacro-iliac joint 仙腸関節 199
Sacrococcygeal joint 仙尾関節 23
Sacrospinous lig. 仙棘靱帯 **201**, 203, 235, 517, 519, 649
Sacrotuberous lig. 仙結節靱帯 **203**, 235, 517, 519, 531, 537, 541, 555, 557, 649
Sacrum 仙骨 3, **23**, 25, 47, 49, 57, 59, 61, 227, 393, 539, 543, 545, 555
Sagittal suture 矢状縫合 679
Salpingopharyngeus 耳管咽頭筋 773

Saphenous n. 伏在神経 633, **639**, 645, 651
Sartorius 縫工筋 521, 527, 551, **553**, 639, 667
Scalenus
- anterior (anterior scalene) 前斜角筋 87, **89**, 461, 815, 817, 839
- medius (middle scalene) 中斜角筋 87, **89**, 815, 817, 843
- posterior (posterior scalene) 後斜角筋 **89**, 815, 817
Scalp 頭皮 857
Scaphoid 舟状骨《手の》 **429**, 433, 445, 487, 493
- fossa 舟状窩 771
Scapula 肩甲骨 **345**, 347, 381, 391, 393
Scapular
- notch 肩甲切痕 347
- part of latissimus dorsi 肩甲骨部《広背筋の》 393
Scapulothoracic joint 肩甲胸郭関節 353
Sciatic n. 坐骨神経 **633**, 635, 641, 653, 667
Sclera 強膜 757
Scrotal skin 陰嚢の皮膚 295
Segmental bronchus 区域気管支 185
Sella turcica トルコ鞍 685
Semicircular ducts 半規管 707
Semilunar line 半月線 215, 337
Semimembranosus 半膜様筋 529, 555, **557**, 575, 643
- tendon 半膜様筋の腱 557
Seminal gland 精嚢 247, 297, 299
Semispinalis
- capitis 頭半棘筋 45, 59, **61**
- cervicis 頸半棘筋 59, **61**
- thoracis 胸半棘筋 59, **61**
Semitendinosus 半腱様筋 529, 555, **557**, 643, 667
Sensory cortex 大脳皮質感覚野 913
Septal
- cusp of right atrioventricular valve 中隔尖《右房室弁の》 155
- nasal cartilage 鼻中隔軟骨 759
Septomarginal trabecula 中隔縁柱 149
Septum pellucidum 透明中隔 871

Serratus
- anterior 前鋸筋 205, 363, 365, 367, 373, **381**
- posterior
-- inferior 下後鋸筋 39, **65**
-- superior 上後鋸筋 65

Sesamoid bones 種子骨 591, 595

Shaft
- of 2nd distal phalanx 体《第2末節骨の》 449, 451, 453
- of clavicle 鎖骨体 343
- of humerus 上腕骨体 389, 391, 397

Short
- head
-- of biceps brachii 短頭《上腕二頭筋の》 367, 395, 499
-- of biceps femoris 短頭《大腿二頭筋の》 533, 555, 557, 641
- saphenous v. 小伏在静脈 645

Shoulder girdle 上肢帯 341

Sigmoid
- aa. S状結腸動脈 313
- colon S状結腸 249, 257
- sinus S状静脈洞 723, 867, 869

Sinu-atrial
- nodal br. 洞房結節枝 157
- node 洞房結節 161

Small cardiac v. 小心臓静脈 159

Soft palate 軟口蓋(口蓋帆) 791, 793

Soleal line of tibia ヒラメ筋線《脛骨の》 587

Soleus ヒラメ筋 573, 577, 579, **585**, 643, 669

Spermatic cord 精索 221, 223

Sphenoid 蝶形骨 675

Sphenoid sinus 蝶形骨洞 763

Sphenopalatine
- a. 蝶口蓋動脈 719, 735
- foramen 蝶口蓋孔 763

Spinal
- arachnoid mater 脊髄クモ膜 907
- br. of thoracic aorta 脊髄枝《胸大動脈の》 67
- cord 脊髄 31, 71
- dura mater 脊髄硬膜 907
- ganglion 脊髄神経節 107, 907, 909, 933
- n. 脊髄神経 907, 909
- part of deltoid 肩甲棘部《三角筋の》 391
- pia mater 脊髄軟膜 907
- root 脊髄根 713
- v. 脊髄静脈 927

Spinalis 棘筋 43, 45
- cervicis 頸棘筋 57
- thoracis 胸棘筋 57

Spine of scapula 肩甲棘 7, 39, **347**, 377, 385, 391, 397, 473

Spinous process 棘突起 5, 9, **11**, 17, 19, 21, 41, 51, 53, 55, 57, 59, 61, 63

Spiral ganglia ラセン神経節 707

Splanchnic n. 内臓神経 909, 933

Spleen 脾臓 241, 251

Splenic
- a. 脾動脈 307, 321
- v. 脾静脈 319, 321

Splenius
- capitis 頭板状筋 45, **51**, 53, 55
- cervicis 頸板状筋 43, **51**, 53, 55

Spongy urethra 尿道の海綿体部 289, 299

Squamous
- part of temporal bone 鱗部《側頭骨の》 675
- suture 鱗状縫合 675

Stapedius アブミ骨筋 775

Stellate ganglion 星状神経節 803, 839

Sternal
- angle of sternum 胸骨角 85, 193
- end of clavicle 胸骨端《鎖骨の》 193
- facet 胸骨関節面 343
- head of sternocleidomastoid 胸骨頭《胸鎖乳突筋の》 379, 845
- part of diaphragm 横隔膜の胸骨部 99

Sternoclavicular joint 胸鎖関節 353

Sternocleidomastoid 胸鎖乳突筋 41, 363, **379**, 713, 727, 795, 825, 841

Sternocostal
- head of pectoralis major 大胸筋の胸肋部 387
- joint 胸肋関節 355
- part of pectoralis major 胸肋部《大胸筋の》 363

Sternohyoid 胸骨舌骨筋 805, **811**, 813
Sternothyroid 胸骨甲状筋 805, **811**, 813, 843
Sternum 胸骨 83, 95, 215, 379, 387
Stomach 胃 237, 239, **253**
Straight
 - head of rectus femoris 大腿直筋の直頭 553
 - sinus 直静脈洞 861, 869
Stria
 - medullaris of thalamus 視床髄条 883
 - terminalis 分界条 885
Striate area 有線野 931
Styloglossus 茎突舌筋 785
Stylohyoid 茎突舌骨筋 705, 799, 801, **807**, 809, 811, 813
Styloid process 茎状突起 689, 769
Stylomastoid foramen 茎乳突孔 705
Stylopharyngeus 茎突咽頭筋 709, 801
Subacromial bursa 肩峰下包 361
Subarachnoid space クモ膜下腔 31, 907
Subcallosal gyrus 梁下野 875
Subclavian
 - a. 鎖骨下動脈 103, 113, **461**, 479, 711, 837, 839
 - v. 鎖骨下静脈 113, **479**, 839
Subclavius 鎖骨下筋 365, **383**
Subcostal plane 肋骨下平面 193
Subcostales 肋下筋 91
Subcutaneous part of external anal sphincter 皮下部《外肛門括約筋の》 261
Subdeltoid bursa 三角筋下包 361
Sublingual gland 舌下腺 797
Submandibular
 - duct 顎下腺管 797
 - ganglion 顎下神経節 789
 - gland 顎下腺 731, **795**, 797, 845
 - triangle 顎下三角 835
Submental triangle オトガイ下三角 835
Suboccipital n. 後頭下神経 73
Subscapular
 - a. 肩甲下動脈 481
 - fossa 肩甲下窩 345
Subscapularis 肩甲下筋 365, 367, 369, **389**
Subsegmental bronchus 亜区域気管支 185
Substantia nigra 黒質 891, 899

Subtalar(talocalcaneal) joint 距骨下関節 593, 595
Subthalamic nucleus 視床下核 891
Sulcal
 - a. 溝動脈 925
 - v. 溝静脈 927
Sulcus of corpus callosum 脳梁溝 875
Superficial
 - br.
 - - of radial n. 浅枝《橈骨神経の》 493, 501, 485
 - - of ulnar n. 浅枝《尺骨神経の》 489
 - dorsal v. of penis 浅陰茎背静脈 289
 - fibular n. 浅腓骨神経 633, **641**, 645, 659, 661
 - head of flexor pollicis brevis 短母指屈筋の浅頭 437, 445
 - inguinal
 - - node 浅鼠径リンパ節 329
 - - ring 浅鼠径輪 205, 211, 337
 - layer
 - - of cervical fascia 浅葉《頸筋膜の》 825
 - - of thoracolumbar fascia 浅葉《胸腰筋膜の》 39, 43
 - palmar arch 浅掌動脈弓 455, 489
 - part
 - - of external anal sphincter 浅部《外肛門括約筋の》 261
 - - of masseter 浅部《咬筋の》 **689**, 693
 - temporal
 - - a. 浅側頭動脈 717, 733
 - - v. 浅側頭静脈 721, 733
 - transverse
 - - metacarpal lig. 浅横中足靱帯 605
 - - perineal m. 浅会陰横筋 225, **233**, 285
Superior
 - angle of scapula 上角《肩甲骨の》 345, 385
 - articular
 - - facet
 - - - of sacrum 上関節面《仙骨の》 25
 - - - of vertebra 上関節面《椎骨の》 17, 19, 21, 37
 - - process 上関節突起 9, 21

-- surface of tibia 上関節面《脛骨の》 559, 561
- belly of omohyoid 上腹《肩甲舌骨筋の》 805, 811, 813
- cerebellar
-- a. 上小脳動脈 865
-- peduncle 上小脳脚 897, 917
- cerebral vv. 上大脳静脈 855
- cervical ganglion 上頚神経節 731, 843
- cluneal nn. 上殿皮神経 75
- colliculi of tectal(quadrigeminal)plate 上丘《蓋板(四丘体板)の》 897
- constrictor 上咽頭収縮筋 799, 801
- costal facet 上肋骨窩 19
- extensor retinaculum 上伸筋支帯 613
- frontal
-- gyrus 上前頭回 873
-- sulcus 上前頭溝 873
- gluteal
-- a. 上殿動脈 653
-- n. 上殿神経 653
-- v. 上殿静脈 653
- head of lateral pterygoid 上頭《外側翼突筋の》 693
- hypogastric plexus 上下腹神経叢 331, 335
- lacrimal
-- canaliculus 上涙小管 755
-- punctum 上涙点 755
- laryngeal
-- a. 上喉頭動脈 819, 833
-- n. 上喉頭神経 711
-- v. 上喉頭静脈 833
- lateral brachial cutaneous n. 上外側上腕皮神経 473
- lobar bronchi 上葉気管支 177, 179
- lobe of left lung 上葉《左肺の》 169, 177, 181
- longitudinal fasciculus 上縦束 879
- medial genicular a. 内側上膝動脈 631
- mediastinum 上縦隔 119
- medullary velum 上髄帆 901
- mesenteric
-- a. 上腸間膜動脈 237, 245, 251, 255, **303**, 321
-- v. 上腸間膜静脈 245, 251, 255, 319, **321**
- nasal concha 上鼻甲介 761
- nuchal line 上項線 41, 51, 63, 377, 679
- oblique 上斜筋 697, 743
-- part of longus colli 上斜部《頚長筋の》 **815**, 817
- ophthalmic v. 上眼静脈 723, 751, 869
- orbital fissure 上眼窩裂 741
- parietal lobule 上頭頂小葉 873
- part
-- of duodenum 上部《十二指腸の》 243
-- of serratus anterior 上部《前鋸筋の》 381
- petrosal sinus 上錐体静脈洞 869
- pubic ramus 恥骨上肢 547
- rectal
-- a. 上直腸動脈 313, 325
-- v. 上直腸静脈 319, 325
- rectus 上直筋 697, 743, 749
- right pulmonary v. 右上肺静脈 189
- root of ansa cervicalis 上根《頚神経ワナの》 821
- sagittal sinus 上矢状静脈洞 855, 857, 859, 861, **867**
- tarsal m. 上瞼板筋 753
- tarsus 上瞼板 753
- temporal
-- gyrus 上側頭回 873
-- sulcus 上側頭溝 873
- thoracic
-- a. 最上胸動脈 103, 481
-- aperture 胸郭上口 81
- thyroid
-- a. 上甲状腺動脈 819, 837, 843
-- v. 上甲状腺静脈 721
- tracheobronchial node 上気管気管支リンパ節 191
- transverse scapular lig. 上肩甲横靱帯 359
- trochlear surface 距骨滑車の上面 615
- vena cava 上大静脈 105, 121, **125**, 131, 133, 135, 141, 143, 147, 151, 163, 165

Supinator 回外筋 407, 409, 413, **425**, 465

Supraclavicular node 鎖骨上リンパ節 115

Supraclavicular nn. 鎖骨上神経 **473**, 477, 715, 821, 841
Supraglenoid tubercle of scapula 関節上結節《肩甲骨の》 345, 395
Supramarginal gyrus 縁上回 873
Supra-orbital
 - aa. 眼窩上動脈 749
 - margin 眼窩上縁 677
 - n. 眼窩上神経 699, 749
Suprapiriform portion of greater sciatic foramen 大坐骨孔《梨状筋上孔の》 649
Suprarenal
 - gland 副腎 273
 - v. 上副腎静脈 315
Suprascapular
 - a. 肩甲上動脈 473, 475, 479
 - n. 肩甲上神経 461, 473, 475
Supraspinatus 棘上筋 369, 373, 375, **389**, 473
Supraspinous
 - fossa 棘上窩 347
 - lig. 棘上靱帯 29, 31, 33
Supratrochlear n. 滑車上神経 699, 725
Sural n. 腓腹神経 645, 659
Surgical neck of humerus 外科頸《上腕骨の》 351
Suspensory (Cooper's) ligs. of breast 乳房提靱帯(クーパー靱帯) 117
Suspensory lig. of ovary 卵巣提靱帯 279
Sustentaculum tali 載距突起 591, 595, 599, 623
Sympathetic
 - ganglion 交感神経幹神経節 71, 107, 933
 - trunk 交感神経幹 129, 137, 333, 803, 839
 - - , middle cervical ganglion 交感神経幹, 中頸神経節 129
 - - , thoracic ganglion 交感神経幹, 胸神経節 135

[T]

T1-T12 vertebrae 第1-12胸椎 3
T1-T4 spinous processes 第1-4胸椎の棘突起 385
T3 vertebra 第3胸椎 7
T7 spinous process 第7胸椎の棘突起 393
T7 vertebra 第7胸椎 7
T8 vertebra 第8胸椎 101
T10 vertebra 第10胸椎 101
T12 spinous process 第12胸椎の棘突起 377
T12 vertebra 第12胸椎 91
Taeniae coli 自由ヒモ 257
Tail of pancreas 膵尾 245, 271
Talonavicular joint 距舟関節 593
Talus 距骨 595, 597, 603, 615
Tarsal
 - bones 足根骨 507
 - glands 瞼板腺 753
 - tunnel 足根管 657
Tarsometatarsal joints 足根中足関節 593
Tectospinal tract 視蓋脊髄路 923
Tectum of midbrain 中脳蓋 899
Tegmentum 中脳被蓋 899
Telencephalon 終脳 853
Temporal
 - brs. of facial n. 側頭枝《顔面神経の》 703, 729
 - lobe 側頭葉 849, 851, 871
 - pole 側頭極 873
Temporalis 側頭筋 689, **691**, 693, 733
Tendinous
 - arch
 - - of levator ani 肛門挙筋腱弓 231
 - - of levator ani 肛門挙筋腱弓 229
 - - of soleus ヒラメ筋腱弓 585
 - cords 腱索 153
 - intersections 腱画 209, 217, 337
Tendon
 - of superior oblique 上斜筋の腱 743
 - of supraspinatus 棘上筋の腱 361
 - sheath 腱鞘 613
Tenia thalami 視床ヒモ 885
Tensor
 - fasciae latae 大腿筋膜張筋 521, 531, 535, **539**, 671
 - tympani 鼓膜張筋 769, 775
 - veli palatini 口蓋帆張筋 737, 773
Tentorial notch テント切痕 859
Tentorium cerebelli 小脳テント 859, 869

Teres
- major 大円筋 367, 371, 375, **393**, 475
- minor 小円筋 375, **389**, 463, 475

Terminal
- bronchiole 終末細気管支 185
- sulcus 分界溝 783

Testicular
- a. 精巣動脈 293, 327
- v. 精巣静脈 293, 315, 327

Testis 精巣 293

Thalamus 視床 883, 889, 913, 915

Thenar
- crease 母指線 503
- eminence 母指球 503
- muscular br. 母指球筋への筋枝 469

Thigh 大腿 507

Third ventricle 第3脳室 863, 885, 889

Thoracic
- aorta 胸大動脈 67, **123**, 137, 169
- aortic plexus 胸大動脈神経叢 163
- duct 胸管 127, 191, 839
- part of esophagus 胸部《食道の》 119, 129, 133

Thoraco-acromial a. 胸肩峰動脈 477, 479

Thoracodorsal
- a. 胸背動脈 103, 455, 481
- n. 胸背神経 481

Thoracolumbar fascia 胸腰筋膜 65, 75, 393, 539

Thymus 胸腺 131

Thyro-arytenoid 甲状披裂筋 833

Thyrocervical trunk 甲状頸動脈 479, 819, 837, 839

Thyrohyoid 甲状舌骨筋 805, 807, 811, **813**, 831
- lig. 甲状舌骨靱帯 829
- membrane 甲状舌骨膜 827

Thyroid
- cartilage 甲状軟骨 183, 805, 811, 813, 823, 827, 845
- gland 甲状腺 825

Tibia 脛骨 507, 539, 555, 557, 571, 595, 671

Tibial
- n. 脛骨神経 633, 643, 655, 657, 669
- tuberosity 脛骨粗面 547, 559, 561, 581

Tibialis
- anterior 前脛骨筋 571, 573, **581**, 641, 661, 669, 671
- anterior tendon 前脛骨筋の腱 663
- posterior 後脛骨筋 579, 587, 655, 657, 669
- - tendon 後脛骨筋の腱 577, 587, 611

Tibiofibular joint 脛腓関節 559, 569

Tonsilla tubaria 耳管扁桃 791

Torus tubarius with lymphatic tissue(tonsilla tubaria) リンパ組織(耳管扁桃)を伴う耳管隆起 791

Trabeculae carneae of interventricular septum 肉柱《心室中隔の》 153

Trachea 気管 131, 133, 167, 823, 825

Tracheal
- bifurcation 気管分岐部 183
- cartilages 気管軟骨 183

Tragus 耳珠 771

Transversalis fascia 横筋筋膜 223

Transverse
- cervical
- - a. 頸横動脈 839
- - n. 頸横神経 715, 821, 841
- colon 横行結腸 239
- costal facet 横突肋骨窩 19
- facial a. 顔面横動脈 725
- head
- - of adductor hallucis 横頭《母趾内転筋の》 611, 621
- - of adductor pollicis 横頭《母指内転筋の》 437, 441, 445
- mesocolon 横行結腸間膜 237, 241
- -, root 横行結腸間膜, 根 243
- part of trapezius 僧帽筋の横行部(水平部) 39, 371, 377
- pericardial sinus 心膜横洞 141

Transverse
- process 横突起 5, 9, 13, 21, 41, 59, 61, 63, 83, 99
- - with sulcus for spinal n. 横突起, 脊髄神経溝 17
- sinus 横静脈洞 867, 869

Transversus
- abdominis 腹横筋 45, 209, **215**, 223

Transversus
- abdominis aponeurosis　腹横筋腱膜　209, 215
- thoracis　胸横筋　87, **93**

Trapezium　大菱形骨　429, 445

Trapezius　僧帽筋　41, 77, 363, **377**, 713, 841, 845

Trapezoid　小菱形骨　429, 449, 451, 453

Triangular part of inferior frontal gyrus　三角部《下前頭回の》　873

Triceps
- brachii　上腕三頭筋　**397**, 411, 465
- surae　下腿三頭筋　585

Trigeminal
- ganglion　三叉神経節　747
- n.(CN V)　三叉神経　701, 895

Trigone of bladder　膀胱三角　277

Triquetrum　三角骨　429, 447

Trochlea　滑車　743
- of humerus　上腕骨滑車　349

Trochlear
- n.(CN IV)　滑車神経　697, **745**, 749, 897
- notch　滑車切痕　399

Tubercle of rib　肋骨結節　83

Tuberosity
- of 5th metatarsal　第5中足骨粗面　583, 591, 619
- of ulna　尺骨粗面　419
- -(brachialis tendon of insertion)　尺骨粗面(上腕筋の停止腱)　395

Tunica
- albuginea　白膜　295
- - of corpora cavernosa　陰茎海綿体白膜　289
- dartos　肉様膜　295
- vaginalis, parietal layer　精巣鞘膜の壁側板　293, 295

Tunnel for fibularis longus tendon　長腓骨筋の腱　599

Tympanic membrane　鼓膜　775

U

Ulna　尺骨　341, 397, 421, 423, 425, 427, 449, 451, 453, 501

Ulnar
- a.　尺骨動脈　455, 485, 487, 491, 501
- collateral lig. of elbow joint　内側側副靱帯《肘関節の》　401, 403
- groove of humerus　尺骨神経溝《上腕骨の》　351
- n.　尺骨神経　**471**, 483, 485, 487, 491, 499, 501
- styloid process　茎状突起《尺骨の》　429, 503

Umbilical
- aa.　臍動脈　171
- ring　臍輪　211
- v.　臍静脈　171

Umbilicus　臍　171, 205

Uncinate process
- of cervical vertebrae　鈎状突起《頸椎の》　11
- of pancreas　鈎状突起《膵臓の》　271

Uncovertebral joint　鈎椎関節　27

Uncus of parahippocampal gyrus　鈎《海馬傍回の》　875, 877

Upper
- eyelid　上眼瞼　753
- subscapular n.　上肩甲下神経　481
- trunk(C5-C6)　上神経幹(第5・6頸神経)　459

Ureter　尿管　259, 277, 279, 305

Ureteric orifice　尿管口　277

Urethra　尿道　277, 297

Urinary bladder　膀胱　247, 249, 273, 275, 297

Urogenital hiatus　尿生殖裂孔　231, 233

Uterine
- a.　子宮動脈　279
- v.　子宮静脈　279
- venous plexus　子宮静脈叢　323

Uterosacral
- fold　直腸子宮ヒダ　279
- lig.　直腸子宮靱帯　279

Uterus　子宮　249

Utricle　卵形嚢　707

Uvula　口蓋垂　773, 793

Vagina　腟　249, 275

Vaginal
- orifice 腟口 283
- venous plexus 腟静脈叢 323
Vagus n.(CN X) 迷走神経 709, **711**, 713, 787, 803, 825, 837, 895, 933
Valve
- of coronary sinus 冠状静脈弁 151
- of inferior vena cava 下大静脈弁 151
Valved orifice
- of coronary sinus 冠状静脈口 151
- of inferior vena cava 下大静脈口 151
Vasa recta 直細動脈 311
Vasocorona 血管冠 925
Vastus
- intermedius 中間広筋 523, 525, **553**, 639
- lateralis 外側広筋 521, 535, **551**, 553, 639, 667, 671
- medialis 内側広筋 521, 527, **551**, 553, 639
Venous ring 静脈輪 927
Ventrolateral thalamic nuclei 視床外側腹側核群 891
Vermis of cerebellum 小脳虫部 903
Vertebra prominens (C7) 隆椎(第7頸椎) 5, 11, 51, 53, 55, 57, 59, 61
Vertebral
- a. 椎骨動脈 73, 717, 907
- arch 椎弓 15, 21
- body 椎体 5, 9, 19, 37
- canal 脊柱管 37
- part
-- of latissimus dorsi 椎骨部《広背筋の》 393
-- of longus colli 垂直部《頸長筋の》 **815**, 817

Vesical plexus 膀胱神経叢 335
Vesico-uterine pouch 膀胱子宮窩 249
Vestibular
- fold 前庭ヒダ 829
- n. (CN VIII) 前庭神経 707, 777
Vestibulospinal tract 前庭脊髄路 923
Visceral
- layer
-- of serous pericardium 漿膜性心膜の臓側板 139
-- of tunica vaginalis 精巣鞘膜の臓側板 293, 295
- pleura 臓側胸膜 109
Vitreous body 硝子体 757
Vocal fold 声帯ヒダ 829
Vomer 鋤骨 759

W・X

White ramus communicans of spinal n. 白交通枝《脊髄神経の》 909, 933
Wrist joint 橈骨手根関節 433
Xiphoid process of sternum 剣状突起《胸骨の》 85, 93, 99, 193, 207, 211, 213, 215, 217, 219

Z

Zygapophyseal joint 椎間関節 27
Zygomatic
- arch 頬骨弓 675, 681, 689, 691
- bone 頬骨 677, 845
- brs. of facial n. 頬骨枝《顔面神経の》 703
- n. 頬骨神経 701
Zygomaticus major 大頬骨筋 687

和文索引

- 索引語は，アルファベット，片仮名，平仮名，漢字（1文字目の読み）の順に配列し，読みが同じ漢字は画数の少ない順で配列している．項目の主要掲載ページは太字で示す．
- 「右」は「う」，「左」は「さ」，「肩」は「けん」，「膝」は「しつ」，「肘」は「ちゅう」に配列している．
- 英文中の a., aa. は artery, arteries を，br., brs. は branch, branches を，lig., ligs. は ligament, ligaments を，m., mm. は mucle, muscles を，n., nn. は nerve, nerves を，v., vv. は vein, veins を表す．

あ

α運動ニューロン　α-motor neuron　919
アキレス腱　Calcaneal (Achilles') tendon　573, 657
アブミ骨筋　Stapedius　775
亜区域気管支　Subsegmental bronchus　185
鞍背　Dorsum sellae　683

い

1次ニューロン　1st neuron　913
― の細胞体　Cell body of 1st neuron　917
― の軸索　Axon of 1st neuron　915
胃　Stomach　237, 239, **253**
胃結腸間膜　Gastrocolic lig.　241
胃十二指腸動脈　Gastroduodenal a.　309
胃底　Fundus of stomach　253
胃脾間膜　Gastrosplenic lig.　241
咽頭口　Pharyngeal orifice　773
咽頭後隙　Retropharyngeal space　825
咽頭神経叢　Pharyngeal plexus　709
陰核　Clitoris　283
陰核亀頭　Glans of clitoris　285
陰核背神経　Dorsal clitoral n.　287
陰核背動脈　Dorsal clitoral a.　287
陰茎海綿体　Corpus cavernosum penis　289, 291, 299
陰茎海綿体白膜　Tunica albuginea of corpora cavernosa　289
陰茎亀頭　Glans penis　291, 293
陰茎脚　Crus of penis　291
陰茎深動脈　Deep penile a.　289
陰茎背神経　Dorsal n. of penis　289, 301, 335
陰茎背動脈　Dorsal a. of penis　289

陰嚢の皮膚　Scrotal skin　295
陰部神経　Pudendal n.　287, 335, **633**, 653

う

右胃大網動脈　Right gastro-omental a.　307
右胃動脈　Right gastric a.　307
右縁枝（鋭角縁枝）《右冠状動脈の》　Right marginal br.　157
右横隔神経　Right phrenic n.　143, 163
右下下腹神経叢　Right inferior hypogastric plexus　333
右下副腎動脈　Right inferior suprarenal a.　317
右下葉気管支　Right inferior lobar bronchus　183
右肝管　Right hepatic duct　267
右冠状動脈　Right coronary a.　157, 159
右脚
― 《横隔膜の》　Right crus of diaphragm　97
― 《房室束の》　Right bundle br. of atrioventricular bundle　161
右結腸曲　Right colic flexure　241
右結腸動脈　Right colic a.　311
右後側壁枝　Right posterolateral a.　159
右鎖骨下静脈　Right subclavian v.　191
右臍動脈　Right umbilical a.　323
右子宮静脈　Right uterine v.　323
右子宮腟神経叢　Right uterovaginal plexus　333
右子宮動脈　Right uterine br.　323
右主気管支　Right main bronchus　121, 183
右上行腰静脈　Right ascending lumbar v.　125

右上肺静脈　Superior right pulmonary v. 189
右上副腎動脈　Right superior suprarenal a. 317
右上葉気管支　Right superior lobar bronchus 183
右心耳　Right auricle 145
右心室　Right ventricle 143, 157, 165
右心房　Right atrium 147, 149, 165, 169
右腎動脈　right renal a. 251
右精巣静脈　Right testicular v. 273, 317
右精巣動脈　Right testicular a. 273, 317
右総腸骨静脈　Right common iliac v. 247, 325
右総腸骨動脈　Right common iliac a. 247, 273, **303**, 325
右大内臓神経　Right greater splanchnic n. 331
右中直腸静脈　Right middle rectal v. 323
右中直腸動脈　Right middle rectal a. 323
右中副腎動脈　Right middle suprarenal a. 317
右内陰部静脈　Right internal pudendal v. 325
右内頸静脈　Right internal jugular v. 125, 191
右内腸骨動脈　Right internal iliac a. 303, 323
右肺　Right lung
　— の斜裂　Oblique fissure of right lung 167, 169
　— の水平裂　Horizontal fissure of right lung 167
右肺静脈　Right pulmonary vv. 141, 177
　— の枝　Brs. of right pulmonary vv. 179
右肺動脈　Right pulmonary a. 135, 139, 149, 177, **189**
　— の枝　Brs. of right pulmonary a. 179
右反回神経　Right recurrent laryngeal n. 163, 711
右半月弁《大動脈弁の》　Right semilunar cusp of aortic valve 155
右閉鎖静脈　Right obturator v. 323
右閉鎖動脈　Right obturator a. 323
右辺縁静脈　Right marginal v. 157
右房室口　Right atrioventricular orifice 151
右房室弁　Right atrioventricular valve 151, 155
右迷走神経　Right vagus n. 135, 163
右葉《甲状腺の》　Right lobe of Thyroid gland 823
右腰リンパ本幹　Right lumbar trunk 329
右卵巣静脈　Right ovarian v. 317
右卵巣動脈　Right ovarian a. 317
右腕頭静脈　Right brachiocephalic v. 105
烏口肩峰靱帯　Coraco-acromial lig. 353, 359
烏口鎖骨靱帯　Coracoclavicular lig. 359
烏口突起　Coracoid process 345, 357, 365, 381, 383, 387, 389, 395, 397
烏口腕筋　Coracobrachialis 369, **387**, 467
運動性脳神経核　Motor cranial n. nuclei 919
運動前野　Premotor cortex 929

え

S状結腸　Sigmoid colon 249, 257
S状結腸動脈　Sigmoid aa. 313
S状静脈洞　Sigmoid sinus 723, 867, 869
S状洞溝　Groove for sigmoid sinus 685
会陰腱中心　Perineal body 233, 235
会陰神経　Perineal nn. 287
会陰縫線　Perineal raphe 283
会陰膜　Perineal membrane 225
鋭角縁枝《右冠状動脈の》　Right marginal br. of right coronary a. 157
腋窩陥凹　Axillary recess 359
腋窩静脈　Axillary v. 113, 479
腋窩神経　Axillary n. 459, 463, 475, 481, 473
腋窩動脈　Axillary a. 113, 459, 463, 479
腋窩リンパ叢　Axillary lymphatic plexus 115
円回内筋　Pronator teres 405, 407, **415**, 501
　— の上腕頭　Humeral head of pronator teres 469
円錐靱帯結節　Conoid tubercle 343

延髄　Medulla oblongata　849，851，853，893
— の錐体　Pyramid of medulla oblongata　895
延髄根　Cranial root　713
遠位指節間（DIP）関節　Distal interphalangeal joint　433
遠位手根線　Distal wrist crease　503
縁上回　Supramarginal gyrus　873

お

オトガイ下三角　Submental triangle　835
オトガイ孔　Mental foramen　677，701，779
オトガイ神経　Mental n.　701，725
オトガイ舌筋　Genioglossus　785，791
オトガイ舌骨筋　Geniohyoid　785，797，**809**
オリーブ　Olive　895，901
黄色靱帯　Ligamenta flava　33，35
横隔胸膜　Diaphragmatic part of parietal pleura　109，175
横隔神経　Phrenic n.　**111**，131，135，461，821，839
横隔膜　Diaphragm　**95**，97，**99**，101，109，119，135
— の右天蓋　Right dome of diaphragm　99
— の胸骨部　Sternal part of diaphragm　99
— の左天蓋　Left dome of diaphragm　99
— の腰椎部　Lumbar part of diaphragm　99
— の肋骨部　Costal part of diaphragm　95，99
横隔膜円蓋　Diaphragm leaflet　167
横筋筋膜　Transversalis fascia　223
横行結腸　Transverse colon　239
横行結腸間膜　Transverse mesocolon　237，241
—，根　Transverse mesocolon, root　243
横静脈洞　Transverse sinus　867，869
横頭《母趾内転筋の》　Transverse head of adductor hallucis　611，621
横洞溝　Groove for transverse sinus　685
横突間靱帯　Intertransverse ligs.　35

横突起　Transverse process　5，9，13，21，41，59，61，63，83
—，脊髄神経溝　Transverse process with sulcus for spinal n.　17
横突孔　Foramen transversarium　11，15，17
横突肋骨窩　Transverse costal facet　19

か

下咽頭収縮筋　Inferior constrictor　799，801，831
下角
—《肩甲骨の》　Inferior angle of scapula　347，381，385，389
—《側脳室の》　Inferior horn of lateral ventricle　863
下顎縁枝《顔面神経の》　Marginal mandibular br. of facial n.　703，729
下顎窩　Mandibular fossa　681
下顎角　Angle of mandible　779，845
下顎孔　Mandibular foramen　779，809
下顎後静脈　Retromandibular v.　721
下顎骨　Mandible　675
下顎枝　Ramus of mandible　779，809
下顎神経　Mandibular n.（CN V₃）　701，735，**737**，781
下顎切痕　Mandibular notch　779
下顎頭　Head of mandible　809
—，関節面　Head of mandible, articular surface　693
下関節突起　Inferior articular process　9
下関節面　Inferior articular facet
—《胸椎の》　Inferior articular facet of thoracic vertebra　19
—《軸椎の》　Inferior articular facet of axis　15
—《腰椎の》　Inferior articular facet of lumber vertebra　21
下眼窩裂　Inferior orbital fissure　739，741
下眼静脈　Inferior ophthalmic v.　751
下気管気管支リンパ節　Inferior tracheobronchial lymph node　191
下丘《蓋板（四丘体板）の》　Inferior colliculi of quadrigeminal plate　897
下瞼板　Inferior tarsus　753
下甲状腺静脈　Inferior thyroid v.　131，837

(かかんりゅうき《けいこつの》) *971*

下甲状腺動脈　Inferior thyroid a.　803, 831, 843
下行結腸　Descending colon　251
下行口蓋動脈　Descending palatine a.　767
下行大動脈　Descending aorta　121, 137, 169
下後鋸筋　Serratus posterior inferior　39, **65**
下後腸骨棘　Posterior inferior iliac spine　509, 515
下後鼻枝, 外側後鼻枝　Posterior inferior nasal brs., lateral posterior nasal aa.　767
下喉頭神経　Inferior laryngeal n.　833
下項線《頸神経ワナの》　Inferior nuchal line　63
下根《頸神経ワナの》　Inferior root of ansa cervicalis　821
下肢帯　Pelvic girdle　507
下肢の受容野　Receptive field of leg　915
下歯槽神経　Inferior alveolar n.　701, 733, 781
下歯槽動脈　Inferior alveolar a.　719, 733
下斜筋　Inferior oblique　697
下斜部《頸長筋の》　Inferior oblique part of longus colli　**815**, 817
下尺側側副動脈　Inferior ulnar collateral a.　483
下小脳脚　Inferior cerebellar peduncle　897, 917
下伸筋支帯　Inferior extensor retinaculum　613
下神経幹　Lower trunk　461
下垂体　Pituitary gland　851, 853, 883, 893
下垂体窩　Hypophyseal fossa　685, 761
下膵十二指腸動脈　Inferior pancreaticoduodenal a.　309
下前腸骨棘　Anterior inferior iliac spine　201, 547, 551
下前頭回　Inferior frontal gyrus　873
下前頭溝　Inferior frontal sulcus　873
下双子筋　Gemellus inferior　541, 543, **545**
下側頭回　Inferior temporal gyrus　873, 877
下側頭溝　Inferior temporal sulcus　873
下腿　Lower leg　507

下腿交叉　Crural chiasm　587
下腿骨間膜　Interosseous membrane of leg　539, 559, 583
下腿三頭筋　Triceps surae　585
下大静脈　Inferior vena cava　101, 105, 111, 133, 141, 145, 159, 189, 245, 251, 265, 269, **307**, 321, 325
下大静脈口　Valved orifice of inferior vena cava　151
下大静脈弁　Valve of inferior vena cava　151
下腸間膜静脈　Inferior mesenteric v.　319, 321, 325
下腸間膜動脈　Inferior mesenteric a.　303, 313, 325
下腸間膜動脈神経節　Inferior mesenteric ganglion　331
下直筋　Inferior rectus　697
下直腸神経　Inferior rectal nn.　287, 301, 335
下直腸動脈神経叢　Inferior rectal plexus　335
下椎切痕　Inferior vertebral notch　21
下頭《外側翼突筋の》　Inferior head of lateral pterygoid　693
下頭斜筋　Obliquus capitis inferior　41, **63**, 73
下頭頂小葉　Inferior parietal lobule　873
下橈尺関節　Distal radio-ulnar joint　433
下尿生殖隔膜筋膜　Perineal membrane　225
下鼻甲介　Inferior nasal concha　755, 761
下鼻道　Inferior nasal meatus　763
下腹壁静脈　Inferior epigastric v.　327
下腹壁動脈　Inferior epigastric a.　327
下葉《左肺の》　Inferior lobe of left lung　169, 181
下葉気管支　Inferior lobar bronchi　177
下涙小管　Inferior lacrimal canaliculus　755
下涙点　Inferior lacrimal punctum　755
架橋静脈　Bridging v.　857
蝸牛　Cochlea　707, 769, 777
蝸牛神経　Cochlear n. (CN VIII)　707
顆間窩《大腿骨の》　Intercondylar notch of femur　511, 563
顆間隆起《脛骨の》　Intercondylar eminence of tibia　563

鵞足　Pes anserinus　553, 557
介在ニューロン　Interneuron　919
回外筋　Supinator　407, 409, 413, **425**, 465
回結腸動脈　Ileocolic a.　311
回旋枝《左冠状動脈の》　Circumflex br. of left coronary a.　157, 159
回腸　Ileum　239, 243
回腸口　Ileocecal orifice　257
回腸動脈　Ileal aa.　311
灰白交通枝　Gray ramus communicans　333, 909, 933
海馬　Hippocampus　881
海馬傍回　Parahippocampal gyrus　875, 877
海綿静脈洞　Cavernous sinus　723, 747, 869
解剖学的嗅ぎタバコ入れ　Anatomic snuffbox　503
解剖頸《上腕骨の》　Anatomical neck of humerus　349
外果　Lateral malleolus　**559**, 573, 575, 583, 585, 595, 601
外頸静脈　External jugular v.　477, **721**, 727, 841
外頸動脈　External carotid a.　717
外肛門括約筋　External anal sphincter　225, **235**, 247, 261
外後頭隆起　External occipital protuberance　377, 679, 867
外子宮口　External os of uterus　281
外枝　External br.
—《上喉頭神経の》　External br. of superior laryngeal n.　711, 831
—《副神経の》　External br. of accessory n.(CN XI)　843
外耳孔　External acoustic opening　689
外耳道　External acoustic meatus　769, 771
外精筋膜　External spermatic fascia　295
外節《淡蒼球の》　Lateral segment of globus pallidus　889
外側縁《肩甲骨の》　Lateral border of scapula　389, 393, 397
外側顆　Lateral condyle
—《脛骨の》　Lateral condyle of tibia　581, 583

—《大腿骨の》　Lateral condyle of femur　511, 561, 563
外側顆上稜《上腕骨の》　Lateral supracondylar ridge of humerus　351
外側塊《環椎(第1頸椎)の》　Lateral masses　13
外側脚《浅鼠径輪の》　Lateral crus of superficial inguinal ring　647
外側弓状靱帯　Lateral arcuate lig.　97
外側嗅条　Lateral stria　877, 887
外側胸筋神経　Lateral pectoral nn.　477, 479
外側胸静脈　Lateral thoracic v.　113
外側胸動脈　Lateral thoracic a.　113, 455, 481
外側頸三角部　Lateral cervical resion　835
外側楔状骨　Lateral cuneiform　589
外側広筋　Vastus lateralis　521, 535, **551**, 553, 639, 667, 671
外側後頭側頭回　Lateral occipitotemporal gyrus　875, 877
外側溝　Lateral sulcus　849, 871, 873
外側骨半規管　Lateral semicircular canal　769
外側枝《眼窩上神経の》　Lateral brs. of Supra-orbital n.　725
外側膝蓋支帯　Lateral patellar retinaculum　551
外側膝状体　Lateral geniculate body　885, 931
外側種子骨　Lateral sesamoid　617, 621
外側上顆　Lateral epicondyle
—《上腕骨の》　Lateral epicondyle of humerus　351, 397, 421, 423, 425, 427
—《大腿骨の》　Lateral epicondyle of femur　565, 585
外側上腕筋間中隔　Lateral intermuscular septum of arm　499
外側神経束《腕神経叢の》　Lateral cord of brachial plexus　459, 461, 467
外側唇《粗線の》　Lateral lip of linea aspera　511
外側靱帯　Lateral lig.　689, 691
外側脊髄視床路　Lateral spinothalamic tract　913, 921
外側前腕皮神経　Lateral antebrachial cutaneous n.　467, 485

(かっしゃしんけい)

外側足根動脈　Lateral tarsal a.　663
外側足底静脈　Lateral plantar v.　665
外側足底神経　Lateral plantar n.　633, 657, 665
外側足底動脈　Lateral plantar a.　657, 665
外側側副靭帯
　—《膝関節の》　Lateral collateral lig. of knee　565, 569
　—《肘関節の》　Radial collateral lig. of elbow joint　401, 403
外側大腿回旋動脈の上行枝　Ascending br. of lateral circumflex femoral a.　651
外側大腿筋間中隔　Lateral femoral intermuscular septum　667
外側大腿皮神経　Lateral cutaneous n. of thigh　635, **645**, 647, 651
外側直筋　Lateral rectus　697, 743, 751
外側頭　Lateral head
　—《短母趾屈筋の》　Lateral head of Flexor hallucis brevis　611, 617
　—《腓腹筋の》　Lateral head of Gastrocnemius　529, 573, 575, 585
　—《上腕三頭筋の》　Lateral head of triceps brachii　375, 397, 475, 499
外側頭直筋　Rectus capitis lateralis　815, **817**
外側突起《踵骨隆起の》　Lateral process of calcaneal tuberosity　617, 619
外側半月　Lateral meniscus　567, 569
外側板《翼状突起の》　Lateral plate of pterygoid process　681
外側皮枝　Lateral cutaneous br.
　—《胸大動脈の》　Lateral cutaneous br. of thoracic aorta　67
　—《脊髄神経の》　Lateral cutaneous br. of spinal n.　107
外側皮質脊髄路　Lateral corticospinal tract　919, 923
外側腓腹皮神経　Lateral sural cutaneous n.　659
外側部　Lateral part
　—《小脳の》　Lateral part of cerebellum　903
　—《腟円蓋の》　Lateral part of vaginal fornix　281
外側面《脛骨の》　Lateral surface of tibia　583

外側翼突筋　Lateral pterygoid　691, **693**, 733
外側輪状甲状筋　Lateral crico-thyroid　833
外腸骨静脈　External iliac v.　259
外腸骨動脈　External iliac a.　259, 629
外腸骨リンパ節　External iliac node　329
外椎骨静脈叢　External vertebral venous plexus　867
外転軸　Axis of abduction　539
外転神経　Abducent n.(CN VI)　697, **745**, 751, 895
外尿道括約筋　External urethral sphincter　235
外尿道口　External urethral orifice　283
外腹斜筋　External oblique　77, 205, **211**, 337
外腹斜筋腱膜　External oblique aponeurosis　205, 211, 221, 223, 647
外閉鎖筋　Obturator externus　525, **547**, 637
外肋間筋　External intercostal mm.　45, 87, **91**, 109, 207
角回　Angular gyrus　873
角膜　Cornea　757
顎下三角　Submandibular(digastric)triangle　835
顎下神経節　Submandibular ganglion　789
顎下腺　Submandibular gland　731, **795**, 797, 845
顎下腺管　Submandibular duct　797
顎静脈　Maxillary v.　723
顎舌骨筋　Mylohyoid　805, **809**, 811, 813
顎舌骨筋枝《下歯槽動脈の》　Mylohyoid br. of inferior alveolar a.　719
顎舌骨筋神経　Mylohyoid n.　737
顎舌骨筋線　Mylohyoid line　809
顎舌骨筋縫線　Mylohyoid raphe　811, 813
顎動脈　Maxillary a.　717, 719, 735
顎二腹筋　Digastric　807
　—の後腹　Posterior belly of digastric　705, 799, 801, 803, 807, 809, 811, 813
　—の前腹　Anterior belly of digastric　799, 805, 807, 811, 813
滑車　Trochlea　743
滑車上神経　Supratrochlear n.　699, 725
滑車神経　Trochlear n.(CN IV)　697, **745**, 749, 897

滑車切痕　Trochlear notch　399
肝胃間膜　Hepatogastric lig.　237, 253
肝円索　Round lig. of liver　173, 263
肝冠状間膜　Coronary lig.　263
肝十二指腸間膜　Hepatoduodenal lig.　245, 253
肝静脈　Hepatic vv.　269, 315
肝臓　Liver　171, **263**, 265
　— の右葉, 横隔面　Right lobe of liver, diaphragmatic surface　263
　— の左葉　Left lobe of liver　239
肝鎌状間膜　Falciform lig.　263
冠状静脈口　Valved orifice of coronary sinus　151
冠状静脈洞　Coronary sinus　147, 159
冠状静脈弁　Valve of coronary sinus　151
冠状縫合　Coronal suture　675
間脳　Diencephalon　853, 893
寛骨臼　Acetabulum　233, 509
寛骨臼縁　Acetabular margin　513
寛骨臼蓋　Acetabular roof　551
幹神経節　Ganglion of sympathetic trunk　909
関節円板　Articular disc
　—《顎関節の》　Articular disc of temporomandibular joint　693
　—《下橈尺関節の》　Articular disc of distal radio-ulnar joint　433
　—《胸鎖関節の》　Articular disc of sternoclavicular joint　355
関節下結節　Infraglenoid tubercle　345, 397
関節窩《肩甲骨の》　Glenoid cavity of scapula　345, 357, 361, 381
関節枝《脊髄神経の》　Articular br. of spinal n.　71
関節上結節《肩甲骨の》　Supraglenoid tubercle of scapula　345, 395
関節突起　Condylar process　779
関節包　Joint capsule
　—, 関節上腕靱帯　Joint capsule, glenohumeral ligs.　359
　—《顎関節の》　Joint capsule of temporomandibular joint　689, 691
環軸関節　Atlantoaxial joint　27
環椎 (第 1 頸椎)　Atlas (C1)　**5**, 29, 41, 57, 63, 385, 815, 817, 89
　— の後弓　Posterior arch of atlas　11

環椎後頭関節　Atlanto-occipital joint　27
岩様部《側頭骨の》　Petrous part of temporal bone　769, 777
眼窩下孔　Infra-orbital foramen　677, 701, 781
眼窩下神経　Infra-orbital n.　701, 725, **739**, 781
眼窩下動脈　Infra-orbital a.　719, 725
眼窩回　Orbital gyri　877
眼窩隔膜　Orbital septum　753
眼窩溝　Orbital sulci　877
眼窩上縁　Supra-orbital margin　677
眼窩上神経　Supra-orbital n.　699, 749
眼窩上動脈　Supra-orbital aa.　749
眼窩板《篩骨の》　Orbital plate of ethmoid bone　741
眼窩部　Orbital part
　—《下前頭回の》　Orbital part of inferior frontal gyrus　873
　—《涙腺の》　Orbital part of lacrimal gland　755
眼窩面《頰骨の》　Orbital surface of zygomatic bone　741
眼角静脈　Angular v.　723, 725
眼角動脈　Angular a.　725
眼瞼部《眼輪筋の》　Palpebral part of orbicularis oculi　753
眼神経　Ophthalmic n. (CN V₁)　699, 745
眼輪筋　Orbicularis oculi　687
顔面横動脈　Transverse facial a.　725
顔面静脈　Facial v.　**723**, 725, 731, 795, 843
顔面神経　Facial n. (CN VII)　703, **705**, 729, 775, 777, 787
　— の耳下腺神経叢　Parotid plexus of facial n. (CN VII)　729
顔面動脈　Facial a.　717, 725, 731, 795, 843

き

キヌタ骨　Incus　775
気管　Trachea　131, 133, 167, 823, 825
気管支縦隔リンパ本幹　Bronchomediastinal trunk　127
気管支肺リンパ節　Bronchopulmonary node　191

(きょうようきんまくのせんよう) 975

気管前葉《頸筋膜の》 Pretracheal layer of cervical fascia 825
気管軟骨 Tracheal cartilages 183
気管分岐部 Tracheal bifurcation 183
気管傍リンパ節 Paratracheal node 191
奇静脈 Azygos v. 69, 111, **125**, 127, 135, 315
亀頭冠 Corona of glans 291
脚間窩 Interpeduncular fossa 899
弓状線 Arcuate line 197, 215
弓状動脈 Arcuate a.
— 《腎臓の》 Arcuate a. of kidney 305
— 《足背動脈の》 Arcuate a. 663
球海綿体筋 Bulbospongiosus 225, **235**, 285, 291, 301
球形嚢 Saccule 707
球状核 Globose nuclei 903
嗅球 Olfactory bulb (CN I) 695, 767, 851, 877
嗅溝 Olfactory sulcus 877
嗅索 Olfactory tract 695, 851, 877
嗅神経糸 Olfactory nn. 695, 765
嗅傍野 Paraolfactory area 875
距骨 Talus 595, 597, 603, 615
距骨下関節 Subtalar (talocalcaneal) joint 593, 595
—, 後区 (距踵関節) Posterior compartment of subtalar joint 597
—, 前区 (距踵舟関節) Anterior compartment of subtalar joint 597
距骨滑車の上面 Superior trochlear surface 615
距骨後突起 Posterior process of talus 623
距骨頭 Head of talus 589
距舟関節 Talonavicular joint 593
距腿関節 Ankle joint 593, 595
共通頭 Common head
— 《尺側手根伸筋の》 Common head of carpi ulnaris 423
— 《小指伸筋の》 Common head of digiti minimi 423
— 《前腕屈筋の》 Common head of flexors 405, 415, 417
— 《[総] 指伸筋の》 Common head of extensor digitorum 423
— 《半腱様筋の》 Common head of semitendinosus 555
胸横筋 Transversus thoracis 87, **93**

胸郭下口 Inferior thoracic aperture 81
胸郭上口 Superior thoracic aperture 81
胸管 Thoracic duct 127, 191, 839
胸棘筋 Spinalis thoracis 57
胸筋腋窩リンパ節 Pectoral axillary lymph node 115
胸筋筋膜 Pectoral fascia 117
胸肩峰動脈 Thoraco-acromial a. 477, 479
胸骨 Sternum 83, 95, 215, 379, 387
胸骨角 Sternal angle of sternum 85, 193
胸骨関節面 Sternal facet 343
胸骨甲状筋 Sternothyroid 805, **811**, 813, 843
胸骨舌骨筋 Sternohyoid 805, **811**, 813
胸骨体 Body of sternum 85, 93, 167
胸骨頭《胸鎖乳突筋の》 Sternal head of sternocleidomastoid 845
胸骨柄 Manubrium of sternum 85, 87, 93, 355
胸鎖関節 Sternoclavicular joint 353
胸鎖乳突筋 Sternocleidomastoid 41, 363, 379, 713, 727, 795, 825, 841
— の胸骨頭 Sternal head of sternocleidomastoid 379
— の鎖骨頭 Clavicular head of sternocleidomastoid 379, 845
胸最長筋 Longissimus thoracis 47, **49**
胸腺 Thymus 131
胸大動脈 Thoracic aorta 137, 169
胸大動脈 Thoracic aorta 67, **123**, 137, 169
胸大動脈神経叢 Thoracic aortic plexus 163
胸腸肋筋 Iliocostalis thoracis 47, 49
胸内筋膜 Endothoracic fascia 109, 111
胸背神経 Thoracodorsal n. 481
胸背動脈 Thoracodorsal a. 103, 455, 481
胸半棘筋 Semispinalis thoracis 59, **61**
胸部《食道の》 Thoracic part of esophagus 119, 129, **133**
胸膜頂 Cervical pleura 175
胸腰筋膜 Thoracolumbar fascia 65, 75, 393, 539
— の浅葉 Superficial layer of thoracolumbar fascia 39, 43

胸肋関節　Sternocostal joint　355
胸肋部《大胸筋の》　Sternocostal part of pectoralis major　363
強膜　Sclera　757
橋　Pons　851, 853, 893, 895, 901
頬筋　Buccinator　795, 799
頬筋枝　Buccal brs.　703
—《顔面神経の》　Buccal brs. of facial n.　729
頬骨　Zygomatic bone　677, 845
頬骨弓　Zygomatic arch　675, 681, 689, 691
頬骨枝《顔面神経の》　Zygomatic brs. of facial n.　703
頬骨神経　Zygomatic n.　701
頬神経　Buccal n.　701, 733, 781
頬動脈　Buccal a.　719, 733
棘下窩　Infraspinous fossa　347
棘下筋　Infraspinatus　373, 375, **389**, 475
棘間靱帯　Interspinous ligs.　33
棘筋　Spinalis　43, 45
棘上窩　Supraspinous fossa　347
棘上筋　Supraspinatus　369, 373, 375, **389**, 473
— の腱　Tendon of supraspinatus　361
棘上靱帯　Supraspinous lig.　29, 31, 33
棘突起　Spinous process　5, 9, **11**, 17, 19, 21, 41, 51, 53, 55, 57, 59, 61, 63
近位指節間（PIP）関節　Proximal interphalangeal joint　433, 503
筋　Muscle　919
筋横隔動脈　Musculophrenic a.　103
筋三角　Muscular triangle　835
筋層《膀胱の》　Muscular coat of urinary bladder　277
筋突起　Coronoid process　691, 731, 779, 809
筋皮神経　Musculocutaneous n.　**467**, 485, 499

く

クーパー靱帯（乳房提靱帯）　Cooper's (suspensory) ligs. of breast　117
クモ膜下腔　Subarachnoid space　31, 907
クモ膜顆粒　Arachnoid granulations　855, 861
クモ膜絨毛　Arachnoid villi　855
区域気管支　Segmental bronchus　185
空腸動脈　Jejunal aa.　311
屈筋支帯　Flexor retinaculum　435, **437**, 487, 489, 657

け

外科頸《上腕骨の》　Surgical neck of humerus　351
茎状突起　Styloid process　689, 769
—《尺骨の》　Ulnar styloid process　429
—《橈骨の》　Radial styloid process　399, 421, 431
茎突咽頭筋　Stylopharyngeus　709, 801
茎突舌筋　Styloglossus　785
茎突舌骨筋　Stylohyoid　705, 799, 801, **807**, 809, 811, 813
茎乳突孔　Stylomastoid foramen　705
脛骨　Tibia　507, 539, 555, 557, 571, 595, 671
— の外側面　Lateral surface of tibia　583
— の後面　Posterior surface of tibia　587
— の内側顆　Medial condyle of tibia　555, 561, 563, 581
脛骨神経　Tibial n.　633, 643, 655, 657, 669
脛骨粗面　Tibial tuberosity　547, 559, 561, 581
脛腓関節　Tibiofibular joint　559, 569
頸横神経　Transverse cervical n.　715, 821, 841
頸横動脈　Transverse cervical a.　839
頸棘間筋　Interspinales cervicis　57
頸棘筋　Spinalis cervicis　57
頸後横突間筋　Posterior cervical intertransversarii　51, **53**, 55
頸最長筋　Longissimus cervicis　47, **49**
頸枝《顔面神経の》　Cervical br.　703
頸静脈孔　Jugular foramen　681, 713, 869
頸心臓枝《迷走神経の》　Cervical cardiac brs.　711
頸神経叢　Cervical plexus　729
頸神経ワナ　Ansa cervicalis　843
頸切痕　Jugular notch　81, 85, 193, 845

頸長筋　Longus colli　815，817
頸腸肋筋　Iliocostalis cervicis　47，49
頸動脈管　Carotid canal　681
頸動脈三角　Carotid triangle　835
頸動脈洞　Carotid sinus　709
頸動脈洞枝　Carotid br.　709
頸半棘筋　Semispinalis cervicis　59，61
頸板状筋　Splenius cervicis　43，51，53，55
頸膨大　Cervical enlargement　905
鶏冠　Crista galli　761
血管冠　Vasocorona　925
結節間滑液鞘　Intertubercular synovial sheath　359
結節間溝《上腕骨の》　Intertubercular sulcus of humerus　349，357，387，395
結腸辺縁動脈　Marginal a.　311
結腸傍溝　Paracolic gutter　245
結腸膨起　Haustra of colon　257
楔状束　Cuneate fasciculus　897，915，921
楔状束核　Cuneate nucleus　897，915
楔状束結節　Cuneate tubercle　897
楔前部　Precuneus　875
楔部　Cuneus　875
月状溝　Lunate sulcus　873
月状骨　Lunate　431，447
肩関節（肩甲上腕関節）　Glenohumeral joint　353
肩甲下窩　Subscapular fossa　345
肩甲下筋　Subscapularis　365，367，369，389
肩甲下動脈　Subscapular a.　481
肩甲回旋動脈　Circumflex scapular a.　475，481
肩甲挙筋　Levator scapulae　39，373，385
肩甲胸郭関節　Scapulothoracic joint　353
肩甲棘　Spine of scapula　7，39，347，377，385，391，397，473
肩甲棘部，三角筋の　Spinal part of deltoid　391
肩甲骨　Scapula　**345**，347，381，391，393
　— の下角　Inferior scapular angle　7
　— の後面　Posterior surface of scapula　385，397

— の内側縁　Medial border of scapula　373
— の肋骨面　Costal surface of scapula，395
肩甲骨部《広背筋の》　Scapular part of latissimus dorsi　393
肩甲鎖骨三角　Omoclavicular triangle　835
肩甲上神経　Suprascapular n.　461，473，475
肩甲上動脈　Suprascapular a.　473，475，479
肩甲切痕　Scapular notch　347
肩甲舌骨筋　Omohyoid　379，805，811，**813**
— の下腹　Inferior belly of omohyoid　805，811，**813**
— の上腹　Superior belly of omohyoid　805，811，**813**
肩鎖関節　Acromioclavicular joint　353
肩鎖靱帯　Acromioclavicular lig.　353，359
肩峰　Acromion　345，347，357，361，377，379，381，383，385，387，389，391，397
肩峰下包　Subacromial bursa　361
肩峰関節面　Acromial facet　343
肩峰端《鎖骨の》　Acromial end of clavicle　343
肩峰部《三角筋の》　Acromial part of deltoid　391
剣状突起《胸骨の》　Xiphoid process of sternum　85，93，99，193，207，211，213，215，217，219
腱画　Tendinous intersections　209，217，337
腱間結合《[総]指伸筋の》　Intertendinous connections of extensor digitorum　423
腱索　Tendinous cords　153
腱鞘　Tendon sheath　613
腱中心《横隔膜の》　Central tendon of diaphragm　95，99
瞼板腺　Tarsal glands　753

こ

呼吸細気管支　Respiratory bronchiole　185，187

固有肝動脈　Hepatic a. proper　245, 265, 309
固有掌側指神経　Proper palmar digital nn. 471, 489
固有掌側指動脈　Proper palmar digital aa. 489
固有底側趾神経　Proper plantar digital nn. 665
固有底側趾動脈　Proper plantar digital aa. 665
固有卵巣索　Lig. of ovary　279
鼓索神経　Chorda tympani　705, 775
鼓膜　Tympanic membrane　775
鼓膜張筋　Tensor tympani　769, 775
口蓋咽頭弓　Palatopharyngeal arch　783, 793
口蓋咽頭筋　Palatopharyngeus　803
口蓋骨　Palatine bone　681
口蓋垂　Uvula　773, 793
口蓋舌弓　Palatoglossal arch　783, 793
口蓋舌筋　Palatoglossus　785
口蓋突起《上顎骨の》　Palatine process of maxilla　681, 759
口蓋帆　Soft palate　791, 793
口蓋帆挙筋　Levator veli palatini　773
口蓋帆張筋　Tensor veli palatini　737, 773
口蓋帆張筋神経　N. to tensor veli palatini　737
口蓋扁桃　Palatine tonsil　783
口角下制筋　Depressor anguli oris　687
口輪筋　Orbicularis oris　687
広背筋　Latissimus dorsi　39, 77, 367, 371, **393**, 483
— の肩甲骨部　Scapular part of latissimus dorsi　393
— の腸骨部　Iliac part of latissimus dorsi　393
— の椎骨部　Vertebral part of latissimus dorsi　393
甲状頸動脈　Thyrocervical trunk　479, 819, 837, 839
甲状舌骨筋　Thyrohyoid　805, 807, 811, **813**, 831
甲状舌骨靱帯　Thyrohyoid lig.　829
甲状舌骨膜　Thyrohyoid membrane　827
甲状腺　Thyroid gland　825
甲状腺峡部　Isthmus of thyroid gland　823
甲状軟骨　Thyroid cartilage　183, 805, 811, 813, 823, 827, 845
甲状披裂筋　Thyro-arytenoid　833
交感神経幹　Sympathetic trunk　129, 137, 333, 803, 839
—, 胸神経節　Sympathetic trunk, thoracic ganglion　135
—, 中頸神経節　Sympathetic trunk, middle cervical ganglion　129
交感神経幹神経節　Sympathetic ganglion　71, 107, 933
肛門挙筋　Levator ani　225, 227, **231**, 249, 259, 285
肛門挙筋腱弓　Tendinous arch of levator ani　229, 231
肛門櫛（白帯）　Anal pecten（white zone）　261
肛門柱　Anal columns　261
肛門尾骨靱帯　Anococcygeal lig.　227, 235
肛門裂孔　Anal aperture　231
岬角《仙骨の》　Promontory　3, **23**, 199, 203, 527, 547
後陰唇交連　Posterior commissure　283
後陰唇神経　Posterior labial nn.　287
後陰嚢神経　Posterior scrotal nn.　301
後縁《尺骨の》　Posterior border of ulna　425
後下行枝　Posterior interventricular br.　159
後角《脊髄の》　Posterior horn of spinal cord　925
後弓《環椎（第1頸椎）の》　Posterior arch of atlas　13
後距腓靱帯　Posterior talofibular lig.　603
後脛骨筋　Tibialis posterior　579, **587**, 655, 657, 669
— の腱　Tibialis posterior tendon　577, 587, 611
後脛骨静脈　Posterior tibial v.　669
後脛骨動脈　Posterior tibial a.　**631**, 655, 657, 669
後脛腓靱帯　Posterior tibiofibular lig.　603
後結節《環椎（第1頸椎）の》　Posterior tubercle of atlas　13, 63
後結節間束　Posterior internodal bundles　161
後交通動脈　Posterior communicating a.　865

(こうじょうとっき《しゃくこつの》) 979

後骨間神経 Posterior interosseous n. 501
後骨間動脈 Posterior interosseous a. 455
後根《脊髄神経の》 Dorsal root of spinal n. 107, 907
後根糸 Posterior rootlets 909
後根静脈 Posterior radicular v. 927
後索《脊髄の》 Posterior funiculus of spinal cord 911
後枝 Posterior ramus
—《胸大動脈の》 Posterior ramus of thoracic aorta 67
—《脊髄神経の》 Posterior ramus of spinal n. 71, 107, 909
後篩骨神経 Posterior ethmoidal n. 699, 749
後篩骨洞の開口部 Orifices of posterior ethmoidal cells 763
後篩骨動脈 Posterior ethmoidal a. 749
後耳介神経 Posterior auricular n. 703, 705
後耳介動脈 Posterior auricular a. 717
後室間枝 Posterior interventricular br. 159
後室間静脈 Posterior interventricular v. 159
後斜角筋 Posterior scalene **89**, 815, 817
後十字靱帯 Posterior cruciate lig. 567, 569
後縦隔 Posterior mediastinum 119
後縦靱帯 Posterior longitudinal lig. 31, 33, 35, **37**
後上歯槽枝《上歯槽神経の》 Posterior superior alveolar brs. of superior alveolar nn. 739
後上歯槽動脈 Posterior superior alveolar aa. 719
後上腕回旋動脈 Posterior circumflex humeral a. 455, 475
後神経束 Posterior cord 461, 463
後髄節動脈 Posterior segmental medullary a. 925
後脊髄小脳路 Posterior spinocerebellar tract 917, 921
後脊髄静脈 Posterior spinal v. 927
後脊髄動脈 Posterior spinal aa. 925
後仙腸靱帯 Posterior sacro-iliac ligs. 519
後尖《右房室弁の》 Posterior cusp of right atrioventricular valve 155
後[前腕]骨間神経 Posterior interosseous n. 465

後前腕皮神経 Posterior antebrachial cutaneous n. 465
後大腿皮神経 Posterior femoral cutaneous n. 633, 645, 653
後大脳動脈 Posterior cerebral a. 865
後中心傍回 Posterior paracentral gyrus 875
後柱 Posterior column 911
後殿筋線 Posterior gluteal line 543, 545
後頭下神経 Suboccipital n. 73
後頭顆 Occipital condyle 681
後頭蓋窩 Posterior cranial fossa 683
後頭極 Occipital pole 873
後頭骨 Occipital bone 679
後頭側頭溝 Occipitotemporal sulcus 877
後頭頂野 Posterior parietal cortex 929
後頭動脈 Occipital a. 73, 717
後頭葉 Occipital lobe 849, 871
後内椎骨静脈叢 Posterior internal vertebral venous plexus 69, 907
後乳頭筋 Posterior papillary m. 153
後半月弁《大動脈弁の》 Posterior semilunar cusp of aortic valve 155
後鼻孔 Choana 759
後部《腕神経叢の》 Posterior divisions of brachial plexus 459
後面 Posterior surface
—《脛骨の》 Posterior surface of tibia 587
—《腓骨の》 Posterior surface of fibula 587
後輪状披裂筋 Posterior crico-arytenoid 803, 833
虹彩 Iris 757
咬筋 Masseter 687, **689**, 691, 727, 735, 795
— の深部 Deep part of masseter **689**, 693
— の浅部 Superficial part of masseter **689**, 693
鉤《海馬傍回の》 Uncus of parahippocampal gyrus 875, 877
鉤状突起
—《頸椎の》 Uncinate process of cervical vertebrae 11
—《尺骨の》 Coronoid process of ulna 399, 419

鉤状突起《膵臓の》 Uncinate process of pancreas 271
鉤椎関節 Uncovertebral joint 27
鉤突窩《上腕骨の》 Coronoid fossa 403
喉頭蓋 Epiglottis 783, 791, 827, 829, 833
喉頭隆起 Laryngeal prominence 827
硬口蓋 Hard palate 793
硬膜 Dura mater 855, 857
硬膜枝《脊髄神経の》 Meningeal br. of spinal n. 909
項靱帯 Nuchal lig. 29, 31, 377
溝静脈 Sulcal v. 927
溝動脈 Sulcal a. 925
黒質 Substantia nigra 891, 899
骨間距踵靱帯 Interosseous talocalcanean lig. 597
骨間筋《手の》 Interossei of hand 471
骨盤内臓神経 Pelvic splanchnic nn. 335

さ

3次ニューロン 3rd neuron 913
― の軸索 Axon of 3rd neuron 915
左胃静脈 Left gastric v. 319, 321
左胃大網静脈 Left gastro-omental v. 319, 321
左胃大網動脈 Left gastro-omental a. 321
左胃動脈 Left gastric a. 307, 321
左横隔神経 Left phrenic n. 137
左下横隔動脈 Left inferior phrenic a. 303, 317
左下直腸動脈 Left inferior rectal a. 325
左下腹神経 Left hypogastric n. 335
左下葉気管支 Left inferior lobar bronchus 183
左外側大動脈リンパ節 Left lateral aortic node 329
左冠状動脈 Left coronary a. 157
左気管支縦隔リンパ本幹 Left bronchomediastinal trunk 191
左結腸曲 Left colic flexure 257
左結腸動脈 Left colic a. 313
左鎖骨下静脈 Left subclavian v. 133
左鎖骨下動脈 Left subclavian a. 123, 129, 133, 819
左主気管支 Left main bronchus 121, 123, 137, **183**

左心耳 Left auricle 145
左心室 Left ventricle 143, **147**, 165
左心房 Left atrium 139, **147**, 153, 165, 169, 173
左腎静脈 Left renal v. 311, 317
左腎動脈 Left renal a. 303, 305, 317
左精巣静脈 Left testicular v. 317
左精巣動脈 Left testicular a. 317
左総頸動脈 Left common carotid a. 123, 145
左中直腸動脈 Left middle rectal a. 325
左内陰部静脈 Left internal pudendal v. 323
左内陰部動脈 Left internal pudendal a. 323
左肺静脈 Left pulmonary vv. 133, 147
左肺動脈 Left pulmonary a. 137, 147
左反回神経 Left recurrent laryngeal n. 129, 163, **711**, 803
左半月弁《大動脈弁の》 Left semilunar cusp of aortic valve 155
左副腎静脈 Left suprarenal v. 273, 317
左閉鎖動脈 Left obturator a. 325
左房室弁 Left atrioventricular valve 153
左迷走神経 Left vagus n. 129, 137
左腰リンパ本幹 Left lumbar trunk 127
左卵巣静脈 Left ovarian v. 317
左卵巣動脈 Left ovarian a. 303, 317
左腕頭静脈 Left brachiocephalic v. 127, 143, 177, **721**
鎖骨 Clavicle 343, 355, 357, 379, 383, 385, 387, 391
― の胸骨端 Sternal end of clavicle 193
鎖骨下筋 Subclavius 365, **383**
鎖骨下筋溝 Groove for subclavius 343
鎖骨下静脈 Subclavian v. 113, **479**, 839
鎖骨下動脈 Subclavian a. 103, 113, **461**, 479, 711, 837, 839
鎖骨胸筋筋膜 Clavipectoral fascia 477
鎖骨上神経 Supraclavicular nn. **473**, 477, 715, 821, 841
鎖骨上リンパ節 Supraclavicular node 115
鎖骨切痕 Clavicular notch 81, 85
鎖骨体 Shaft of clavicle 343
鎖骨中線 Midclavicular line (MCL) 193
鎖骨頭《胸鎖乳突筋の》 Clavicular head of sternocleidomastoid 379, 845

鎖骨部　Clavicular part
― 《大胸筋の》　Clavicular part of pectoralis major　363
― 《三角筋の》　Clavicular part of deltoid　391
坐骨　Ischium　555
坐骨海綿体筋　Ischiocavernosus　225, **235**, 285, 291
坐骨棘　Ischial spine　**197**, 199, 203, 227, 229, 235, 509, 515, 537, 543, 545
坐骨結節　Ischial tuberosity　197, 233, 509, **515**, 531, 541, 557
坐骨肛門窩(坐骨直腸窩)　Ischio-anal fossa　259
坐骨枝　Ramus of ischium　197, 233
坐骨神経　Sciatic n.　**633**, 635, 641, 653, 667
坐骨大腿靱帯　Ischiofemoral lig.　519
細気管支　Bronchiole　185
細胞体　Cell body
― ，1次ニューロンの　Cell body of 1st neuron　917
― ，2次ニューロンの　Cell body of 2nd neuron　917
最上胸動脈　Superior thoracic a.　103, 481
最長筋　Longissimus　43
最内肋間筋　Innermost intercostal m.　87
載距突起　Sustentaculum tali　591, 595, 599, 623
臍　Umbilicus　171, 205
臍静脈　Umbilical v.　171
臍動脈　Umbilical a.　171
― の遺残(内側臍索)　Obliterated umbilical aa.(medial umbilical ligs.)　173
臍輪　Umbilical ring　211
三角筋　Deltoid　361, 363, 369, 371, **391**, 463, 477
― の肩甲棘部　Spinal part of deltoid　391
― の肩峰部　Acromial part of deltoid　391
― の鎖骨部　Clavicular part of deltoid　391
三角筋下包　Subdeltoid bursa　361
三角筋粗面《上腕骨の》　Deltoid tuberosity of humerus　349, 391

三角骨　Triquetrum　429, 447
三角靱帯　Deltoid lig.　603
三角部《下前頭回の》　Triangular part of inferior frontal gyrus　873
三叉神経　Trigeminal n.(CN V)　701, 895
― ，下顎神経　Mandibular division of trigeminal n.　715
― ，眼神経　Ophthalmic division of trigeminal n.　715
― ，上顎神経　Maxillary division of trigeminal n.　715
三叉神経節　Trigeminal ganglion　747

し

子宮　Uterus　249
子宮間膜　Mesometrium　279
子宮筋層　Myometrium　281
子宮頸　Cervix of uterus　275
子宮頸管　Cervical canal　281
子宮静脈　uterine v.　279
子宮静脈叢　Uterine venous plexus　323
子宮底　Fundus of uterus　275, 279
子宮動脈　uterine a.　279
四丘体板　Quadrigeminal plate　883
矢状縫合　Sagittal suture　679
指骨(指節骨)　Phalanges　341
指背腱膜　Dorsal digital expansion　411, 423
脂肪被膜《腎臓の》　Perirenal fat capsule of kidney　273
視蓋脊髄路　Tectospinal tract　923
視交叉　Optic chiasm(CN II)　699, 747, 887, **931**
視索　Optic tract　889, 931
視床　Thalamus　883, 889, 913, 915
視床下核　Subthalamic nucleus　891
視床下部　Hypothalamus　883
視床外側腹側核群　Ventrolateral thalamic nuclei　891
視床室傍核群　Paraventricular nuclei　891
視床髄条　Stria medullaris of thalamus　883
視床前核群　Anterior thalamic nuclei　891
視床枕　Pulvinar　885
視床内側核群　Medial thalamic nuclei　891
視床ヒモ　Tenia thalami　885
視神経　Optic n.(CN II)　699, **745**, 747, 751, 757, 851, 931

視神経管　Optic canal　685, 741
視神経乳頭(視神経円板)　Optic disk　757
視放線　Optic radiation　879, 931
歯状回　Dentate gyrus　875, 881
歯状核　Dentate nucleus　903
歯突起《軸椎(第2頸椎)の》　Dens of axis (C2)　15, 29
歯突起窩　Facet for dens　13
篩骨胞　Ethmoid bulla　763
篩板　Cribriform plate　685, 695, 763
示指伸筋　Extensor indicis　413, **427**
　— の腱　Extensor indicis tendon　443
耳下腺　Parotid gland　795
耳下腺管　Parotid duct　725, 727, 795
耳介側頭神経　Auriculotemporal n.　701, 727, **737**, 781
耳管　Pharyngotympanic (auditory) tube　769
耳管咽頭筋　Salpingopharyngeus　773
耳管咽頭口　Pharyngeal opening of auditory tube　791
耳管骨部　Pharyngotympanic tube, bony part　773
耳管扁桃　tonsilla tubaria　791
耳甲介　Concha of auricle　771
耳甲介舟　Cymba conchae　771
耳珠　Tragus　771
耳状面《仙骨の》　Auricular surface of sacrum　25
耳神経節　Otic ganglion　737
耳垂　Lobule of auricle　771
耳輪　Helix　771
自由ヒモ　Taeniae coli　257
軸索　Axon
　—, 1次ニューロンの　Axon of 1st neuron　915
　—, 2次ニューロンの　Axon of 2nd neuron　915
　—, 3次ニューロンの　Axon of 3rd neuron　915
軸椎(第2頸椎)　Axis(C2)　**5**, 11, 29, 41, 57, 63, 385, 89
　— の歯突起　Dens of axis(C2)　791
室間孔　Interventricular foramen　863
室頂核　Fastigial nucleus　903
膝窩　Posterior part of knee　529
膝窩筋　Popliteus　**555**, 557, 577, 579
膝窩静脈　Popliteal v.　653, 655

膝窩動脈　Popliteal a.　629, **631**, 653, 655
膝蓋下枝《伏在神経の》　Infrapatellar br. of saphenous n.　639
膝蓋骨　Patella　507, 547, 561, 567, 581, 583
膝蓋靱帯　Patellar lig.　523, 551, 565, 569
膝蓋大腿関節　Femoropatellar joint　565
膝神経節　Geniculate ganglion　705, 777
櫛状筋　Pectinate mm.　151
射精管　Ejaculatory duct　299
斜台　Clivus　685
斜頭《母趾内転筋の》　Oblique head of adductor hallucis　611, 621
斜裂　Oblique fissure
　—《右肺の》　Oblique fissure of right lung　179
　—《左肺の》　Oblique fissure of left lung　181
尺骨　Ulna　341, 397, 421, 423, 425, 427, 449, 451, 453, 501
　— の茎状突起　Ulnar styloid process　429, 503
尺骨神経　Ulnar n.　**471**, 483, 485, 487, 491, 499, 501
　— の掌枝　Palmar br. of ulnar n.　495
　— の背側枝　Dorsal br. of ulnar n.　497
尺骨神経溝《上腕骨の》　Ulnar groove of humerus　351
尺骨粗面　Tuberosity of ulna　419
　—（上腕筋の停止腱）　Tuberosity of ulna (brachialis tendon of insertion)　395
尺骨動脈　Ulnar a.　455, 485, 487, 491, 501
尺側手根屈筋　Flexor carpi ulnaris　405, 411, **417**, 435, 471, 501
尺側手根伸筋　Extensor carpi ulnaris　411, **423**, 443, 501
尺側皮静脈　Basilic v.　457
手根骨　Carpal bones　341
手根中央関節　Midcarpal joint　433
手掌腱膜　Palmar aponeurosis　415, 435
手背静脈網《手の》　Dorsal venous network of hand　457
種子骨　Sesamoid bones　591, 595
受容野　Receptive field　913, 917
　—《下肢の》　Receptive field of leg　915

(しょうこつりゅうき) 983

― 《上肢の》 Receptive field of arm 915
― 1 Receptive field 1 917
― 2 Receptive field 2 917
舟状窩 Scaphoid fossa 771
舟状骨
― 《足の》 Navicular **589**, 591, 595, 597, 599, 615
― 《手の》 Scaphoid **429**, 433, 445, 487, 493
終脳 Telencephalon 853
終板傍回 Paraterminal gyrus 875
終末細気管支 Terminal bronchiole 185
十二指腸 Duodenum 253, **255**, 313
― の下行部 Descending part of duodenum 255
― の上部 Superior part of duodenum 243
― の水平部 Horizontal part of duodenum 245, 255
十二指腸空腸曲 Duodenojejunal flexure 243
縦隔胸膜 Mediastinal part of parietal pleura 131, 175
鋤骨 Vomer 759
小陰唇 Labium minus 283
小円筋 Teres minor 375, **389**, 463, 475
小胸筋 Pectoralis minor 365, **383**, 479
小結節《上腕骨の》 Lesser tubercle of humerus 349, 357, 387
小口蓋神経 Lesser palatine nn. 767
小後頭神経 Lesser occipital n. 715, 821, 841
小後頭直筋 Rectus capitis posterior minor 63
小坐骨孔 Lesser sciatic foramen 203, 649
小指外転筋 Abductor digiti minimi 437, **447**
小指球 Hypothenar eminence 503
小指伸筋 Extensor digiti minimi **423**, 501
小指対立筋 Opponens digiti minimi 441, **447**
小趾外転筋 Abductor digiti minimi 607, **619**
小趾対立筋 Opponens digiti minimi 619

小十二指腸乳頭 Minor duodenal papilla 255
小心臓静脈 Small cardiac v. 159
小錐体神経 Lesser petrosal n. 737, 777
小舌《肺の》 Lingula of lung 181
小節 Nodule 901
小帯回 Fasciolar gyrus 875
小転子《大腿骨の》 Lesser trochanter of femur 219, 511, 513, 537, 541, 543, 545, 549, 553, 557
小殿筋 Gluteus minimus 531, 543, 545, 653
小内転筋 Adductor minimus 547
小脳 Cerebellum 849, 851, 853, 893
小脳延髄槽 Cerebellomedullary cistern 861
小脳虫部 Vermis of cerebellum 903
小脳テント Tentorium cerebelli 859, 869
小伏在静脈 Short saphenous v. 645
小網 Lesser omentum 253
小翼《蝶形骨の》 Lesser wing of sphenoid 683
小菱形筋 Rhomboid minor 373, **385**
小菱形骨 Trapezoid 429, 449, 451, 453
小弯《胃の》 Lesser curvature of stomach 253
松果体 Pineal gland 883, 885
掌枝《尺骨神経の》 Palmar br. of ulnar n. 495
掌側指神経 Palmar digital nn. 495
― の背側枝 Dorsal brs. of palmar digital nn. 497
掌側手根靱帯 Palmar carpal lig. 487, 489
掌側中手動脈 Palmar metacarpal aa. 491
硝子体 Vitreous body 757
漿膜性心膜 Serous pericardium
― の臓側板 Visceral layer of serous pericardium 139
― の壁側板 Parietal layer of serous pericardium 139
踵骨 Calcaneus 575, 583, 591, 597, 615
踵骨腱 Calcaneal (Achilles') tendon 573, 575, 585, 657
踵骨隆起 Calcaneal tuberosity 585, 605, 617, 619, 623

踵腓靱帯　Calcaneofibular lig.　603
上咽頭収縮筋　Superior constrictor　799, 801
上腋窩リンパ節　Apical axillary node　115
上外側上腕皮神経　Superior lateral brachial cutaneous n.　473
上角《肩甲骨の》　Superior angle of scapula　345, 385
上顎骨　Maxilla　675, 677
上顎神経　Maxillary n.(CN V₂)　701, **739**, 781
上顎洞　Maxillary sinus　741
上顎洞裂孔　Maxillary hiatus　763
上関節突起　Superior articular process　9, 21
上関節面
　―《脛骨の》　Superior articular surface of tibia　559, 561
　―《仙骨の》　Superior articular facet of sacrum　25
　―《椎骨の》　Superior articular facet of vertebra　17, 19, 21, 37
上眼窩裂　Superior orbital fissure　741
上眼瞼　Upper eyelid　753
上眼瞼挙筋　Levator palpebrae superioris　697, **743**, 749, 753
上眼静脈　Superior ophthalmic v.　723, 751, 869
上気管気管支リンパ節　Superior tracheobronchial node　191
上丘《蓋板(四丘体板)の》　Superior colliculi of tectal(quadrigeminal) plate　897
上下腹神経叢　Superior hypogastric plexus　331, 335
上頸神経節　Superior cervical ganglion　731, 843
上肩甲横靱帯　Superior transverse scapular lig.　359
上肩甲下神経　Upper subscapular n.　481
上瞼板　Superior tarsus　753
上瞼板筋　Superior tarsal m.　753
上甲状腺静脈　Superior thyroid v.　721
上甲状腺動脈　Superior thyroid a.　819, 837, 843
上行咽頭動脈　Ascending pharyngeal a.　819

上行結腸　Ascending colon　239, 245, 257
上行大動脈　Ascending aorta　121, **123**, 139, 141, 145, 165, 189
上行腰静脈　Ascending lumbar v.　315
上後鋸筋　Serratus posterior superior　65
上後腸骨棘　Posterior superior iliac spine　515, 519, 649
上喉頭静脈　Superior laryngeal v.　833
上喉頭神経　Superior laryngeal n.　711
上喉頭動脈　Superior laryngeal a.　819, 833
上項線　Superior nuchal line　41, 51, 63, 377, 679
上根《頸神経ワナの》　Superior root of ansa cervicalis　821
上矢状静脈洞　Superior sagittal sinus　855, 857, 859, 861, **867**
上肢帯　Shoulder girdle　341
上肢の受容野　Receptive field of arm　915
上歯槽神経の後上歯槽枝　Posterior superior alveolar a. of superior alveolar nn.　701
上斜筋　Superior oblique　697, 743
―の腱　Tendon of superior oblique　743
上斜部《頸長筋の》　Superior oblique part of longus colli　**815**, 817
上縦隔　Superior mediastinum　119
上縦束　Superior longitudinal fasciculus　879
上小脳脚　Superior cerebellar peduncle　897, 917
上小脳動脈　Superior cerebellar a.　865
上伸筋支帯　Superior extensor retinaculum　613
上神経幹(第5・6頸神経)　Upper trunk (C5-C6)　459
上唇小帯　Frenulum of upper lip　793
上錐体静脈洞　Superior petrosal sinus　869
上髄帆　Superior medullary velum　901
上前区動脈《腎臓の》　Anterior superior segmental a. of kidney　305
上前腸骨棘　Anterior superior iliac spine　**197**, 207, 211, 213, 215, 337, 509, 513, 535, 541, 547, 551, 649
上前頭回　Superior frontal gyrus　873
上前頭溝　Superior frontal sulcus　873

上双子筋　Gemellus superior　541, 543, **545**
上側頭回　Superior temporal gyrus　873
上側頭溝　Superior temporal sulcus　873
上大静脈　Superior vena cava　105, 121, **125**, 131, 133, 135, 141, 143, 147, 151, 163, 165
上大脳静脈　Superior cerebral vv.　855
上腸間膜静脈　Superior mesenteric v.　245, 251, 255, 319, **321**
上腸間膜動脈　Superior mesenteric a.　237, 245, 251, 255, **303**, 321
上直筋　Superior rectus　697, 743, 749
上直腸静脈　Superior rectal v.　319, 325
上直腸動脈　Superior rectal a.　313, 325
上殿静脈　Superior gluteal v.　653
上殿神経　Superior gluteal n.　653
上殿動脈　Superior gluteal a.　653
上殿皮神経　Superior cluneal nn.　75
上頭《外側翼突筋の》　Superior head of lateral pterygoid　693
上頭斜筋　Obliquus capitis superior　41, **63**
上頭頂小葉　Superior parietal lobule　873
上橈尺関節　Proximal radio-ulnar joint　399
上鼻甲介　Superior nasal concha　761
上部《十二指腸の》　Superior part of duodenum　243
上副腎静脈　Suprarenal v.　315
上葉《左肺の》　Superior lobe　169, 177, 181
上葉気管支　Superior lobar bronchi　177, 179
上涙小管　Superior lacrimal canaliculus　755
上涙点　Superior lacrimal punctum　755
上肋骨窩　Superior costal facet　19
上腕　Arm　341
上腕筋　Brachialis　369, 395, 407, 467, 499
上腕骨　Humerus　341, 387, 393, 421, 499
— の内側上顆　Medial epicondyle of humerus　419
上腕骨滑車　Trochlea of humerus　349
上腕骨小頭　Capitulum of humerus　349, 403
上腕骨体　Shaft of humerus　389, 391, 397
上腕骨頭　Head of humerus　351, 397
上腕三頭筋　Triceps brachii　**397**, 411, 465
— の外側頭　Lateral head of triceps brachii　375, 397, 475, 499
— の長頭　Long head of triceps brachii　371, 375, 397, 499
— の内側頭　Medial head of triceps brachii　375, 397, 499
上腕静脈　Brachial v.　499
上腕深動脈　Deep a. of arm　455, 475
上腕動脈　Brachial a.　455, 481, **483**, 485, 499
上腕二頭筋　Biceps brachii　363, **395**, 405, 467, 483
— の短頭　Short head of biceps brachii　367, 395, 499
— の長頭　Long head of biceps brachii　367, 369, 395, 499
— の停止腱　Biceps brachii tendon of insertion　395
上腕二頭筋腱膜　Bicipital aponeurosis　367, 395
静脈管　Ductus venosus　171
静脈管索　Ligamentum venosum　173
静脈洞交会　Confluence of sinuses　859, 861, 867
静脈輪　Venous ring　927
食道　Esophagus　101, 111, 123, **133**, 135, 169, 253, 801, 831
— の胸部　Thoracic part of esophagus　119, 129, **133**
食道静脈　esophageal vv.　319
食道神経叢　Esophageal plexus　129
食道裂孔《横隔膜の》　Esophageal hiatus of diaphragm　95, 97, 99
心圧痕　Cardiac impression　181
心室中隔　Interventricular septum　161, 169
心尖　Apex of heart　143, 167
心臓神経叢　Cardiac plexus　163
心房間束　Interatrial bundle　161
心房中隔　Interatrial septum　151, 153
心膜　Pericardium　111
心膜横隔静脈　Pericardiacophrenic v.　111, 131, 135

心膜横隔動脈　Pericardiacophrenic a.　111, 131, 135
心膜横洞　Transverse pericardial sinus　141
心膜腔　Pericardial cavity　139
心膜斜洞　Oblique pericardial sinus　141
伸筋支帯《手の》　Extensor retinaculum of hand　443
深陰茎背静脈　Deep dorsal v. of penis　289
深会陰横筋　Deep transverse perineal m.　229, **233**, 285
深横中手靱帯　Deep transverse metacarpal lig.　437
深頸動脈　Deep cervical a.　73
深枝　Deep br.
　—《尺骨神経の》　Deep br. of ulnar n.　471
　—《橈骨神経の》　Deep br. of radial n.　485
深指屈筋　Flexor digitorum profundus　409, **419**, 439, 469, 471, 501
　— の腱　Flexor digitorum profundus tendons　407, 441, 449, 487
深掌動脈弓　Deep palmar arch　491
深錐体神経　Deep petrosal n.　739
深鼡径リンパ節　Deep inguinal node　329
深層の屈筋群　Deep flexors　643
深足底動脈弓　Deep plantar arch　665
深側頭静脈　Deep temporal vv.　721
深側頭神経　Deep temporal nn.　733
深側頭動脈　Deep temporal aa.　719, 733
深腓骨神経　Deep fibular n.　**645**, 659, 661, 669
　— の皮枝　Cutaneous br. of deep fibular n.　663
深部《外肛門括約筋の》　Deep part of external anal sphincter　261
人中　Philtrum　845
腎静脈　Renal v.　315
腎錐体　Renal pyramids　305
腎臓　Kidney　251

す

水晶体　Lens　757
水平板《口蓋骨の》　Horizontal plate of Palatine bone　759
水平部《十二指腸の》　Horizontal part of duodenum　245, 255
水平裂　Horizontal fissure
　—《右肺の》　Horizontal fissure of right lung　179
　—《小脳の》　Horizontal fissure of cerebellum　901
垂直板　Perpendicular plate
　—《口蓋骨の》　Perpendicular plate of palatine bone　763
　—《篩骨の》　Perpendicular plate of ethmoid bone　741, 759, 695, 677
垂直部《頸長筋の》　Vertical part of longus colli　**815**, 817
錐体筋　Pyramidalis　209, **217**
錐体交叉　Decussation of pyramids　919
錐体上縁　Petrous ridge　683
錐体葉《甲状腺の》　Pyramidal lobe of thyroid gland　823
錐体路　Pyramidal tract　919
膵管　Pancreatic duct　267, 271
膵臓　Pancreas　237, 241, 245, 251, 255, **271**, 307
膵体　Body of pancreas　245, 271
膵頭　Head of pancreas　271
膵尾　Tail of pancreas　245, 271
髄核《椎間円板の》　Nucleus pulposus of intervertebral disc　33

せ

正中弓状靱帯　Median arcuate lig.　97
正中臍ヒダ　Median umbilical fold　239
正中神経　Median n.　459, **469**, 483, 485, 487, 489, 497, 499, 501
　— の固有領域　Exclusive area of median n.　497
　— の掌枝　Palmar br. of median n.　495
正中仙骨動脈　Median sacral a.　303
正中仙骨稜　Median sacral crest　25
正中部《小脳の》　Median part of cerebellum　903
声帯ヒダ　Vocal fold　829
星状神経節　Stellate ganglion　803, 839
精管　Ductus deferens　273, 297, 327
精索　Spermatic cord　221, 223
精巣　Testis　293
精巣挙筋　Cremaster　293, 295
精巣挙筋膜　Cremasteric (cremaster) fascia　293, 295

（せんそくとうどうみゃく） *987*

精巣鞘膜　Tunica vaginalis
— の臓側板　Visceral layer of tunica vaginalis　293, 295
— の壁側板　Parietal layer of tunica vaginalis
精巣上体の体　Body of epididymis　293
精巣静脈　Testicular v.　293, 315, 327
精巣動脈　Testicular a.　293, 327
精嚢　Seminal gland　247, 297, 299
赤核　Red nucleus　899
赤核脊髄路　Rubrospinal tract　923
脊髄　Spinal cord　31, 71
脊髄円錐　Conus medullaris of spinal cord　905
脊髄クモ膜　Spinal arachnoid mater　907
脊髄硬膜　Spinal dura mater　907
脊髄根　Spinal root　713
脊髄枝《胸大動脈の》　Spinal br. of thoracic aorta　67
脊髄静脈　Spinal v.　927
脊髄神経　Spinal n.　907, 909
脊髄神経溝　Groove for spinal n.　11
脊髄神経節　Spinal ganglion　107, 907, 909, 933
— の後枝　Posterior ramus/i of spinal n.　715
— の後枝（内側皮枝）　Posterior ramus/i (medial cutaneous brs.) of spinal n.　75
脊髄軟膜　Spinal pia mater　907
脊柱管　Vertebral canal　37
切歯管　Incisive canal　759
舌咽神経　Glossopharyngeal n.(CN IX)　709, 787
舌下神経　Hypoglossal n.(CN XII)　731, **789**, 821, 843, 895
舌下腺　Sublingual gland　797
舌骨　Hyoid bone　379, **785**, 789, 791, 805, 809, 811, 813, 827, 833
— の大角　Greater horn of hyoid bone　801
舌骨喉頭蓋靱帯　Hyo-epiglottic lig.　829
舌骨舌筋　Hyoglossus　785
舌状回　Lingual gyrus　875, 877
舌神経　Lingual n.(CN V₃)　701, 733, 737, 781, 787, **789**
舌深動脈　Deep lingual a.　789
舌動脈　Lingual a.　717, 789, 797

舌扁桃　Lingual tonsil　783
舌盲孔　Foramen cecum of tongue　783
仙棘靱帯　Sacrospinous lig.　**201**, 203, 235, 517, 519, 649
仙結節靱帯　Sacrotuberous lig.　**203**, 235, 517, 519, 531, 537, 541, 555, 557, 649
仙骨　Sacrum　3, **23**, 25, 47, 49, 57, 59, 61, 227, 393, 539, 543, 545, 555
仙骨角　Sacral horn　25
仙骨管　Sacral canal　25, 203
仙骨神経叢　Sacral plexus　331, 333, 651
仙骨尖　Apex of sacrum　23
仙骨翼　Ala of sacrum　23, 199
仙骨裂孔　Sacral hiatus　25
仙腸関節　Sacro-iliac joint　199
仙尾関節　Sacrococcygeal joint　23
浅陰茎背静脈　Superficial dorsal v. of penis　289
浅会陰横筋　Superficial transverse perineal m.　225, **233**, 285
浅横中足靱帯　Superficial transverse metacarpal lig.　605
浅枝　Superficial br.
—《尺骨神経の》　Superficial br. of Ulnar n.　489
—《橈骨神経の》　Superficial br. of Radial n.　493, 501, 485
浅指屈筋　Flexor digitorum superficialis　407, **417**, 469, 501
— の腱　Flexor digitorum superficialis tendons　441, 487
— の上腕尺骨頭　Humero-ulnar head of flexor digitorum superficialis　409
— の橈骨頭　Radial head of flexor digitorum superficialis　409
浅掌動脈弓　Superficial palmar arch　455, **489**
浅鼡径リンパ節　Superficial inguinal node　329
浅鼡径輪　Superficial inguinal ring　205, 211, 337
浅側頭静脈　Superficial temporal v.　721, 733
浅側頭動脈　Superficial temporal a.　717, 733

浅腓骨神経 Superficial fibular n. 633, **641**, 645, 659, 661
浅部《外肛門括約筋の》 Superficial part of external anal sphincter 261
浅葉《頸筋膜の》 Superficial layer of cervical fascia 825
栓状核 Emboliform nucleus 903
腺下垂体の前葉 Anterior lobe of adenohypophysis 883
線維性心膜 Fibrous pericardium 131, 133, 175
線維輪《椎間円板の》 Anulus fibrosus of intervertebral disc 33
前下行枝 Anterior interventricular br. 157
前下腿筋間中隔 Anterior intermuscular septum of leg 659
前外椎骨静脈叢 Anterior external vertebral venous plexus 69
前角《脊髄の》 Anterior horn of spinal cord 925
前関節面《軸椎の》 Anterior articular facet of axis 15
前眼房 Anterior chamber of eyeball 757
前弓《環椎(第1頸椎)の》 Anterior arch of atlas(C1) 29
前距腓靱帯 Anterior talofibular lig. 601
前鋸筋 Serratus anterior 205, 363, 365, 367, 373, **381**
— の下部 Inferior part of serratus anterior 381
— の上部 Superior part of serratus anterior 381
— の中間部 Intermediate part of serratus anterior 381
前胸鎖靱帯 Anterior sternoclavicular lig. 353, 355
前脛骨筋 Tibialis anterior 571, 573, **581**, 641, 661, 669, 671
前脛骨筋の腱 Tibialis anterior tendon 663
前脛骨静脈 Anterior tibial v. 661, 669
前脛骨動脈 Anterior tibial a. **629**, 631, 661, 663, 669
前脛腓靱帯 Anterior tibiofibular lig. 601
前頸静脈 Anterior jugular v. 721
前結節《環椎(第1頸椎)の》 Anterior tubercle of atlas 13
前結節間束 Anterior internodal bundles 161
前交連 Anterior commissure 883, 887, 913
前骨間静脈 Anterior interosseous v. 501
前骨間神経 Anterior interosseous n. 501
前骨間動脈 Anterior interosseous a. 491, 501
前根《脊髄神経の》 Anterior root of spinal n. 909, 933
前根糸 Anterior rootlets 909
前根静脈 Anterior radicular v. 927
前索《脊髄の》 Anterior funiculus of spinal cord 911
前枝 Anterior rumus/i
—《胸大動脈の》 Anterior ramus of thoracic aorta 67
—《脊髄神経の》 Anterior ramus of spinal n. 71, 909, 933
—《腰神経の》 anterior rami of Lumbar nn. 333
—《肋間神経の》 Anterior(ventral) ramus (intercostal n.) 107
前篩骨動脈 Anterior ethmoidal a. 765, 767
前室間溝 Anterior interventricular sulcus 145
前室間枝 Anterior interventricular br. 157
前斜角筋 Scalenus anterior (anterior scalene) 87, **89**, 461, 815, 817, 839
前十字靱帯 Anterior cruciate lig. 567, 569
前縦隔 Anterior mediastinum 119
前縦靱帯 Anterior longitudinal lig. 31, **33**, 35, 201, 517
前床突起 Anterior clinoid process 685
前上歯槽動脈 Anterior superior alveolar aa. 719
前上腕回旋動脈 Anterior circumflex humeral aa. 455
前正中裂 Anterior median fissure 919
前脊髄視床路 Anterior spinothalamic tract 913, 921
前脊髄小脳路 Anterior spinocerebellar tract 917, 921
前脊髄静脈 Anterior spinal v. 927
前脊髄動脈 Anterior spinal a. 865, 925
前仙骨孔 Anterior sacral foramina 23

(そくとうし《がんめんしんけいの》) *989*

前仙腸靱帯　Anterior sacro-iliac lig.　201, 517
前尖《右房室弁の》　Anterior cusp of right atrioventricular valve　149, 155
前大脳動脈　Anterior cerebral a.　865
前中心傍回　Anterior paracentral gyrus　875
前柱　Anterior column　911
前庭球　Bulb of vestibule　285
前庭神経　Vestibular n. (CN VIII)　707, 777
前庭脊髄路　Vestibulospinal tract　923
前庭ヒダ　Vestibular fold　829
前頭蓋窩　Anterior cranial fossa　683
前頭極　Frontal pole　873
前頭筋（後頭前頭筋）　Occipitofrontalis, frontal belly　687
前頭骨　Frontal bone　675, 677, 689
前頭神経　Frontal n.　699, 745, 749
前頭前野　Prefrontal cortex　929
前頭側頭束　Frontotemporal fasciculus　879
前頭直筋　Rectus capitis anterior　815, **817**
前頭洞　Frontal sinus　685, 695, 741
前頭突起《上顎骨の》　Frontal process of maxilla　761
前頭葉　Frontal lobe　849, 851, 871
前内椎骨静脈叢　Anterior internal vertebral venous plexus　69
前乳頭筋　Anterior papillary m.　149, 153
前皮枝《脊髄神経の》　Anterior cutaneous br. of spinal n.　107
前皮質脊髄路　Anterior corticospinal tract　919, 923
前迷走神経幹　Anterior vagal trunk　129, 331
前立腺　Prostate　247, 297, 299
前肋間静脈　Anterior intercostal vv.　105
前肋間静脈　Anterior intercostal v.　69
前腕　Forearm　341
前腕骨間膜　Interosseous membrane of forearm　399, 419, 421, 501

鼠径靱帯　Inguinal lig.　**201**, 205, 211, 213, 215, 217, 221, 223, 647

粗線《大腿骨の》　Linea aspera of femur　515, 555
僧帽筋　Trapezius　41, 77, 363, 713, 841, 845
　— の横行部（水平部）　Transverse part of trapezius　39, 371, **377**
　— の下行部　Descending part of trapezius　371, **377**, 473
　— の上行部　Ascending part of trapezius　371, **377**
総肝管　Common hepatic duct　267
総肝動脈　Common hepatic a.　269, 309
総頸動脈　Common carotid a.　103, 803, **819**, 837
総腱輪　Common tendinous ring　743
［総］指伸筋　Extensor digitorum　411, **423**, 443, 501
　— の腱　Extensor digitorum tendon　411, 465
総掌側指動脈　Common palmar digital aa.　489
総胆管　Bile duct　245, 265, 267, 269
総腸骨静脈　Common iliac v.　315
総腸骨リンパ節　Common iliac node　329
総腓骨神経　Common fibular n.　633, **641**, 655, 659
臓側胸膜　Visceral pleura　109
足関節窩　Ankle mortise　559
足根管　Tarsal tunnel　657
足根骨　Tarsal bones　507
足根中足関節　Tarsometatarsal joints　593
足底筋　Plantaris　577, **585**
　— の腱　Plantaris tendon　585
足底腱膜　Plantar aponeurosis　605
足底交叉　Plantar chiasm　587
足底方形筋　Quadratus plantae　609, **623**, 625, 627, 665
足背動脈　Dorsal pedal a.　629, 663
側索《脊髄の》　Lateral funiculus of spinal cord　911
側柱《脊髄の》　Lateral column of spinal cord　911
側頭極　Temporal pole　873
側頭筋　Temporalis　689, **691**, 693, 733
側頭骨の岩様部　Petrous part of temporal bone　685
側頭枝《顔面神経の》　Temporal brs. of facial n.　703, 729

側頭葉　Temporal lobe　849，851，871
側脳室　Lateral ventricle　887
側副溝　Collateral sulcus　877

た

手綱　Habenula　885
多裂筋　Multifidus　59，**61**
体《第2末節骨の》　Shaft of 2nd distal phalanx　449，451，453
帯状回　Cingulate gyrus　875
帯状溝　Cingulate sulcus　875
大陰唇　Labium majus　283
大円筋　Teres major　367，371，375，**393**，475
大胸筋　Pectoralis major　117，363，369，**387**
　— の胸肋部　Sternocostal head of pectoralis major　387
　— の鎖骨部　Clavicular head of pectoralis major　387，477
　— の腹部　Abdominal part of pectoralis major　387
大頬骨筋　Zygomaticus major　687
大結節《上腕骨の》　Greater tubercle of humerus　351，357，387，389，397
大結節稜《上腕骨の》　Crest of greater tubercle of humerus　387
大口蓋神経　Greater palatine n.　739，767
大口蓋動脈　Greater palatine a.　767
大後頭孔　Foramen magnum　681，683
大後頭神経　Greater occipital n.　73，715，727
大後頭直筋　Rectus capitis posterior major　41，**63**
大坐骨孔　Greater sciatic foramen　203
　—《梨状筋下孔の》　Infrapiriform portion of greater sciatic foramen　649
　—《梨状筋上孔の》　Suprapiriform portion of greater sciatic foramen　649
大坐骨切痕　Greater sciatic notch　509
大耳介神経　Great auricular n.　73，715，727，**821**，841
大十二指腸乳頭　Major duodenal papilla　255，267
大静脈孔《横隔膜の》　Caval opening of diaphragm　95，97，99
大心臓静脈　Great cardiac v.　157，159

大腎杯　Major calyces　305
大錐体神経　Greater petrosal n.　705，739，777
大槽　Cisterna magna　861
大腿　Thigh　507
大腿筋膜　Fascia lata　223
大腿筋膜張筋　Tensor fasciae latae　521，531，535，**539**，671
大腿骨　Femur　507，547
　— の外側上顆　Lateral epicondyle of femur　585
　— の内側顆　Medial condyle of femur　561
　— の内側上顆　Medial epicondyle of femur　585
大腿骨頸　Neck of femur　511，513
大腿骨頭　Head of femur　511，513
大腿四頭筋　Quadriceps femoris　553
　— の腱　Quadriceps femoris tendon　521，565
　— の停止腱　Quadriceps femoris tendon of insertion　551
大腿静脈　Femoral v.　221，303，327，647，**651**，667
大腿神経　Femoral n.　221，633，635，**639**，645，647，651
大腿深静脈　Deep v. of thigh　667
大腿深動脈　Deep a. of thigh　629，651，667
大腿直筋　Rectus femoris　521，**551**，553，639，667，671
　— の直頭　Straight head of rectus femoris　553
　— の反転頭　Reflected head of rectus femoris　553
大腿動脈　Femoral a.　221，303，327，**629**，647，651，667
大腿二頭筋　Biceps femoris　555，655
　— の腱　Biceps femoris tendon　573，575
　— の短頭　Short head of biceps femoris　533，555，557，641
　— の長頭　Long head of biceps femoris　529，535，555，557，643
大腿方形筋　Quadratus femoris　531，541，543，**545**

大転子《大腿骨の》 Greater trochanter of femur 511, 513, 515, 541, 543, 545, 549, 551, 553, 557
大殿筋 Gluteus maximus 77, 225, 529, 533, 535, **539**
大動脈 Aorta 101
大動脈弓 Aortic arch **123**, 133, 143, 165, 167
大動脈腎動脈神経節 Aorticorenal ganglia 331
大動脈弁 Aortic valve 155
大動脈隆起 aortic knob 165
大動脈裂孔《横隔膜の》 Aortic hiatus of diaphragm 97, 99
大内臓神経 Greater splanchnic n. 135
大内転筋 Adductor magnus 525, 527, 533, **547**, 549, 629, 637, 667
― の筋性の停止部 Adductor magnus, muscular insertion 643
― の腱 Adductor magnus tendon 631
― の腱性の停止部 Adductor magnus, tendon of insertion 547
大脳鎌 Falx cerebri 857, 859
大脳脚 Cerebral peduncle 879, 895, 899
大脳弓状線維 Cerebral arcuate fibers(U fibers) 879
大脳縦裂 Longitudinal cerebral fissure 877
大脳皮質運動野 Motor cortex 919
大脳皮質感覚野 Sensory cortex 913
大伏在静脈 Great saphenous v. 645
大網 Greater omentum 237, 239
大腰筋 Psoas major 97, 99, 219, 273, 521, **537**
大翼《蝶形骨の》 Greater wing of sphenoid 675, 741
大菱形筋 Rhomboid major 39, 373, 385
大菱形骨 Trapezium 429, 445
大弯《胃の》 Greater curvature 253
第1貫通動脈 1st perforating a. 653
第1基節骨 1st proximal phalanx 445, 591
第1頸椎(環椎) C1(Atlas) 5, 29, 41, 57, 63, 89, 385, 815, 817
第1掌側骨間筋 1st palmar interosseous 453
第1中手骨 1st metacarpal 425, 429, 451

第1中足骨 1st metatarsal 623, 627
第1中足骨底 Base of 1st metatarsal 589
第1中足骨頭 Head of 1st metatarsal 589
第1虫様筋 1st lumbrical **449**, 469
第1背側骨間筋 1st dorsal interosseous 437, 443, **451**, 493, **627**
第1末節骨 1st distal phalanx 445, 589
第1腰静脈 1st lumbar v. 105
第1腰椎 L1 5, 99, 251, 635
第1肋骨 1st rib 89, 93, 355, 383
第1-3貫通動脈 1st through 3rd perforating aa. 629
第1-3底側骨間筋 1st through 3rd plantar interossei 627
第1-4胸椎の棘突起 T1-T4 spinous processes 385
第1-4頸椎の横突起 C1-C4 transverse processes 385
第1-4虫様筋 1st through 4th lumbricals 625
第1-4背側骨間筋 1st through 4th dorsal interossei 627
第1-5仙椎 S1-S5 3
第1-5中足骨 1st through 5th metatarsals 615
第1-5末節骨 1st through 5th distal phalanges 581
第1-5腰椎 L1-L5 3, 49
第1-5腰椎体 Vertebral bodies, L1-5 99
第1-7頸椎 C1-C7 3
第1-9肋骨 1st through 9th ribs 381
第1-12胸椎 T1-T12 vertebrae 3
第一裂 Primary fissure 901
第2貫通動脈 2nd perforating a. 653
第2基節骨 2nd proximal phalanx 449, 453
第2頸椎(軸椎) Axis (C2) 5, 11, 29, 41, 57, 63, 89, 385
第2掌側骨間筋 2nd palmar interosseous 441, 453
第2中手骨 2nd metacarpal 425, 449, 453
第2中節骨 2nd middle phalanx 429, 449, 451, 453
第2虫様筋 2nd lumbrical **449**, 469
第2背側骨間筋 2nd dorsal interosseous 451
第2肋骨 2nd rib 815, 817

第2-5基節骨　2nd through 5th proximal phalanges　451
第2-5中手骨　2nd through 5th metacarpals　451, 453
第2-5中節骨　2nd through 5th middle phalanges　415, 417
第3胸椎　T3　7
第3後頭神経　3rd occipital n.　73
第3掌側骨間筋　3rd palmar interosseous　441, 453
第3虫様筋　3rd lumbrical　449
第3底側骨間筋　3rd plantar interosseous　627
第3脳室　Third ventricle　863, 885, 889
第3脳室脈絡叢　Choroid plexus of third ventricle　861
第3背側骨間筋　3rd dorsal interosseous　451
第3腓骨筋　Fibularis tertius　573, **583**
第3腰椎　L3　99
第3-5肋骨　3rd through 5th ribs　383
第4虫様筋　4th lumbrical　449
第4脳室　Fourth ventricle　853, 863, 893, 901
第4脳室外側陥凹　Lateral recess of fourth ventricle　897
第4脳室正中口　Median aperture　861
第4脳室脈絡叢　Choroid plexus of fourth ventricle　861
第4背側骨間筋　4th dorsal interosseous　451
第4末節骨　4th distal phalanx　419
第4腰椎　L4　7, 637
第5基節骨　5th proximal phalanx　615
第5中手骨　5th metacarpal　447
第5中節骨　5th middle phalanx　615
第5中足骨　5th metatarsal　599
第5中足骨粗面　Tuberosity of 5th metatarsal　583, 591, 619
第5末節骨　5th phalanx　615
第5腰椎　L5 vertebra　237, 537, 905
第5肋骨　5th rib　47, 55, 211, 217
第7胸椎　T7　7
── の棘突起　T7 spinous process　393
第7頸神経　C7 spinal n.　459
第7頸椎（隆椎）　C7 (vertebra prominens)　5, 7, 11, 51, 53, 55, 57, 59, 61, 89
── の棘突起　C7 spinous process　377, 385
第8胸椎　T8 vertebra　101
第10胸椎　T10 vertebra　101
第10肋骨　10th rib　99, 213
第12胸椎　T12　91
── の棘突起　T12 spinous process　377
第12肋骨　12th rib　7, 99, 537
胆膵管　Hepatopancreatic duct　269
胆嚢　Gallbladder　251, 265, 269
胆嚢管　Cystic duct　267, 269
胆嚢底　Fundus of gallbladder　267
短回旋筋　Rotatores breves　**59**, 61
短趾屈筋　Flexor digitorum brevis　607, **623**, 625, 627
短趾伸筋　Extensor digitorum brevis　613, 615
── の腱　Extensor digitorum brevis tendons　615
短小指屈筋　Flexor digiti minimi brevis　439, **447**
短小趾屈筋　Flexor digiti minimi brevis　607, **619**
短掌筋　Palmaris brevis　435
短頭《上腕二頭筋の》　Short head of biceps brachii　367, 395, 499
短橈側手根伸筋　Extensor carpi radialis brevis　413, **421**, 501
短内転筋　Adductor brevis　523, 525, **549**, 637
短腓骨筋　Fibularis brevis　573, **583**, 669
── の腱　Fibularis brevis tendon　583
短母指外転筋　Abductor pollicis brevis　437, **445**
短母指屈筋の浅頭　Superficial head of flexor pollicis brevis　437, **445**
短母指伸筋　Extensor pollicis brevis　**427**, 501
── の腱　Extensor pollicis brevis tendon　493
短母趾屈筋　Flexor hallucis brevis　617
短母趾伸筋　Extensor hallucis brevis　571, **615**
── の腱　Extensor hallucis brevis tendon　615, 663
短肋骨挙筋　Levatores costarum breves　53, **55**

ち

恥丘　Mons pubis　283
恥骨下肢　Inferior pubic ramus　233, 235
恥骨筋　Pectineus　523, 547, **549**, 639
恥骨筋線　Pectineal line　197
恥骨結合　Pubic symphysis　201, 213, 215, 217, 219, 229, 233, 235, 275
恥骨結節　Pubic tubercle　197, 219, 509, 513
恥骨櫛　Pecten pubis　199
恥骨上肢　Superior pubic ramus　547
恥骨大腿靱帯　Pubofemoral lig.　517
恥骨直腸筋　Puborectalis　227, **231**
恥骨尾骨筋　Pubococcygeus　227, **231**
腟　Vagina　249, 275
腟円蓋の外側部　Lateral part of vaginal fornix　281
腟口　Vaginal orifice　283
腟静脈叢　Vaginal venous plexus　323
中咽頭収縮筋　Middle constrictor　799, 801
中隔縁柱　Septomarginal trabecula　149
中隔後鼻枝　Posterior septal brs.　765
中隔尖《右房室弁の》　Septal cusp of right atrioventricular valve　155
中隔前鼻枝　Anterior septal brs.　765
中間楔状骨　Intermediate cuneiform　615
中間広筋　Vastus intermedius　523, 525, **553**, 639
中間部《小脳の》　Intermediate part of cerebellum　903
中頸神経節　Middle cervical ganglion　803
中結節間束　Middle internodal bundles　161
中結腸動脈　Middle colic a.　311
中硬膜動脈　Middle meningeal a.　735
中斜角筋　Middle scalene　87, **89**, 815, 817, 843
中手骨　Metacarpals　341
中手指節（MCP）関節　Metacarpophalangeal joint　433
中縦隔　Middle mediastinum　119
中小脳脚　Middle cerebellar peduncle　897
中心腋窩リンパ節　Central nodes　115
中心管　Central canal　863
中心後回　Postcentral gyrus　849, 873, 915, 929
中心後溝　Postcentral sulcus　873, 875
中心溝　Central sulcus　849, 871, 873, 875, 929
中心前回　Precentral gyrus　849, 873, 929
中心前溝　Precentral sulcus　873, 875
中心臓静脈　Descending v.　159
中心傍溝　Paracentral sulcus　875
中心傍小葉　Paracentral lobule　875
中前頭回　Middle frontal gyrus　873
中足趾節関節　Metatarsophalangeal joints　593
― の関節包　Metatarsophalangeal joint capsules　617, 619, 621
中側頭回　Middle temporal gyri　873
中大脳動脈　Middle cerebral a.　865
中直腸横ヒダ　Middle transverse rectal fold　261
中殿筋　Gluteus medius　77, 529, 533, 535, 539, **541**
中殿皮神経　Middle cluneal nn.　75
中頭蓋窩　Middle cranial fossa　683, 747
中脳　Mesencephalon　853, 893, 901
中脳蓋　Tectum of midbrain　899
中脳水道　Cerebral aqueduct　863, 893, 899
中脳被蓋　Tegmentum　899
中鼻道　Middle nasal meatus　761
中葉《右肺の》　Middle lobe of right lung　177, 179
虫様筋　Lumbricals　439, 609
肘筋　Anconeus　**397**, 411
肘正中皮静脈　Median cubital v.　457
肘頭　Olecranon　397, 399, 421, 423, 425, 427
肘頭窩《上腕骨の》　Olecranon fossa of humerus　351
長回旋筋　Rotatores longi　**59**, 61
長胸神経　Long thoracic n.　461, 481
長趾屈筋　Flexor digitorum longus　579, **587**, 625, 655, 657
― の腱　Flexor digitorum longus tendon　577, 587, 609, 623, 625
長趾伸筋　Extensor digitorum longus　571, **581**, 613, 641, 661

長趾伸筋の腱　Extensor digitorum longus tendon　581
長掌筋　Palmaris longus　405，**415**，501
— の腱　Palmaris longus tendon　435
長足底靱帯　Long plantar lig.　599，619
長頭　Long head
— 《上腕三頭筋の》　Long head of triceps brachii　371，375，397，499
— 《上腕二頭筋の》　Long head of biceps brachii　367，369，395，499
長橈側手根伸筋　Extensor carpi radialis longus　411，413，**421**，501
— の腱　Extensor carpi radialis longus tendon　443
長内転筋　Adductor longus　523，**549**，637，671
長腓骨筋　Fibularis longus　573，**583**，641，659
— の腱　Fibularis longus tendon　577，583，599，611，619，623，625
長腓骨筋腱溝　Groove for fibularis longus tendon　591
長母指外転筋　Abductor pollicis longus　413，**425**，427，443，465，501
— の腱　Abductor pollicis longus tendon　493
長母指屈筋　Flexor pollicis longus　409，**419**，469，501
— の腱　Flexor pollicis longus tendon　407，439，487
長母指伸筋　Extensor pollicis longus　413，**427**，501
— の腱　Extensor pollicis longus tendon　443，493，503
長母趾屈筋　Flexor hallucis longus　579，**587**
— の腱　Flexor hallucis longus tendon　575，587，607
長母趾伸筋　Extensor hallucis longus　571，**581**，613
— の腱　Extensor hallucis longus tendon　581，663，671
長毛様体神経　Long ciliary nn.　745，751
長肋骨挙筋　Levatores costarum longi　53，**55**
鳥距溝　Calcarine sulcus　875
腸間膜　Mesentery　243
腸間膜根　Root of mesentery　245

腸間膜動脈間神経叢　Intermesenteric plexus　331
腸脛靱帯　Iliotibial tract　529，535，539，659
腸骨　Ilium　393
腸骨下腹神経　Iliohypogastric n.　635
腸骨窩　Iliac fossa　199，217
腸骨筋　Iliacus　219，525，**537**
腸骨鼡径神経　Ilio-inguinal n.　633，635
腸骨大腿靱帯　Iliofemoral lig.　517，519
腸骨尾骨筋　Iliococcygeus　227，**231**
腸骨尾骨筋縫線　Iliococcygeal raphe　231
腸骨部《広背筋の》　Iliac part of latissimus dorsi　393
腸骨稜　Iliac crest　7，47，49，197，219，393，509，539，541，543，545，547
— の外唇　Outer lip of iliac crest　211
— の中間線　Intermediate zone of iliac crest　213
腸恥筋膜弓　Iliopectineal arch　537，647
腸腰筋　Iliopsoas　219，521，537，639
腸腰靱帯　Iliolumbar lig.　201，517，519
腸肋筋　Iliocostalis　43
蝶形骨洞　Sphenoid sinus　763
蝶口蓋孔　Sphenopalatine foramen　763
蝶口蓋動脈　Sphenopalatine a.　719，735
直回　Gyrus rectus　877
直細動脈　Vasa recta　311
直静脈洞　Straight sinus　861，869
直腸　Rectum　247，257，259，275
直腸子宮窩　Recto-uterine pouch　249
直腸子宮靱帯　Uterosacral lig.　279
直腸子宮ヒダ　Uterosacral fold　279
直腸静脈叢　Rectal venous plexus　261
直腸前線維　Prerectal fibers　231
直腸膀胱窩　Rectovesical pouch　247，299

つ

ツチ骨　Malleus　769，775
対輪　Antihelix　771
椎間円板　Intervertebral disc　3，5，37
椎間関節　Zygapophyseal joint　27
椎間孔　Intervertebral foramen　3，37，907
椎弓　Vertebral arch　15，21

（どうぼうけっせつし） 995

椎弓根　Pedicle of vertebral arch　9, 19, 37
椎弓板　Lamina of vertebral arch　9, **17**, 19, 35
椎骨動脈　Vertebral a.　73, 717, 907
椎骨動脈溝　Groove for vertebral a.　13
椎骨部《広背筋の》　Vertebral part of latissimus dorsi　393
椎前神経節　Prevertebral ganglion　933
椎体　Vertebral body　5, 9, 19, 37
椎体間関節　Intervertebral joint　27
蔓状静脈叢　Pampiniform plexus　293, 327

て

テント切痕　Tentorial notch　859
底　Base
　—《第1基節骨の》　Base of 1st proximal phalanx　427
　—《第1中手骨の》　Base of 1st metacarpal　425
　—《第1末節骨の》　Base of 1st distal phalanx　419, 427
　—《第2中手骨の》　Base of 2nd metacarpal　417, 421
　—《第2末節骨の》　Base of 2nd distal phalanx　449
　—《第3中手骨の》　Base of 3rd metacarpal　421, 445
　—《第5基節骨の》　Base of 5th proximal phalanx　423, 447
　—《第5中手骨の》　Base of 5th metacarpal　417, 423
　—《中手骨の》　Base of metacarpal　431
底側骨間筋　Plantar interossei　611
底側踵舟靱帯　Plantar calcaneonavicular lig.　597, 599
底側中足動脈　Plantar metatarsal aa.　665
転子間線《大腿骨の》　Intertrochanteric line of femur　553
転子間稜《大腿骨の》　Intertrochanteric crest of femur　511, 541, 543, 545
殿筋粗面《大腿骨の》　Gluteal tuberosity of femur　541
殿筋面《腸骨の》　Gluteal surface of ilium　543, 545

と

トルコ鞍　Sella turcica　685
豆状骨　Pisiform　419, 431, 447, 449, 451
透明中隔　Septum pellucidum　871
頭　Head
　—《第1中手骨の》　Head of 1st metacarpal　445
　—《第2末節骨の》　Head of 2nd distal phalanx　449
　—《中手骨の》　Head of metacarpal　431
頭最長筋　Longissimus capitis　47, **49**
頭長筋　Longus capitis　**815**, 817
頭頂間溝　Intraparietal sulcus　873
頭頂後頭溝　Parieto-occipital sulcus　873, 875
頭頂骨　Parietal bone　679, 689
頭頂葉　Parietal lobe　871
頭半棘筋　Semispinalis capitis　45, 59, **61**
頭板状筋　Splenius capitis　45, **51**, 53, 55
頭皮　Scalp　857
橈骨　Radius　341, 397, 419, 421, 423, 425, 427, 449, 451, 453, 501
　— の茎状突起　Radial styloid process　421
橈骨手根関節　Wrist joint　433
橈骨神経　Radial n.　**465**, 475, 481, 499
　—, 浅枝　Radial n., superficial br.　465, 497
　—, 背側指神経　Radial n., dorsal digital n.　495, 497
橈骨粗面　Radial tuberosity　395, 399, 417, 419
橈骨動脈　Radial a.　**455**, 485, 491, 493, 501
橈骨頭　Head of radius　399, 403
橈骨輪状靱帯　Annular lig. of radius　401, 403
橈側手根屈筋　Flexor carpi radialis　405, **417**, 469, 501
　— の腱　Flexor carpi radialis tendon　487
橈側皮静脈　Cephalic v.　457, 477
洞房結節　Sinu-atrial node　161
洞房結節枝　Sinu-atrial nodal br.　157

動眼神経　Oculomotor n.(CN III)　697, **745**, 747, 895, 899
動脈円錐　Conus arteriosus　149
動脈管　Ductus arteriosus　171
動脈管索　Ligamentum arteriosum　137, 141, 149, 173
導出静脈　Emissary v.　857

な

内陰部静脈　Internal pudendal v.　259, 287, 301
内陰部動脈　Internal pudendal a.　259, 287, 301
内果　Medial malleolus　559, 571
内胸静脈　Internal thoracic v.　69, 105, 113, 131
内胸動脈　Internal thoracic a.　103, 113, 131
― の前肋間枝　Anterior intercostal brs. of internal thoracic a.　103
内頸静脈　Internal jugular v.　105, 127, **721**, 723, 729, 803, 825, 837, 867
内頸動脈　Internal carotid a.　731, 745, 747, 773, 775, **819**, 843, 865
内頸動脈神経叢　Internal carotid plexus　745
内肛門括約筋　Internal anal sphincter　261
内子宮口《子宮峡部の》　Internal os(at uterine isthmus)　281
内枝《上喉頭神経の》　Internal br. of superior laryngeal n.　831, 833
内唇《腸骨稜の》　Inner lip of iliac crest　215
内精筋膜　Internal spermatic fascia　293, 295
内節《淡蒼球の》　Medial segment of globus pallidus　889
内臓神経　Splanchnic n.　909, 933
内側縁《肩甲骨の》　Medial border of scapula　347, 381, 385
内側顆　Medial condyle
―《脛骨の》　Medial condyle of tibia　555, 561, 563, 581, 559
―《大腿骨の》　Medial condyle of femur　511, 563

内側脚《浅鼡径輪の》　Medial crus of superficial inguinal ring　647
内側嗅条　Medial stria　877
内側胸筋神経　Medial pectoral nn.　477, 479
内側楔状骨　Medial cuneiform　**589**, 591, 597, 599, 615, 623
内側広筋　Vastus medialis　521, 527, **551**, 553, 639
内側後頭側頭回　Medial occipitotemporal gyrus　875, 877
内側枝
　―《脊髄神経の》　Medial brs. of spinal n.　71
　―《眼窩上神経の》　Medial brs. of supra-orbital n.　725
内側膝蓋支帯　Medial patellar retinaculum　551
内側膝状体　Medial geniculate body　885
内側種子骨　Medial sesamoid　617, 621
内側上顆　Medial epicondyle
　―《上腕骨の》　Medial epicondyle of humerus　**349**, 397, 401, 403, 405, 415, 417, 421, 425, 427
　―《大腿骨の》　Medial epicondyle of femur　511, 549, 561, 563, 585
内側上膝動脈　Superior medial genicular a.　631
内側上腕筋間中隔　Medial intermuscular septum of arm　483, 499
内側神経束《腕神経叢の》　Medial cord of brachial plexus　459, 471
内側唇《粗線の》　Medial lip of linea aspera　511
内側足底神経　Medial plantar n.　633, 657, 665
内側足底動脈　Medial plantar a.　657, 665
内側側副靱帯
　―《膝関節の》　Medial collateral lig. of knee　565, 567, 569
　―《肘関節の》　Ulnar collateral lig. of elbow joint　401, 403
内側大腿回旋動脈　Medial circumflex femoral a.　629, 651
内側直筋　Medial rectus　697, 743
内側頭　Medial head
　―《上腕三頭筋の》　Medial head of triceps brachii　375, 397, 499

(はいかんまく) *997*

―《短母趾屈筋の》 Medial head of flexor hallucis brevis 611, 617
―《腓腹筋の》 Medial head of gastrocnemius 529, 575, 579, 585, 669
内側突起《踵骨隆起の》 Medial process of calcaneal tuberosity 617, 619
内側半月 Medial meniscus 565, 567
内側板《翼状突起の》 Medial plate of pterygoid process 681, 761
内側皮枝《胸大動脈の》 Medial cutaneous br. of thoracic aorta 67
内側毛帯 Medial lemniscus 915
内側翼突筋 Medial pterygoid **693**, 735
内腸骨静脈 Internal iliac v. 327
内腸骨動脈 Internal iliac a. 327
内腸骨リンパ節 Internal iliac lymph node 329
内転筋管 Adductor canal 629
内転筋結節 Adductor tubercle 511
[内転筋]腱裂孔 Adductor hiatus 525, 549, 631
内転軸 Axis of adduction 539
内腹斜筋 Internal oblique 45, 207, **213**, 221, 223
内腹斜筋腱膜 Internal oblique aponeurosis 213
内閉鎖筋 Obturator internus 225, 231, 259, 527, 531, 541, 543, **545**
内閉鎖筋筋膜 Obturator internus fascia 229
内包 Internal capsule 879, 887, 919
内肋間筋 Internal intercostal m. 87, **91**, 93, 207
軟口蓋 Soft palate 791, 793
軟骨部《耳管の》 Cartilaginous part of pharyngotympanic tube 773
軟膜 Pia mater 855

に

2次ニューロン 2nd neuron 913
― の細胞体 Cell body of 2nd neuron 917
― の軸索 Axon of 2nd neuron 915
肉柱《心室中隔の》 Trabeculae carneae of interventricular septum 153
肉様膜 Tunica dartos 295

乳管 Lactiferous duct 117
乳管洞 Lactiferous sinus 117
乳頭 Nipple 117
乳頭体 Mammillary body 881, 891
乳頭突起《腰椎の》 Mammillary process of lumbar vertebrae 21, 53, 55
乳ビ槽 Cisterna chyli 127, 329
乳房提靱帯(クーパー靱帯) Suspensory (Cooper's) ligs. of breast 117
乳様突起《側頭骨の》 Mastoid process of temporal bone 49, 51, 679, 689
尿管 Ureter 259, 277, 279, 305
― の骨盤部 Pelvic ureter 297
― の腹部 Abdominal part of ureter 273
尿管間ヒダ Interureteric fold 277
尿管口 Ureteric orifice 277
尿生殖裂孔 Urogenital hiatus 231, 233
尿道 Urethra 277, 297
― の海綿体部 Spongy urethra 289, 299
尿道海綿体 Corpus spongiosum penis 291
尿道球 Bulb of penis 291
尿道球腺 Bulbo-urethral gland 297, 301

の

脳幹 Brain stem 919
脳弓 Fornix 853, 871, 883, 889
脳弓脚 Crus of fornix 881
脳弓体 Body of fornix 881
脳底動脈 Basilar a. 865
脳梁 Corpus callosum 853, 871, 875, 879, 881, 887
脳梁溝 Sulcus of corpus callosum 875

は

馬尾 Cauda equina 905
背側結節《橈骨の》 Dorsal tubercle of radius 411, 425, 427
背側骨間筋《足の》 Dorsal interossei of foot 611
背側枝, 尺骨神経の Dorsal br. of ulnar n. 497
背側指神経 Dorsal digital n. 497
背側足根靱帯 Dorsal tarsal ligs. 601
背側中足動脈 Dorsal metatarsal aa. 663
肺間膜 Pulmonary lig. 179

肺神経叢　Pulmonary plexus　163
肺尖　Apex of lung　177，179，181
肺動脈　Pulmonary aa.　173
肺動脈幹　Pulmonary trunk　123，141，145，153，165，177，**189**
肺動脈弁　Pulmonary valve　149
肺胞　Alveolus　187
肺胞嚢　Alveolar sac　187
肺門　Hilum of lung　181
排尿筋　Detrusor　277
白交通枝《脊髄神経の》　White ramus communicans of spinal n.　909，933
白線　Linea alba　205，211，213，215，217，219，337
白膜　Tunica albuginea　295
薄筋　Gracilis　525，527，533，**549**，637
　─ の停止腱　Gracilis tendon of insertion　549
薄束　Gracile fasciculus　897，915，921
薄束核　Gracile nucleus　897，915
薄束結節　Gracile tubercle　897
反回神経　Recurrent laryngeal n.　839
半奇静脈　Hemi-azygos v.　125，137，315
半規管　Semicircular ducts　707
半月線　Semilunar line　215，337
半腱様筋　Semitendinosus　529，555，**557**，643，667
半膜様筋　Semimembranosus　529，555，**557**，575，643
　─ の腱　Semimembranosus tendon　557
板間層　Diploë of cranial bone　857

ひ

ヒラメ筋　Soleus　573，577，579，**585**，643，669
ヒラメ筋腱弓　Tendinous arch of soleus　585
ヒラメ筋線《脛骨の》　Soleal line of tibia　587
皮下部《外肛門括約筋の》　Subcutaneous part of external anal sphincter　261
皮枝《閉鎖神経の》　Cutaneous br. of obturator n.　637
皮質核線維　Corticonuclear fibers　919
皮質脊髄線維　Corticospinal fibers　919
披裂喉頭蓋ヒダ　Ary-epiglottic fold　829
被殻　Putamen　889

脾静脈　Splenic v.　319，321
脾臓　Spleen　241，251
脾動脈　Splenic a.　307，321
腓骨　Fibula　507，539，555，557
　─ の後面　Posterior surface of fibula　587
腓骨静脈　Fibular v.　669
腓骨頭　Head of fibula　535，557，559，581，583，585，587，641，659
腓骨動脈　Fibular a.　631，655，669
腓腹筋　Gastrocnemius　**585**，643，671
　─ の内側頭　Medial head of gastrocnemius　579，669
腓腹神経　Sural n.　645，659
尾骨　Coccyx　3，25，233，235
尾骨筋　Coccygeus　227，229
尾状核　Caudate nucleus　887，891
尾状葉《肝臓の》　Caudate lobe of liver　265
鼻口蓋神経　Nasopalatine n.　765
鼻骨　Nasal bone　677
鼻根点　Nasion　677
鼻中隔　Nasal septum　695
鼻中隔軟骨　Septal nasal cartilage　759
鼻毛様体神経　Nasociliary n.　699，751
鼻涙管　Nasolacrimal duct　755

ふ

付着板　Lamina affixa　885
伏在神経　Saphenous n.　633，**639**，645，651
副神経　Accessory n.（CN XI）　75，**713**，731，839，895
副腎　Suprarenal gland　273
副膵管　Accessory pancreatic duct　271
副半奇静脈　Accessory hemi-azygos v.　125
腹横筋　Transversus abdominis　45，209，**215**，223
腹横筋腱膜　Transversus abdominis aponeurosis　209，215
腹腔神経節　Celiac ganglion　331
腹腔動脈　Celiac trunk　237，269，303，**309**，321
腹腔リンパ節　Celiac node　329
腹大動脈　Abdominal aorta　307

(もうのう) 999

腹直筋　Rectus abdominis　209, **217**, 221, 337
腹直筋鞘　Rectus sheath
　— の後葉　Posterior layer of rectus sheath 215
　— の前葉　Anterior layer of rectus sheath 207, 215, 221
腹部《大胸筋の》　Abdominal part of pectoralis major　363
腹膜垂　Omental appendices　257
噴門　Cardia　253
分界溝　Terminal sulcus　783
分界条　Stria terminalis　885
分界稜　Crista terminalis　151

へ

閉鎖管　Obturator canal　227
閉鎖孔　Obturator foramen　197, 509
閉鎖神経　Obturator n.　635, 637, 651
閉鎖膜　Obturator membrane　201, 203
壁側胸膜
　— の横隔部　Diaphragmatic part of parietal pleura　109
　— の縦隔部　Mediastinal part of parietal pleura　131
　— の肋骨部　Costal part of parietal pleura　111
壁側腹膜　Parietal peritoneum　223
壁内部《尿管の》　intramural part of ureter　277
辺縁葉　Limbic lobe　871
扁桃体　Amygdaloid body　889
弁蓋部《下前頭回の》　Opercular part of inferior frontal gyrus　873

ほ

ボクダレク三角　Bochdalek's triangle　97
母指球　Thenar eminence　503
母指球筋への筋枝　Thenar muscular br.　469
母指線　Thenar crease　503
母指対立筋　Opponens pollicis　439, **445**
母指内転筋　Adductor pollicis　445
　— の横頭　Transverse head of adductor pollicis　437, 441, 445
　— の斜頭　Oblique head of adductor pollicis　441, 445
母趾外転筋　Abductor hallucis　605, **617**, 657, 665
母趾内転筋　Adductor hallucis　621
　— の横頭　Transcerse head of adductor hallucis　611, 621
　— の斜頭　Oblique head of adductor hallucis　611, 621
方形回内筋　Pronator quadratus　409, **419**
方形筋弓　Quadratus arcade　99
方形葉《肝臓の》　Quadrate lobe of liver　265
放線冠　Corona radiata　879
縫工筋　Sartorius　521, 527, 551, **553**, 639, 667
房室結節　Atrioventricular node　161
房室束　Atrioventricular bundle　161
帽状腱膜　Galea aponeurotica（epicranial aponeurosis）　687
膀胱　Urinary bladder　247, 249, 273, 275, 297
膀胱頸　Neck of bladder　277
膀胱三角　Trigone of bladder　277
膀胱子宮窩　Vesico-uterine pouch　249
膀胱神経叢　Vesical plexus　335
膀胱体　Body of bladder　299

み

脈絡叢　Choroid plexus　883, 901
脈絡ヒモ　Choroid line　885

む・め

無漿膜野（横隔面）　Bare area（diaphragmatic surface of liver）　263
迷走神経　Vagus n.（CN Ⅹ）　709, **711**, 713, 787, 803, 825, 837, 895, 933

も

毛様体　Ciliary body　757
毛様体筋　Ciliary m.　757
毛様体神経節　Ciliary ganglion　699, 745
盲腸　Cecum　257
網嚢　Omental bursa　251

網嚢孔　Omental foramen　241
網膜　Retina　757
網様体脊髄路　Reticulospinal tract　923
門脈　Hepatic portal v.　245, 265, 319, 321

ゆ

有鈎骨　Hamate　429, 447
有鈎骨鈎　Hook of hamate　417, 419, 431, 447, 449
有線野　Striate area　931
有頭骨　Capitate　431, 445
幽門括約筋　Pyloric sphincter　255
幽門洞　Pyloric antrum　253
幽門部《胃の》　Pyloric part of stomach　251

よ

葉間動脈　Interlobar a.　305
腰外側横突間筋　Intertransversarii laterales lumborum　**53**, 55
腰棘間筋　Interspinales lumborum　57
腰筋弓　Psoas arcade　99
腰三角, 内腹斜筋　Lumbar triangle, internal oblique　39
腰静脈　Lumbar vv.　125, 315
腰神経節　lumbar ganglia　333
腰仙骨神経幹　Lumbosacral trunk　635
腰腸肋筋　Iliocostalis lumborum　**47**, 49
腰内臓神経　Lumbar splanchnic n.　333
腰内側横突間筋　Intertransversarii mediais lumborum　**53**, 55
腰方形筋　Quadratus lumborum　99, **219**
腰膨大　Lumbosacral enlargement　905
腰肋三角　Lumbocostal triangle　97
翼口蓋神経節　Pterygopalatine ganglion　701, 767, 781
翼突管神経　N. of pterygoid canal　739
翼突筋静脈叢　Pterygoid plexus　721, 723

ら

ラセン神経節　Spiral ganglia　707
ラムダ縫合　Lambdoid suture　679
卵円窩　Oval fossa　151

卵円孔　Foramen ovale　171, 173, **681**, 685, 737
卵管間膜　Mesosalpinx　279
卵管峡部　Isthmus of uterine tube　281
卵管膨大部　Ampulla　281
卵管漏斗　Infundibulum　281
卵形嚢　Utricle　707
卵巣　Ovary　279
卵巣静脈　Ovarian v.　279, 315
卵巣提索帯　Suspensory lig. of ovary　279
卵巣動脈　Ovarian a.　279

り

リンパ組織(耳管扁桃)を伴う耳管隆起　Torus tubarius with lymphatic tissue (tonsilla tubaria)　791
梨状陥凹　Piriform recess　829
梨状筋　Piriformis　227, 229, 527, 531, 541, **543**, 545, 649
立方骨　Cuboid　589, 599
隆椎(第7頸椎)　Vertebra prominens(C7)　5, 11, 51, 53, 55, 57, 59, 61
梁下野　Subcallosal gyrus　875
菱形窩　Rhomboid fossa　893, 897
輪状甲状筋　Cricothyroid　711, 799, 831
輪状甲状靱帯　Cricothyroid lig.　827
輪状軟骨　Cricoid cartilage　183, 827, 829
鱗状縫合　Squamous suture　675
鱗部《側頭骨の》　Squamous part of temporal bone　675

る

涙丘　Lacrimal caruncle　755
涙腺　Lacrimal gland　749, 755
涙腺神経　Lacrimal n.　749
涙腺動脈　Lacrimal a.　749
涙嚢　Lacrimal sac　755

ろ

肋下筋　Subcostales　91
肋鎖靱帯　Costoclavicular lig.　355
肋鎖靱帯圧痕　Impression for costoclavicular lig.　343

肋軟骨　Costal cartilage　81, 83, 87, 93, 355
肋間静脈　Posterior intercostal vv.　69, **105**, 109, 111, 125
肋間神経　Intercostal n.　75, 109, 129
肋間動脈　Posterior intercostal aa.　67, **103**, 109, 111
肋骨　Rib　95
肋骨横隔洞　Costodiaphragmatic recess　109, 177
肋骨下平面　Subcostal plane　193
肋骨角　Angle of rib　83
肋骨弓　Costal margin(arch)　81
肋骨挙筋　Levatores costarum　45
肋骨頸　Neck of rib　83
肋骨結節　Tubercle of rib　83
肋骨溝　Costal groove　109
肋骨頭　Head of rib　83
肋骨突起　Costal process/es　35, 49, 53, 55, 59, 61, 99
肋骨部　Costal part　175

腕神経叢　Brachial plexus　**479**, 837
腕頭動脈　Brachiocephalic trunk　143, 147
腕橈骨筋　Brachioradialis　405, **421**, 485, 501
　― の停止腱　Brachioradialis tendon of insertion　421